IADVL

INDIAN ASSOCIATION OF DERMATOLOGISTS VENEREOLOGISTS & LEPROLOGISTS IADVL 1973

Practical Manual of Leprosy

IADVL

Practical Manual of Leprosy

Chief Editor

P Narasimha Rao MD DD PhD
Professor
Department of Dermatology
Bhaskar Medical College
Hyderabad, Telangana, India

Associate Editor

Santoshdev P Rathod MD DNB
Professor and Deputy Medical Superintendent
Department of Dermatology, STD and Leprosy
Smt SCL Hospital
Smt NHL Municipal Medical College
Ahmedabad, Gujarat, India

Assistant Editors

Neel Prabha MD
Associate Professor
Department of Dermatology
All India Institute of Medical Sciences
Raipur, Chhattisgarh, India

Shekhar N Pradhan MD
Professor and Head
Department of Dermatology
BJ Government Medical College
Pune, Maharashtra, India

CBSPD

CBS Publishers & Distributors Pvt Ltd

New Delhi • Bengaluru • Chennai • Kochi • Kolkata • Lucknow • Mumbai
Gujarat • Hyderabad • Jharkhand • Nagpur • Patna • Pune • Uttarakhand

Disclaimer

Science and technology are constantly changing fields. New research and experience broaden the scope of information and knowledge. The editors have tried their best in giving information available to them while preparing the material for this book. Although all efforts have been made to ensure optimum accuracy of the material, yet it is quite possible some errors might have been left uncorrected. The publisher, printer and the editors will not be held responsible for any inadvertent errors or inaccuracies.

IADVL

Practical Manual of

Leprosy

ISBN: 978-93-5466-913-2

First Edition: 2026

Published by **Satish Kumar Jain** and produced by **Varun Jain** for

CBS Publishers & Distributors Pvt Ltd

4819/XI Prahlad Street, 24 Ansari Road, Daryaganj, New Delhi 110 002, India
Ph: 011-23289259, 23266838 Website: www.cbspd.com
e-mail: delhi@cbspd.com

Corporate Office: 204 FIE, Industrial Area, Patparganj, Delhi 110 092, India
Ph: 011-49344934 Fax: 011-49344935 e-mail: publishing@cbspd.com; publicity@cbspd.com

Branches

- **Bengaluru:** Seema House 2975, 17th Cross, K.R. Road, Banasankari 2nd Stage, Bengaluru 560 070, Karnataka, India
  Ph: +91-80-26771678/79 Fax: +91-80-26771680 e-mail: bangalore@cbspd.com
- **Chennai:** 18/8B, Subbarayan Street, Shenoy Nagar, Chennai 600 030, Tamil Nadu, India
  Ph: +91-44-42032115, 26681266 e-mail: chennai@cbspd.com
- **Kochi:** 42/1325, 1326, Power House Road, Opposite KSEB, Power House, Ernakulam 682018, Kochi, Kerala, India
  Ph: +91-484-4059061–65 Fax: +91-484-4059065 e-mail: kochi@cbspd.com
- **Kolkata:** 147, Hind Ceramics Compound, 1st Floor, Nilgunj Road, Belghoria, Kolkata 700056, West Bengal, India
  Ph: +91-33-25330055/56 e-mail: kolkata@cbspd.com
- **Lucknow:** Basement, Khushuma Complex, 7 Meerabai Marg (behind Jawahar Bhawan), Lucknow 226001, UP, India
  Ph: +91-522-4000032 e-mail: tiwari.lucknow@cbspd.com
- **Mumbai:** PWD Shed, Gala No. 25/26, Ramchandra Bhatt Marg, Next JJ Hospital, Gate No. 2, Opp. Union Bank of India Noorbaug, Mumbai 400009, Maharashtra, India
  Ph: +91-22-66661880/89 e-mail: mumbai@cbspd.com

Representatives

- **Gujarat** • **Hyderabad** • **Jharkhand** • **Nagpur** • **Patna** • **Pune** • **Uttarakhand**

For trade terms please contact customercare@cbspd.com
For general enquiries please contact info@cbspd.com

Printed at: Goyal Offset Works Pvt. Ltd, Kundli, Sonipat, Haryana

Contributors

Abhishek Bhardwaj MD
Professor and Head
Department of Dermatology, Venereology and Leprosy, AIIMS, Jodhpur, Rajasthan, India
e-mail: dr.abhishekbhardwaj@gmail.com

Ajeet Singh MD DNB
Senior Resident
Department of Dermatology, AIIMS, Raipur
Chhattisgarh, India
e-mail: a.ajityadav@gmail.com

Akshay Ambasana MD
Assistant Professor
Department of Dermatology
GMERS Medical College and Hospital
Junagadh, Gujarat, India
e-mail: akshayambasana@gmail.com

Anil Patki MD DNB
Senior Consultant, Department of Dermatologist
Deenanath Mangeshkar Hospital, Pune
Maharashtra, India

Ankit Bharti MD
Consultant Dermatologist and Dermatopathologist
Aura Skin Clinic, Vyara, Surat, Gujarat, India
e-mail: dr.ankithbharti@gmail.com

Anupama Gopalan MD
Associate Professor
Department of Dermatology, STD and Leprosy
Shimoga Institute of Medical Sciences
Shimoga, Karnataka, India
e-mail: dranu82@yahoo.co.in

Ashwini PK MD
Associate Professor
Department of Dermatology, STD and Leprosy
JSS Medical College and Hospital
Mysuru, Karnataka, India
e-mail: drashwinipk@gmail.com

Bela Shah MD
Professor and Head
Department of Dermatology, STD and Leprosy
BJ Medical College and Civil Hospital
Ahmedabad, Gujarat, India
e-mail: shah.drbela@gmail.com

Bhumesh Kumar Katakam DCH MD
Associate Professor and Head
Department of Dermatology, STD and Leprosy
Government Medical College
Suryapet, Telangana, India
e-mail: Drbhumesh124@gmail.com

Bikash Ranjan Kar MD
Professor and Head
Department of Dermatology, STD and Leprosy
Institute of Medical Sciences and SUM Hospital
Bhubaneswar, Odisha, India
e-mail: karbikash@gmail.com

Biswanath Behera MD DNB
Assistant Professor
Department of Dermatology, STD and Leprosy
AIIMS, Bhubaneswar, Odisha, India
e-mail: biswanathbehera61@gmail.com

Brahmaiah Upputuri DDVL
Consultant in LEPRA Society
Blue Peter Public Health and Research Centre and
Oliva Skin and Hair Clinic
Hyderabad, Telangana, India
e-mail: brahmaiah2red@gmail.com

Chirag Desai DDVL
Consultant Dermatopathologist
Divya Sparsh Dermatopathology Services
Mumbai, Maharashtra, India
e-mail: 83.chirag@gmail.com

David Prakash Kumar MPT (Ortho) MSc (Medical Sociology)
Head, Training and Principal
College of Health Sciences, SIHRLC, Karigiri
Vellore, Tamil Nadu, India
e-mail: sihrlctraining@gmail.com

Deepali Tarate DVD DNB
Junior Consultant
Nirali Hospital-Larsen and Toubro, Powai, Mumbai
Maharashtra, India
e-mail: drdeepalitarate9@gmail.com

Deepika Pandhi MD
Director Professor
Department of Dermatology
University College of Medical Sciences (UCMS)
New Delhi, India
e-mail: pandhi.deepika@gmail.com

Delicia Roshini MPT (Orthopaedics)
Physiotherapist
Dematology, Venereology and Leprosy
Schiefflin Institute of Health Research and Leprosy Centre, Karigiri, Tamil Nadu, India

Faizan Younus Shah MD
Founder: Skinnic Dermatology Center
Bemina, Srinagar, Jammu and Kashmir, India

Gauri Mahabal MD MRCP
Assistant Professor
Department of Dermatology, STD and Leprosy
Christian Medical College and Hospital
Vellore, Tamil Nadu, India
e-mail: dr.gaurimahabal@gmail.com

Gopikrishnan Anjaneyan MD DNB
Additional Professor
Department of Dermatology, STD and Leprosy
AIMS, Kochi, Kerala, India
e-mail: drgopikrishnana@gmail.com

Hemanta Kumar Kar MD
Professor and Head
Department of Dermatology
Venereology and Leprosy, Kalinga Institute of Medical Sciences, KIIT deemed to be University
Bhubaneswar, Odisha, India
e-mail: hkkar_2000@yahoo.com

Itu Singh PhD
Scientist-In-Charge
Stanley Browne Laboratory
The Leprosy Mission Community Hospital
Nand Nagari, Shahdara, Delhi
e-mail: utpal.sengupta@leprosymission.in

Jerry Joshua MBBS MS MCh
Director
Schiefflin Institute of Health Research and Leprosy Centre, Karigiri
Tamil Nadu, India
e-mail: jerryjoshua@yahoo.com

Mallika Lavania PhD
ICMR-National Institute of Virology, Pune
Enteric Viruses Group, 20A Ambedkar Road
Agarkar Nagar, Pune
e-mail: mallikalavanya@gmail.com

Meghana Phiske DDV MD DNB
Associate Professor
Department of Dermatology, STD and Leprosy
MGM Medical College, Kalamboli, Navi Mumbai
Maharashtra, India
e-mail: phiskemeghana@gmail.com

Mohammad Adil MD
Assistant Professor
Department of Dermatology, STD and Leprosy
Jawaharlal Nehru Medical College and Hospital
Aligarh Muslim University,
Aligarh, Uttar Pradesh, India
e-mail: dr.mohd.adil@gmail.com

Neelakumari M Patel MD
Professor and Head
Department of Dermatology, STD and Leprosy
AMC MET Medical College
Sheth LG General Hospital, Ahmedabad
Gujarat, India
e-mail: patelneela1974@yahoo.co.in

Neelam Kumari Bhatt MBBS MD DNB
Assistant Professor
BJ Medical College, Pune, India
e-mail: drneelambhatt1@gmail.com

Neel Prabha MD
Associate Professor
Department of Dermatology
All India Institute of Medical Sciences
Raipur Chhattisgarh, India
e-mail: ripuneel@gmail.com

Ranugha PSS MD DNB
Assistant Professor
Department of Dermatology, STD and Leprosy
JSS Medical College and Hospital
Mysore, Karnataka, India
e-mail: renukaderm@gmail.com

P Narasimha Rao MD DD PhD
Professor
Department of Dermatology
Bhaskar Medical College, Hyderabad
Andhra Pradesh, India
e-mail: dermarao@gmail.com

Pooja Agarwal MD
Associate Professor
Department of Dermatology, STD and Leprosy
Smt NHL Municipal Medical College
Ahmedabad, Gujarat, India
e-mail: pooja.kgmc@gmail.com

Pragya Nair DVD MD
Professor and Head
Department of Dermatology, STD and Leprosy
Pramukhswami Medical College
Karamsad, Gujarat, India
e-mail: drpragash2000@yahoo.com

Preethi B Nayak
MD DVL DNB FRGUHS (Dermatosurgery) MNAMS
Experia Advanced Skin and Hair Clinic
Bengaluru, Karnataka, India

Priti P Shahk MD Dermatology
Professor and Head
Department of Dermatology Venereology and Leprosy, Swaminarayan Institute of Medical Sciences and Research
Kalol, Gandhinagar
e-mail: pritishah1960@rediffmail.com

Ravindra P Turankar PhD
Senior Research Scientist
Stanley Browne Laboratory
The Leprosy Mission Trust India
Nand Nagari, Shahdara, New Delhi

Reetu Agarwal DVD MD
Classified Specialist
INHS Asvini, Mumbai, Maharashtra, India
e-mail: reetuagarwal@gmail.com

Santoshdev P Rathod MD DNB
Professor and Deputy Medical Superintendent
Department of Dermatology, STD and Leprosy
Smt SCL Hospital
Smt NHL Municipal Medical College
Ahmedabad, Gujarat, India
e-mail: santosh_rathod85@yahoo.com

Sathish Paul BPT M Tech PhD
Head
Physiotherapy and Research, SIHRLC, Karigiri
Vellore, Tamil Nadu, India
e-mail: sathishpaul77@gmail.com

Patnaik Satyadarshi MD
MKCG Medical College
Behrampur, Odisha, India
e-mail: stydrsh@yahoo.co.in

Sejal Thakkar DVD MD
Associate Professor
Department of Dermatology, STD and Leprosy
GMERS Medical College
Gotri, Vadodara, Gujarat, India
e-mail: drsejal98@gmail.com

Shagufta Rather MD FRCP(edin)
Associate Professor
Department of Dermatology, Venereology, and Leprosy, Govt Medical College,
Srinagar, Jammu and Kashmir
India

Shashank Bhargava MD
Assistant Professor
Department of Dermatology, STD and Leprosy
RD Gardi Medical College
Ujjain, Madhya Pradesh, India
e-mail: shashank2811@gmail.com

Shekhar N Pradhan MD
Professor and Head
Department of Dermatology
BJ Government Medical College, Pune
Maharashtra, India
e-mail: drsnpradhan@yahoo.co.in

Shivani Ranjan MD
Lecturer
Department of Dermatology, STD and Leprosy
Government Medical College
Jammu, Jammu and Kashmir, India
e-mail: drshivaniranjan@rocketmail.com

Shylaja Someshwar DVD MD
Professor and Head
Department of Dermatology, STD and Leprosy
MGM Medical College, Kamothe
Navi Mumbai, Maharashtra, India
e-mail: shaila38@yahoo.co.in

S Kingsley Diploma in Physiotherapy
Bombay Leprosy Project, 11 VN Purav Marg,
Sion-Chunabhatti, Mumbai, Maharashtra, India

Smitha Prabhu MD DVD
Associate Professor
Department of Dermatology, STD and Leprosy
Kasturba Medical College
Manipal University, Manipal, Karnataka, India
e-mail: drsmithaprabhu@yahoo.com

Sugat Jawade MD PhD
Professor
Department of Dermatology, STD and Leprosy
Jawaharlal Nehru Medical College
Wardha, Maharashtra, India
e-mail: drsugat09@gmail.com

Sujai Suneetha DCP MPhil PhD
Director, Research and Development
Institute for Specialized Services in Leprosy (INSSIL)
Nireekshana ACET (AIDS Care Education and Training), Hyderabad, Telangana, India
e-mail: drsujai@gmail.com

Swetalina Pradhan MD
Assistant Professor
Department of Dermatology, STD and Leprosy
AIIMS, Patna, Bihar, India
e-mail: dr.swetalinapradhan@gmail.com

Tarun Narang MD
Associate Professor
Department of Dermatology, Venereology
and Leprology, PGIMER
Chandigarh, India
e-mail: narangtarun2012@gmail.com

Usha Khemani DVD MD
Associate Professor and Head
Department of Dermatology, STD and Leprosy
GT Hospital, Grant Government Medical College
Sir JJ Group of Hospitals
Mumbai, Maharashtra, India
e-mail: ushakhemani@gmail.com

Utpal Sengupta MVSc PhD
Consultant
Stanley Browne Laboratory
The Leprosy Mission Community Hospital
Nand Nagari, Shahdara, Delhi, India
e-mail: utpal.sengupta@leprosymission.in

Vaishnavi R Gowda MD
Consultant Dermatologist
Kaya Skin Clinic, Bengaluru, Karnataka
e-mail: vaishnaviramegowda@gmail.com

Vinod Kumar Hanumanthu MD
Senior Resident
Department of Dermatology
Venereology and Leprology
PGIMER, Chandigarh, India

Vivek M Pai MD DNB
Bombay Leprosy Project, 11 VN Purav Marg
Sion-Chunabhatti, Mumbai, Maharashtra, India

Message from the IADVL President

It is a proud moment for me to savour. The book *IADVL Practical Manual of Leprosy*, conceived and designed during my tenure as President, IADVL, is ready for release. There is dearth of books on leprosy covering the Indian context of this age-old disease. There was an urgent need for a book that can be used as a ready reckoner. This manual, covering every aspect of leprosy in 5 sections, will be of immense help to clinicians, postgraduates and researchers. Chapters in all sections are written with utmost dedication and detail by all contributing authors. I am grateful to them for putting in such efforts.

I commend the editorial team of Dr P Narasimha Rao, Dr Santoshdev P Rathod and Dr Neel Prabha for achieving the goal. I am sure your work will be appreciated by everyone.

"Read and learn all about Leprosy."

Jayadev Betkerur
President, IADVL 2021
Professor and Head
Department of Dermatology
Dr Moopen's Medical College
Wayanad, Kerala

Preface

Welcome to this practical manual on leprosy, a comprehensive resource designed to equip healthcare professionals, researchers, and caregivers with the knowledge and tools necessary to address the complexities of this age-old disease. Leprosy, also known as Hansen's disease, has persisted throughout history, often shrouded in misunderstanding and stigma. However, with advances in medical science and increased awareness, we stand at a crucial juncture where we can significantly impact the lives of those affected by leprosy.

While significant strides have been made in leprosy control over the years, challenges persist in understanding the issues and needed responses to various aspects of the disease, including their management. While there is a lot of published information about the etiopathogenesis, clinical aspects, management and rehabilitation of leprosy, there is little published assistance on certain 'How to examine', 'How to diagnose', 'How to manage a particularly difficult situation in leprosy'? This practical manual endeavors to fill that lacuna and to provide simple implementation steps about how to address some such questions in a given leprosy patient.

This manual is a testament to the dedication and expertise of the contributing authors, who have meticulously compiled evidence-based strategies and best practices for managing leprosy across different contexts in five sections. It encompasses various aspects of the disease, including examination and assessment, investigations, treatment and rehabilitation. In addition, it also delves into the management of special scenarios, including those after leprosy reactions. On the whole, this manual aims to bridge the gap between knowledge and practice, offering practical guidance that is adaptable to diverse settings and contexts. By providing up-to-date information and evidence-based strategies, we aspire to enhance the quality of care and support available to individuals affected by leprosy.

We hope this book shall be a 'go to' book when in question about 'addressing a specific concern of a leprosy patient' for healthcare personnel, including dermatologists and leprologists and postgraduate students learning the nuances of leprosy. For an experienced leprologist, this might rekindle the old fond memories of classic leprosy practice.

We commend the contributing authors for their dedication to this endeavour, as well as the IADVL, which has supported the development of this manual. It is our sincere hope that it will serve as a valuable resource to understand the common and less-often-discussed aspects of the disease and to equip healthcare professionals with the tools necessary to identify and treat leprosy effectively.

P Narasimha Rao
Santoshdev P Rathod
Neel Prabha
Shekhar N Pradhan

Contents

Section 3: Drug Therapy and Management of Leprosy

Section 4: Management of Special Scenarios in Leprosy

Section 5: Role of Physiotherapy

Abbreviations

AFB : Acid fast bacilli
ADR : Adverse drug reaction
AMR : Anti-microbial resistance
ASHA : Accredited Social Health Activist
BCG : Bacillus Calmette-Guerin
BI : Bacteriological/bacillary index
BL : Borderline lepromatous leprosy
BT : Borderline tuberculoid leprosy
CBR : Community based rehabilitation
CMI : Cell mediated immunity
CNS : Central nervous system
Covid 19 : Corona virus disease 2019
ENL : Erythema nodosum leprosum
G1D : Grade-1 disability
G2D : Grade-2 disability
HCP : Health care provider
H & E. : Haematoxylin and eosin stain
HLA : Human leucocyte antigen
HRUS : High resolution ultrasonography
IEC : Information, education, communication
IAL : Indian Association of Leprologists
IADVL : Indian Association of Dermatologists, Venereologists and Leprologists
ILEP : International Federation of Anti-Leprosy Associations
LL : Lepromatous leprosy
LAMP assay Loop-mediated isothermal amplification assay
BB : Mid-borderline leprosy
M. leprae : *Mycobacterium leprae*
MB : Multi-bacill*ary*
MDT : *Multi-drug therapy*
MDR : *Multi-drug resistance*
MFT : Monofilament
MI : Morphological index
MIC : Minimum inhibitory concentration
MIP : Mycobacterium indicus pranii
MO : *Medical officer*
MRI : Magnetic resonance imaging
NFI : Nerve function impairment
NGO : Non-governmental organisation
NLEP : National Leprosy Eradication Program

NCDR	:	New case detection rate
NSAID	:	Non-steroidal anti-inflammatory drugs
NTD	:	Neglected tropical disease
PB	:	Pauci-bacillary
PCR	:	Polymerase chain peaction
PEP	:	Post exposure prophylaxis
PNL	:	Pure neural leprosy
POC	:	Point of care
qPCR	:	Quantitative real-time PCR assay
RLEP	:	Leprae-specific repetitive element
ROM	:	Rifampicin, ofloxacin, minocycline
RR	:	Reversal reaction
RT PCR	:	Real time PCR
SOP	:	Standard operative procedure
SDR	:	Single dose rifampicin
SW	:	Semmes-Weinstein (monofilament)
TB	:	Tuberculosis
T1R	:	Type 1 lepra reaction
T2R	:	Type 2 reaction
TNF	:	Tumor necrosis factor-alpha
TT	:	Tuberculoid leprosy
VMT	:	Voluntary muscle testing
UN	:	United Nations
WASH	:	Water, sanitation and hygiene
WHO	:	World Health Organization

Section 1

Examination of a Leprosy Patient

Chapter 1

Classification and Clinical Diagnosis of Leprosy

• Gopikrishnan Anjaneyan • Vaishnavi R Gowda • P Narasimha Rao

INTRODUCTION

Leprosy is a dynamic infection and the presentation of it differs within the individual with changes in the immune response and/or institution of anti-leprosy treatment. Appropriate disease classification is essential for planning treatment and management of the patient. It also helps in systematic recording, analysis, comparing and sharing of information in a standard manner. Classification of the type of leprosy is important in counseling the patient, determining the treatment regimen, prognosticating course and complications. This chapter shall discuss the various classification schemes of leprosy and their clinical presentation.

CLASSIFICATION OF LEPROSY

Various classification systems were proposed and adopted for leprosy over the last century, many named after the city where they were proposed (e.g.) Manila, Cairo, Madrid classifications). Most of them are only of historical interest now. Although earlier classification of leprosy has been primarily based on clinical features, the better understanding of the microbiological, histopathological and immunological characteristics over the years has helped to make it more inclusive. Below we describe in brief the classifications which are relevant and are widely accepted/used at present.

Ridley and Jopling Classification: A Five Group System (1966)

This is the most widely followed classification in scientific communications and research as it is an amalgamation of clinical features, histopathological features, immunological status and bacteriological index (BI). Two stable polar forms are included at either end of the spectrum with the polar tuberculoid leprosy (TT) on one end with low bacterial load, predominant cell-mediated immunity, and low specific antibodies; and the polar lepromatous form (LL) at the other end with high bacterial load, low *M. leprae*–specific cell-mediated immunity and high specific antibodies. The immunological and clinical unstable borderline forms are in-between (Box 1.1).

Box 1.1: Ridley and Jopling classification	
Classification	Tuberculoid leprosy (TT) Borderline tuberculoid leprosy (BT) Mid-borderline leprosy (BB) Borderline lepromatous leprosy (BL) Lepromatous leprosy (LL)

The virtue of this scheme is that its subdivisions correlate with the number of acid-fast bacilli detected on slit skin smear examination, expressed as bacteriologic index (BI), on a logarithmic scale ranging from 0 to 6. The disadvantage of this scheme is the absence of incorporation of indeterminate and pure neuritic forms of leprosy.

Limitations of this classification are the lab investigations involved. Skin smear interpretation is heavily dependent on the skill and technique of the person performing it. Lepromin test as an immunological indicator is seldom performed now.

The IAL Classification (1981)

In this consensus leprosy classification of Indian Association of Leprologists, there are 5 groups, which are Lepromatous (L), Tuberculoid (T), Poly (pure) neuritic (P), Borderline (B) and Indeterminate (I). The maculo-anesthetic leprosy which was previously a separate entity as proposed in 1955 was merged with tuberculoid leprosy.[1] Pure neuritic leprosy, a type of leprosy without skin patches but with peripheral nerve involvement, observed especially in Indian sub-continent is included in this classification. All the borderline leprosy types of RJ classification (BT, BB and BL) are grouped into a single borderline group in this system. Indeterminate leprosy forms an important part of this scheme.

The WHO Classification of Leprosy for Therapeutic Purposes—1982 and 1998

WHO in 1982 with the introduction of MDT for leprosy, proposed a classification for therapeutic purposes dividing leprosy into Paucibacillary (PB) and Multibacillary (MB) groups, based on skin smear status. In 1998, it was further modified [1] and formulated based on the number of skin lesions and presence of AFB in skin smears, to simplify selection of the type of MDT for a leprosy patient. This widely accepted therapeutic classification of leprosy was found very useful for field workers, especially where laboratory facilities are not readily available (Table 1.1).

The 'Single-skin lesion (SSL) Leprosy' patients designated in 1998 for therapeutic purposes, were given a one-day therapy with a single dose regimen of ROM (rifampicin 600 mg, ofloxacin 400 mg and minocycline 100 mg). However, after 2004, this SSL leprosy classification for therapeutic purpose was done away with/withdrawn, including the use of ROM. Post 2005, the term SSL leprosy was abandoned and it was included in PB leprosy.

The drawback of this WHO therapeutic classification based on count of skin lesions is the risk of classifying a smear positive (MB) leprosy wrongly as PB leprosy, thus resulting in undertreatment.

Leprosy Classifications of Present Relevance

At present the classification of leprosy for therapeutic purposes is the most popular and widely accepted classification globally and in national leprosy programs. The recent WHO and NLEP-India definitions of PB and MB leprosy are given below.

Table 1.1 WHO Classification of leprosy for therapeutic purposes (1998)

Single skin lesion (SSL) leprosy	Patients having only a solitary skin lesion without nerve thickening
Paucibacillary (PB) leprosy	2–5 skin lesions without detectable acid-fast bacilli (AFB) on skin smears
Multibacillary (MB) leprosy	≥6 skin lesions and all skin smear positive cases

WHO 2017-Definition of PB and MB Leprosy

The 'monitoring and evaluation guide' of global leprosy strategy for 2016–2020 revised the case definitions of PB and MB leprosy, as follows.[2] Here the neuritis and nerve involvement were given consideration (Table 1.2).

NLEP-India 2019-Definition of PB and MB Leprosy

The NLEP (National Leprosy Eradication Programme), India, in its training manual recommends that[3], after making a diagnosis of leprosy, one should group the patient in to PB and MB based on characteristics given in the table for the purposes of therapy. Note that NLEP classification also gives importance to the number of peripheral nerves involved (Table 1.3).

CLINICAL DIAGNOSIS OF LEPROSY

Despite the recent advancements in the serological and molecular diagnosis of leprosy, the majority of leprosy cases are diagnosed on the basis of clinical criteria (cardinal clinical features of leprosy) and visualization of *Mycobacterium leprae* in slit skin smear. Clinical evaluation is the first step for leprosy diagnosis, which is usually enough in most cases; however, detection of leprosy is becoming increasingly difficult due to the varied clinical manifestations coupled with the lack of highly sensitive tests. Furthermore, simplified classification systems based on count of lesions at times may lead to under and over diagnosis subsequently leading to under and overtreatment of cases. The clinical presentation of leprosy is dictated by the organism's tropism towards skin and peripheral nerves as well as patient's variable susceptivity to *M. leprae* depending on their T cell mediated immunity (CMI). A case of leprosy is an individual who has one of the following cardinal signs of leprosy.

Table 1.2: Definition of PB and MB leprosy (WHO 2017)

Monitoring and evaluation guide, Global leprosy strategy (2016–2020)	
Paucibacillary (PB) case	• A case of leprosy with 1–5 skin lesions, without demonstrated presence of bacilli in a skin smear
Multibacillary (MB) case	• A case of leprosy with more than five skin lesions; or with nerve involvement (pure neuritis, or any number of skin lesions and neuritis)
	• or with the demonstrated presence of bacilli in a slit-skin smear, irrespective of the number of skin lesions.

Table 1.3: NLEP-classification of Leprosy for therapy

(NLEP Training Manual for Medical Officers, 2019)	
Paucibacillary (PB)	• Skin lesions 1–5 • Peripheral nerve involvement: No nerve or only one nerve involvement • Skin smear: Should be negative at all sites
Multibacillary (MB)	• Skin lesions: 6 and above • Peripheral nerve involvement: >1 nerve involvement • Skin smear: Positive at any site • Any one of these features can be sufficient for the diagnosis of MB leprosy

Diagnosis of Leprosy[3]

A case of leprosy is diagnosed by eliciting *cardinal* (unique and very important) *signs of leprosy* through systematic clinical and wherever required bacteriological examination. According to NLEP, India, at least one of the following cardinal signs must be present to diagnose leprosy.

a. Hypopigmented or reddish skin lesion(s) with definite sensory deficit
b. Involvement of the peripheral nerves, as demonstrated by definite thickening with loss of sensation and weakness/paralysis of the corresponding muscles of the hands, feet or eyes
c. Demonstration of *Mycobacterium leprae* in the lesions.

The first two cardinal signs can be identified by clinical examination alone, while the third can be identified by examination of the slit skin smear. A person with at least one cardinal sign of leprosy and yet to complete full course of MDT may be called as a "case of leprosy" (Box 1.2).

Approach Towards a Clinical Diagnosis of the Suspected Case

Clinical diagnosis of a case of leprosy is simple using the cardinal signs mentioned above. However, it becomes difficult when only few clinical signs are present. Usually, leprosy is a slowly progressive disease and all clinical signs do not manifest in the beginning and become more clear with passing of time (Flowchart 1.1).

CLINICAL TYPES OF LEPROSY

Leprosy manifests as a spectrum of different clinical forms determined by the immune status of the host. The spectrum ranges from tuberculoid (TT) and borderline tuberculoid (BT) in patients having a strong cell-mediated immunity (CMI); to borderline lepromatous (BL) and lepromatous (LL) forms in those with a very weak CMI to *M. leprae*. The clinical features of various types of leprosy are detailed below. (Flowchart 1.2)

Indeterminate Leprosy

This is characterized by single asymptomatic, hypopigmented, ill to well demarcated, smooth surfaced (or slightly creased and wrinkled) macule, with absence of infiltration. In fair-skinned individuals, lesions may be erythematous, while in darker skin types, they may be coppery brown[5] (Fig. 1.1). Due to lack of fulfillment of diagnostic criteria, it is termed indeterminate. It is mostly seen in children, usually located in the cooler body parts—face,

Box 1.2: WHO Global Leprosy Strategy (2016–2020 document)

It is of interest to note that in the WHO-Global Leprosy Strategy 2016–2020 document,[4] has updated the definition of case of leprosy to be *more in line with ground reality practices and the need to enhance activities for drug surveillance*. These definitions include autonomic dysfunction and histopathology. The document mentions that the new case definitions listed below are expected to be adopted by national leprosy programs.

A case of leprosy is a patient having one or more of the following:

1. Hypopigmented skin lesions with loss of sensation
2. Impairment or involvement of the peripheral nerves as demonstrated by (a) definite loss of sensation, or (b) weakness of hands/feet or face or, (c) autonomic function disorders such as anhidrosis (dry skin)
3. Presence of visible deformities
4. Signs of the disease with demonstrated presence of bacilli in skin smear or histopathological confirmation

~ AND in need of leprosy treatment as decided by a clinician.

Flowchart 1.1: Algorithm for a clinical diagnosis of the suspected case

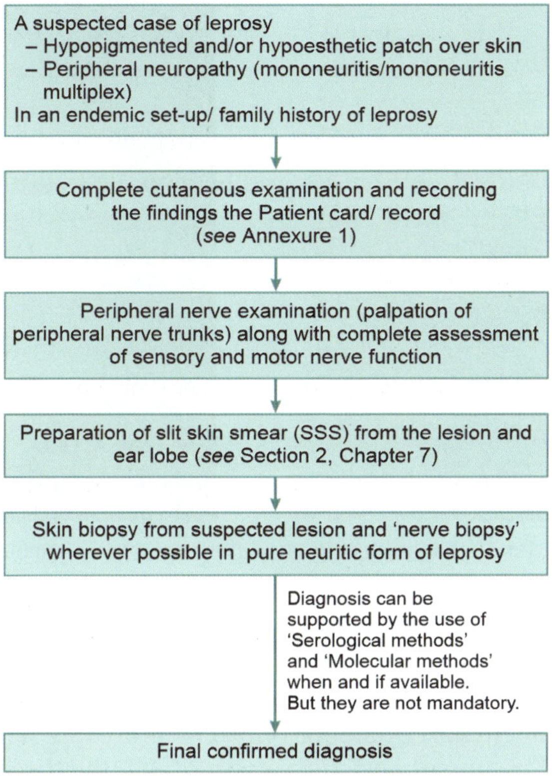

Flowchart 1.2: Clinical types of leprosy—RJ classification

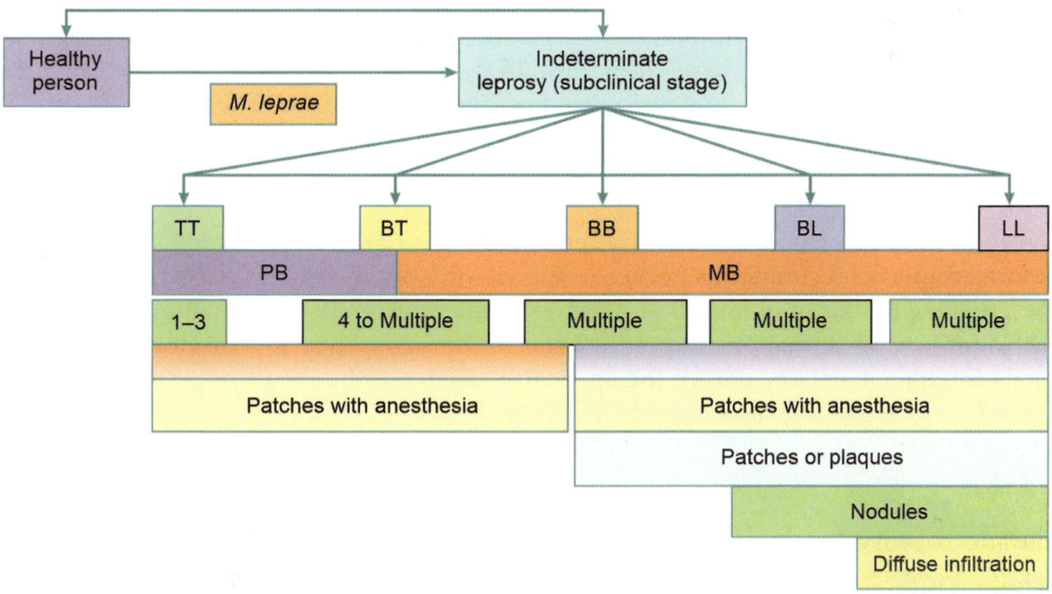

From; *CLTRI Leprosy Training Manual.* (https://cltri.gov.in/TrainingMaterial/4.8–%20Classification%20and%20treatment.pdf)

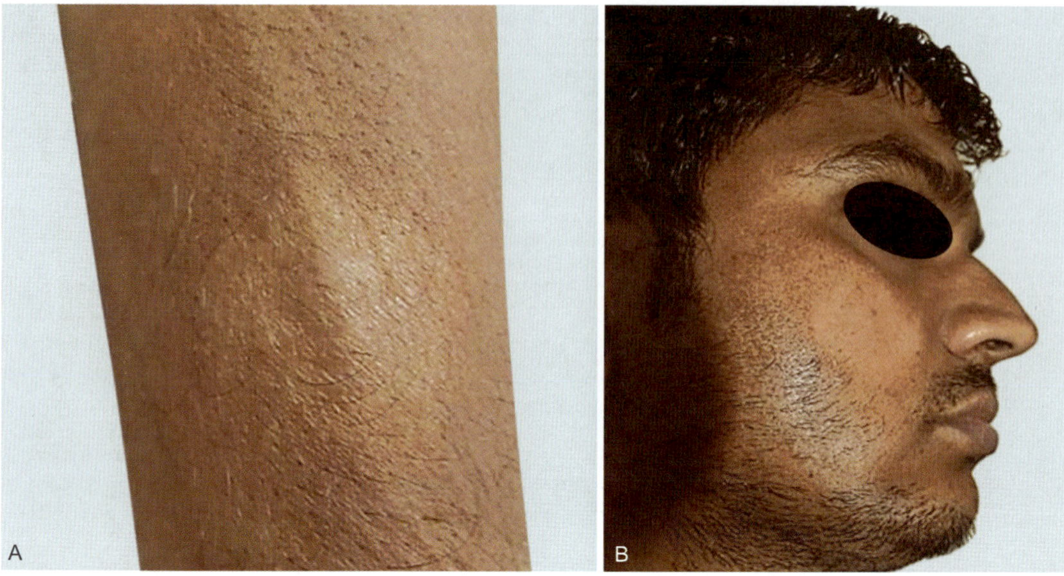

Fig. 1.1: Indeterminate leprosy: Ill-defined hazy patches

extensor aspects of the limbs and buttocks. Some reports mention that this form of leprosy is the earliest clinical presentation in 20% of the patients.[4,5] It can spontaneously heal/regress in the presence of strong CMI or if CMI is moderate will progress to Tuberculoid leprosy. It is not contagious and permanent nerve damage or reactions are rare with adequate treatment.[6] On the contrary, without treatment and with a weak CMI, the disease progresses towards lepromatous spectrum.[5,6]

Tuberculoid (TT) Leprosy

This type usually presents with 1–3 hypopigmented to coppery erythematous, well-defined macules or plaques in an asymmetric distribution (Fig. 1.2A and B). Lesions are dry, scaly, devoid of hair with hypo or anaesthesia due to denervation of the cutaneous appendages and nerve sheath thickening. The lesions may extend up to 10 cm in diameter.[6]

Typical TT lesions are plaques which demonstrate elevated infiltrated borders (Fig. 1.2C to E). Varying degrees of alteration in temperature, touch and pain sensations are noted in that order.

Nerve involvement is usually restricted to a single nerve trunk; acute, prominent and unilateral. Superficial cutaneous nerves in the vicinity of the lesions, also known as serving nerves, may be tender or enlarged or both. Skin smear examination is usually negative.

Although nerve abscesses are seldom seen in leprosy, they are predominantly noted towards the paucibacillary end of the spectrum. They are the result of softening caseating granuloma which forms an abscess, which is palpable as a cystic swelling along a nerve. These changes are more often noted in individuals with higher cell-mediated immune response. Very rarely multiple nerve abscesses along the course of the nerve are also noted.[7]

Borderline Leprosy Group

As per the Ridley-Jopling classification, situated between the two polar types, these unstable intermediate forms constitute the largest leprosy type/group. Whilst the tuberculoid and

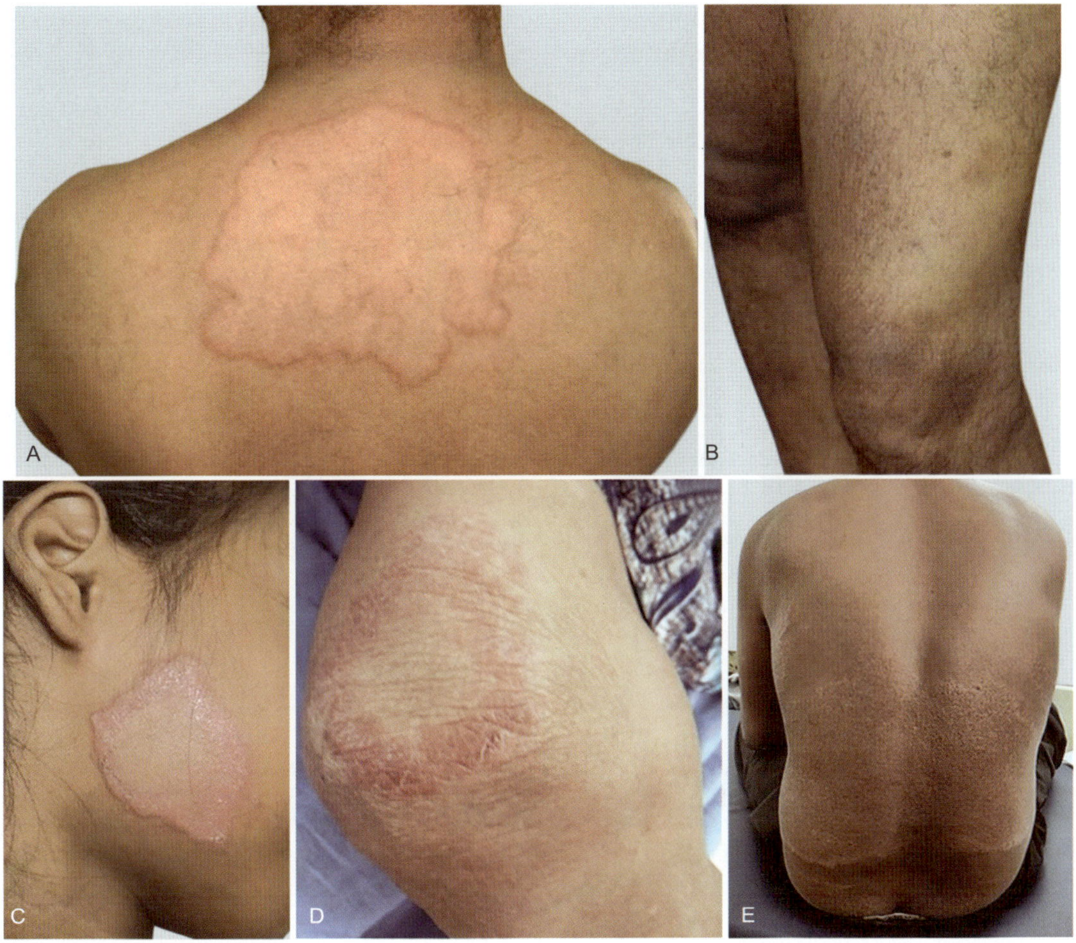

Fig. 1.2: Tuberculoid leprosy: Well-defined erythematous or hypopigmented plaques. Some lesions with scaling with loss of hair

lepromatous poles of the spectrum are stable, cases in this group tend to downgrade toward the lepromatous end when not treated and when offered treatment, they move toward the tuberculoid pole, with reversal reactions.

Borderline Tuberculoid (BT)

Cutaneous lesions have characteristics similar to TT, but they are larger, more extensive, hypoesthetic and asymmetrical, with the number of lesions varying from 4–10 with less infiltrated edges. Smaller newly forming lesions, also known as satellite lesions may be noted near the larger ones and some may have pseudopodia-like (finger-like) extensions. The lesions are dry, scaly and anhidrotic although not as severe as in TT patients. In BT, the lesional edges may be sharp in some areas and ill-defined elsewhere, unlike in TT which has a uniform crisp edge.[8] Occasionally, BT lesions can be flat anesthetic macules (maculoanesthetic patches), either erythematous or hypopigmented associated with nerve enlargement (Fig. 1.3). They most commonly occur on the face, buttocks and lateral aspects of extremities.[9]

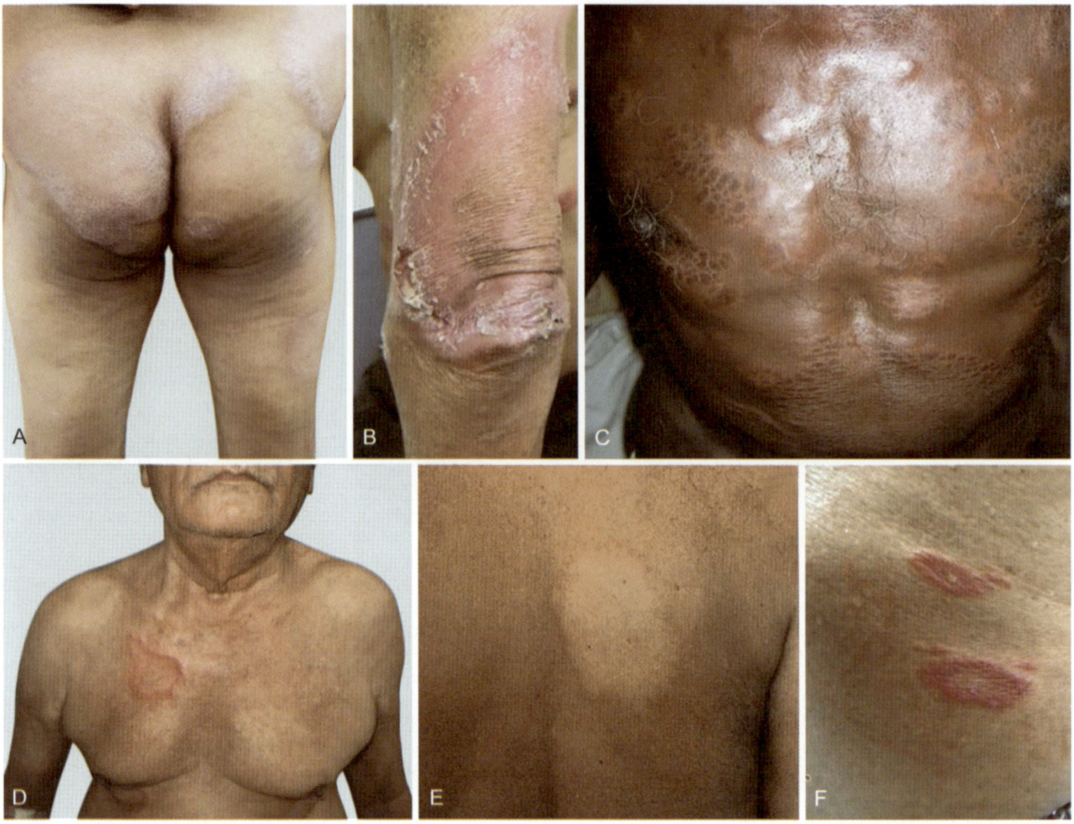

Fig. 1.3: Borderline tuberculoid leprosy: Large-well defined erythematous scaly plaques with mild scaling

Nerve thickening is irregular, asymmetrical and more nerve trunks could be involved but less intense inflammation than in tuberculoid leprosy. BI of Skin smear of BT leprosy varies from being negative to 1+.

Type 1 or reversal reactions occur in BT leprosy not infrequently, as a result of 'reversal' (improvement) of CMI from weak to strong response, manifesting as acute inflammation in the skin lesions and nerves. During reversal reaction, the nerve function could get impaired, which may be the initial stage of presentation of BT in some patients.

Mid Borderline or Borderline Borderline (BB)

Being the most immunologically unstable form, it is transient and very uncommon. In most patients, dimorphic lesions showing features of both tuberculoid and lepromatous types are noted and patients may quickly move towards either pole depending on their immune status and treatment.[5] It is characterized by numerous (10–30), nearly symmetrical non-anesthetic macules, shiny papules, plaques and annular lesions in varying combinations with obscure edges. Hypopigmented macules surrounded by peripheral erythema and edema with a clear inner margin but a sloping outer margin are termed as "punched out" or "inverted saucer" shaped lesions and annular lesions are also seen classically in BB leprosy[9] (Fig. 1.4).

Nerve involvement is widespread and motor and sensory damage occurs in varying proportions. Anhidrosis is seldom noted. If there is downgrading from BT, asymmetric multiple mononeuropathy could be seen and symmetrical nerve enlargement could be

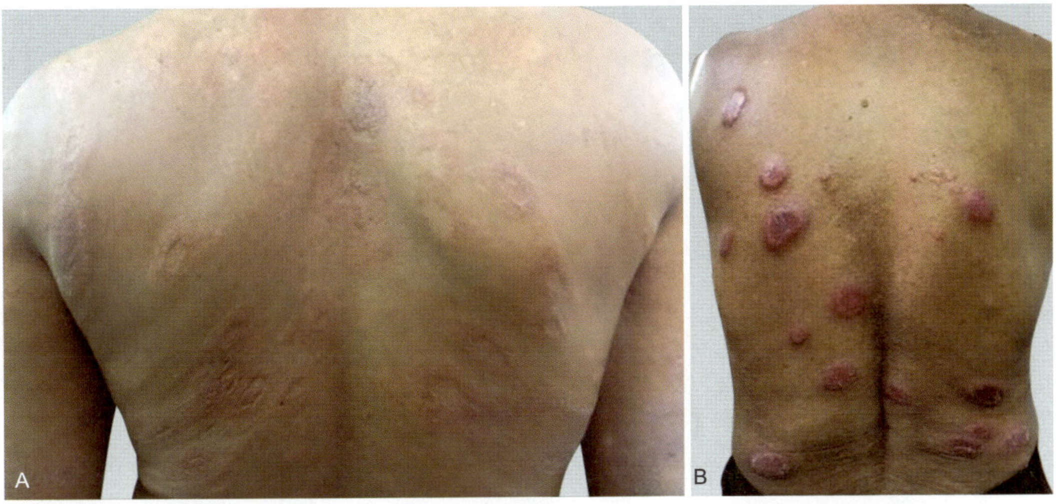

Fig. 1.4: Mid borderline leprosy: Annular lesions with a well-demarcated inner edge which is 'punched out' and the ill-defined sloping outer edge

noted in those upgraded from BL. Reactions in BB usually present with symmetrical polyneuritis.[8]

Lepromin test is negative/weakly positive. Skin smear is positive for AFB, up to 3+.

Borderline Lepromatous (BL)

It is characterized by numerous, (>30), small, mostly symmetrically distributed erythematous macules, papules and nodules with diffuse margins, interspersed with areas of normal skin. Loss of hair and anhidrosis is not very prominent, lesions are in evolutionary phases resembling lepromatous leprosy. However, some lesions may also resemble BT or BB type, indicating downgrading from those types to BL over time. Infiltration is first noted in centre of the macules resulting in the formation of nodules and plaques[5] (Fig. 1.5).

Peripheral nerve involvement is extensive and symmetrical and damage occurs earlier than in LL but not severe as in BT. Motor and sensory impairment does not occur in initial stages. Both type 1 and 2 reactions can occur in these patients. The Lepromin test is negative. BI of skin smears is strongly positive for AFB, reaching up to 4+.

Lepromatous Leprosy

The failure to elicit a successful CMI results in unrestricted multiplication and hematogenous dissemination of *M. leprae* in LL resulting in the production of extensive bilaterally symmetrical (due to the anergic response), numerous hypopigmented and/or copper-red macules, which later progress to shiny papules, tubercles and nodular infiltrates (lepromas/leprous nodules) affecting the skin and mucous membranes. Lepromin test is negative and BI of skin smears are highly positive, reaching up to 6+, including globi formation.

There are two subtypes of LL-subpolar (LLs) which develop as a result of downgrading from borderline spectrum without treatment and polar (LLp) which develops primarily due to the anergic state. In LLs various morphologies of lesions are noted with well-defined borders while in LLp is characterized by diffuse infiltration of the skin with vague edges.[9] With treatment the subpolar group results in faster bacteriological clearance than the polar form.

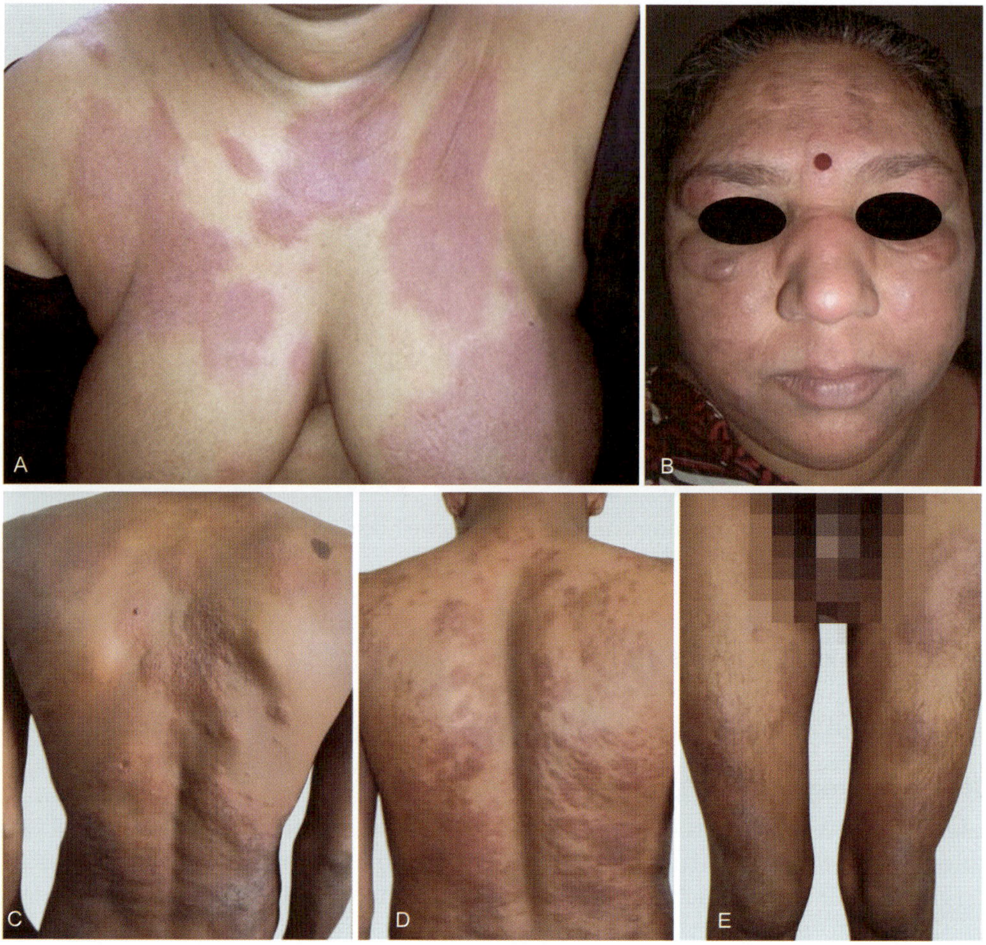

Fig. 1.5: Borderline lepromatous leprosy: Multiple asymmetrically distributed plaques with mild infiltration

Leprous nodules over the face have a symmetrical centrofacial distribution leading to diffuse infiltration, thickening, and nodulation, thus enhancing the skin folds (Fig. 1.6). Infiltration is striking over the face and ears giving rise to a succulent and waxy papules (histoid nodules) appearance which is better appreciated by pinching. On a infiltrated eyebrow ridge, loss of eyebrows starting from the outer third is seen in LL. Loss of eyelashes (ciliary madarosis) is also seen. The convexities of the face become more prominent and with furrowing of creases. This type of appearance is termed as "leonine facies".

Lepromas occurring in the nasal mucosa lead to obstruction, perforation of the nasal septum, bleeding (epistaxis) and resorption of the nasal cartilage and resorption of the anterior nasal spine resulting in collapse of the nose leading to saddle nose deformity.[6]

Nerve involvement is extensive and symmetrical with progressive anesthesia of the hands and feet in a typical glove and stocking distribution. Anhidrosis and ichthyosis of the limbs is noted at a later stage, irrespective of the location of skin lesions. Sensory nerve impairment occurs early in the course of LL, although the patient may be unaware. Motor weakness and atrophy of the muscles develops subsequently. These changes result in trophic ulcers at the pressure bearing sites which may also get infected secondarily.

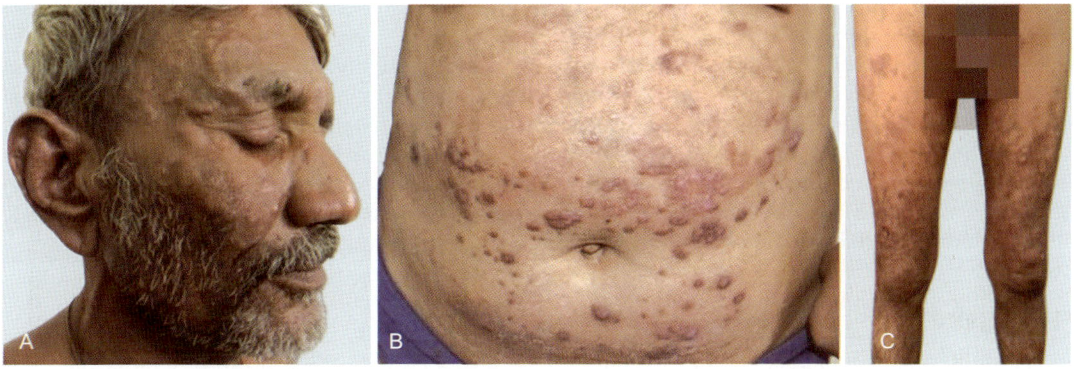

Fig. 1.6: Lepromatous leprosy: Extensive symmetrically distributed small erythematous nodules all over the body

Involvement of ophthalmic division of the trigeminal nerve causes decreased corneal sensitivity. These changes predispose to corneal exposure, dryness, abrasion, uveitis, iritis, ulceration and when unattended can progress to loss of vision and blindness.

Systemic involvement in the form of affection of kidneys manifesting as glomerulonephritis, nephrotic syndrome, and amyloidosis; Lepromatous infiltration of liver in the form of hepatitis, periportal fibrosis and amyloidosis are rarely noted. Testicular involvement in LL results in atrophic testes and/or acute orchitis resulting in hormone imbalance, gynecomastia, and infertility. Osseous involvement mostly of the small bones of the hands and feet leads to bone marrow lepromas and joint effusions. Osteoporosis is also seen in lepromatous leprosy.[10]

Pure Neural Leprosy (PNL)

This type of presentation of leprosy is infrequent (4–7% of all leprosy cases) but not rare. It is characterized by enlarged/thickened nerve trunk with associated symptoms, but without classical leprosy skin lesions anywhere on the body. However, in area of distribution of involved nerve, there will be sensory loss, which may or may not be associated with motor deficit. In PNL, ulnar and popliteal nerves are commonly involved and mononeuritis is the conventional presentation, although rarely multiple (polyneuritic) asymmetrical nerve trunks may also be affected. Nerve involvement causes tenderness, thickening, nodularity or beading of the nerves, pain, and nerve function impairment. In the area of distribution of the affected nerve, sensory, motor and autonomic dysfunction may leads to some or all of these features; hypo/anesthesia, anhidrosis, weakness, atrophy and paralysis of the muscles, fissures, ulcers and rarely deformities.[11]

Although skin lesions are absent, skin biopsies performed along the affected nerve segment very occasionally do reveal granulomas to indicate subclinical involvement. However, skin smears should be always be negative in PNL, and if positive it negates the diagnosis of PNL and indicates lepromatous leprosy. In addition, when followed, up to 4% of PNL cases develop skin lesions, often for the first time during reactions.[10] When nerve biopsy is taken, the spectrum of PNL may range from tuberculoid to lepromatous pattern.[10] Overall, PNL can be considered as a phase of leprosy prior to the appearance of skin lesions, with a predominant nerve involvement.

SUMMARY

Clinical evaluation is the first step for leprosy diagnosis and is usually enough in most cases. It should be supplemented wherever possible, by skin smear examination, to classify it further for therapeutic and academic/research purposes. Strong clinical suspicion along with detailed physical examination is vital, as early detection of leprosy is becoming increasingly difficult due to reduction in expertise and varied clinical presentations, coupled with the lack of highly sensitive laboratory tests. Periodic training of general practitioners and health care providers, especially those practicing in rural areas, on clinical and neurological features of leprosy and their differential diagnoses would help in promoting early diagnosis of leprosy.

REFERENCES

1. WHO Expert Committee on Leprosy, seventh report WHO Technical report series, 874, WHO Geneva 1998.
2. Guidelines for the Diagnosis, Treatment and Prevention of Leprosy WHO 2018.
3. NLEP Training Manual for Medical Officers, CLD, MoHandFW, Govt of India-2019.
4. Monitoring and Evaluation Guide, Global Leprosy Strategy 2016–2020, WHO 2017.
5. Kumar B, Uprety S, Dogra S. (2017). Clinical diagnosis of leprosy, in International Textbook of Leprosy, eds D. M. Scollard and T. P. Gills. Available online at: www.internationaltextbookofleprosy.org
6. Kundakci N, Erdem C. Leprosy: a great imitator. Clin Dermatol. 2019;3(37):200–12.
7. Kamath PR, Rao SS, Shenoy MM. Multiple median nerve abscesses: A rare presentation of leprosy. Arch Med Health Sci 2013;1:57–8.
8. Jopling WH, McDougall AC. Handbook of Leprosy. 5th revised ed. New Delhi: CBS Publishers. 1996.
9. Talhari C, Talhari S, Penna GO. Clinical aspects of leprosy. Clin Dermatol. 2015;33(1):26–37.
10. Fischer M. Leprosy-an overview of clinical features, diagnosis, and treatment. J Dtsch Dermatol Ges. 2017;15(8):801–27.
11. Rao PN, Suneetha S. Pure neuritic leprosy: Current status and relevance. Indian J Dermatol Venereol Leprol. 2016;82(3):252–61.

Chapter 2

Cutaneous Examination

• Bela Shah • Pragya Nair

INTRODUCTION

Leprosy is a chronic infectious disease caused by *Mycobacterium leprae* that mainly affects the peripheral nerves and skin.[1] The presentation of leprosy is highly variable in all its stages, which can mimic a variety of dermatological and neurological conditions. Hence, it is important to be diligent to perform a detailed clinical examination and strict observation of signs and symptoms before making the diagnosis.

Proper baseline documentation of examination findings helps a healthcare provider not only with the diagnosis but also guides to determine the clinical classification of the disease, which in turn helps in deciding the therapeutic schedules and monitoring treatment response. It is important that all the patients' details are recorded in such a pro-forma at every healthcare facility, including by private practitioners treating leprosy. This chapter will outline the salient features of the cutaneous examination of a leprosy patient and their proper documentation.

Cardinal signs of leprosy/Diagnostic criteria[2]

According to NLEP, India, at least one of the following cardinal signs must be present to diagnose leprosy:

a. Hypopigmented or reddish skin lesion(s) with definite sensory deficit
b. Involvement of the peripheral nerves, as demonstrated by definite thickening with loss of sensation and weakness/paralysis of the corresponding muscles of the hands, feet or eyes
c. Demonstration of *M. leprae* in the lesions by skin smear examination.

CHECKLIST BEFORE CUTANEOUS EXAMINATION

Prior explanation of what healthcare provider is going to do will help gain the confidence and cooperation of the patient. Informed consent to be obtained from the patient for examination, unless it is implied. Privacy of the patient is to be maintained at every stage of the management.

- Ensure the presence of an assistant of the same sex as that of the patient to assist you.
- Examine the patient from head to toe in natural light preferably. Examine from a distance initially (general survey), thereafter do a closer examination. Always compare both the sides of the body.
- In case of artificial light, the patient should face the source of light, with the examiner on the same side of the source. The skin lesions (e.g. ill-defined macules and infiltration of skin in LL disease) are better appreciated in an oblique/tangential light.

- General physical examination should precede cutaneous examination. Complete examination of a leprosy patient includes the following mentioned below; only the cutaneous examination part is dealt with in this chapter, rest are described in subsequent chapters of this section. It is recommended that examination finding should be documented in a preformatted leprosy patient record (Annexure 1) with body charting provision, at the time of initial examination and follow-up. However, note that the standard preformatted patient record recommended by NLEP and WHO is concise and focused to record essential details needed from a program point of view and does not have provision to record all the details of clinical examination.
- Cutaneous examination (skin/mucosa)
- Testing for sensations (*see* Section 1, Chapter 5)
- Examination of peripheral nerves (*see* Section 1, Chapter 3)
- Motor examination (*see* Section 1, Chapter 5)
- Examination of eyes (*see* Section 1, Chapter 6)
- Systemic examination (*see* Section 1, Chapter 6)

GENERAL PHYSICAL EXAMINATION

A swift general physical examination is performed to check patients overall health. It also gives healthcare providers a chance to talk to the patient about any ongoing pain or symptoms that they are experiencing or any other health concerns they might have. Presenting complaints and history of present illness should be sought and recorded. Past illnesses, their treatment and medications should also be noted. It helps to determine contraindications or ailments that may preclude the use of drugs recommended in the MDT. Patient's weight, pulse rate and blood pressure should be recorded.

CUTANEOUS EXAMINATION

After a quick general cutaneous survey is done, a detailed examination and recording of skin lesions should be carried out.

1. Site of lesion: Lesions can involve the face, trunk, extremities. Also look for lesions over sites like axillae, groin, genitalia, palms, soles, and buttocks.
2. Number of lesions: Record the number of all skin lesions observed and peripheral nerves involved.

   This helps to classify the type of leprosy (PB or MB), plan type of MDT and the patient follow-up for response. The number of lesions may vary in different types of leprosy; in TT (up to 3), BT (up to 10), BB (10–30), BL (>30), and LL (innumerable). Note that when skin lesions are ≤5, the patient is considered for MDT PB and when they are 6 or more, for MDT MB as per the present guidelines. Hence, appearance of new skin lesions can influence the treatment schedule. It is ideal to record the size of the skin lesions, although not mandatory, when the number is few. This would help to note change in size of lesions (Annexure 2).
3. Note the distribution of lesions: Unilateral, bilateral, symmetrical, asymmetrical. Bilateral symmetrical lesions are observed in lepromatous forms of leprosy.
4. Record morphology of lesions: Note that a variety of skin lesions can be present in a leprosy patient. Common types of skin lesions are macules, papules patches, plaques, and nodules. Occasionally ulcers, vesicles, pustules, fissures and bullae can also be present in a patient.

a. Shape of the lesions can be oval, round, annular or irregular. When it is annular or inverted saucer shaped, it is indicative of mid-borderline leprosy
b. Note the color of lesion: Hypopigmented, erythematous, coppery red or rarely hyperpigmented.
c. Surface of lesions can be dry, scaly, shiny, smooth, edematous, or ulcerated.
d. Margins and the edge of lesions: Well-defined or ill-defined, raised or flat, punched out, sloping.
e. Look for sparseness or absence of hair.
f. Look for infiltration of skin. Infiltrated skin appears shiny, edematous and slightly thickened, with prominent skin pores.

5. Feel for warmth and tenderness of the lesions, especially for those which are erythematous.

   Rarely, well-defined smooth shiny, hemispherical, dome-shaped, non-tender soft to firm papules and nodules of skin colour or with slight erythema, can be seen appearing on otherwise normal-looking skin on trunk and limbs in lepromatous leprosy, which is characteristic of histoid leprosy (Fig. 2.1). Rarely, they can be seen over face, buttocks and over bony prominences, especially around the elbows and knees (Table 2.1).

Examination of nasal cavity: The nasal mucosa is characteristically involved in lepromatous leprosy, and almost never in tuberculoid leprosy. The earliest nasal mucosal changes are oedema, submucosal granulomatous infiltration and crusting of anterior inferior turbinate and nasal septum. This can be associated with increased secretions, sometimes with a blood tinge and occasionally with episodes of frank bleeding (epistaxis). The involvement can rarely progress to septal perforation, especially during ENL reactions. In advanced stages anosmia, atrophic rhinitis and saddle nose deformity can occur.

Oral cavity: Oral mucosal involvement is uncommon in leprosy. However, BT leprosy patch can involve lips, and it can become erythematous and prominent during phases of T1R. Rarely diffuse enlargement of lips in lepromatous leprosy (Macrocheilia) can be observed.[5] Palatal ulceration/perforation is a very rarely encountered complication of lepromatous leprosy, which was more common in pre-MDT era.

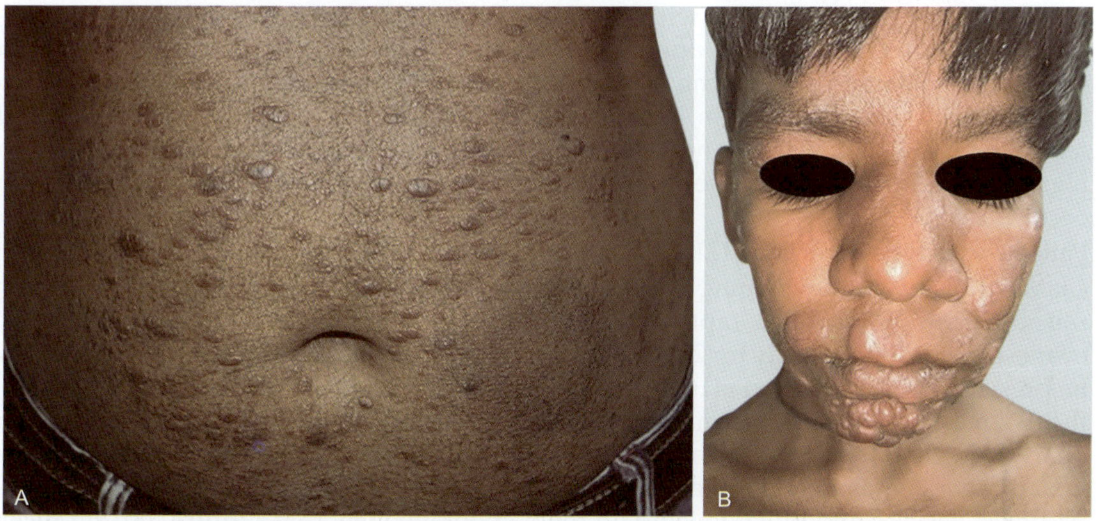

Fig. 2.1: Histoid leprosy: Multiple, discrete, well-defined, shiny, dome shaped papules over: (A) Abdomen; (B) Face

Table 2.1: Characteristics of clinical types of leprosy based on Ridley-Jopling classification[3]

	Indeterminate	*TT (Tuberculoid)*	*BT (Borderline tuberculoid)*	*BB (Mid borderline)*	*BL (Borderline lepromatous)*	*LL (Lepromatous)*
Morphology	Macules	Infiltrated plaques	Infiltrated plaques	Plaques or dome-shaped punched-out lesions	Macules, plaques, papules, infiltration	Macules, papules nodules diffuse infiltration
Number	One or few	Up to 5	Few with satellite lesion or more than 5 (up to 10)	Several (10–30)	Many, >30	Numerous
Distribution	Variable	Localized, asymmetrical	Not diffuse, asymmetrical	Evident asymmetry	Tendency to symmetry	Symmetrical
Size	Small to moderate	Variable, usually large	Variable, some are large	Variable	Small, some can be large	Small
Border	Not always defined	Well-defined with sharp borders	Well-defined with sharp borders	Vague, poorly defined borders	Vague, less well defined border	Vague, difficult to distinguish normal and affected skin
Surface	Normal	Very dry, scaly, turgid	Dry, scaly, bright and infiltrated	Dull/slightly shiny	Shiny	Shiny
Sensation	Absent	Absent	Markedly diminished	Moderately diminished	Slightly diminished	Minimally diminished, not affected
Hair growth	Absent	Absent	Markedly diminished	Moderately diminished	Slightly diminished	Not affected initially

Note that pure neuritic leprosy (PNL) and indeterminate leprosy are not included in R-J classification.

Clinical Examination Findings in Patients with Lepra Reactions

1. Patients with type 1 reaction (T1R)[4] (Fig. 2.2)
   History usually corroborates with patches becoming swollen recently or becoming erythematous. Occasionally, appearance of new skin lesions is also observed. On examination, some or all of the existing leprosy lesions in T1R show signs of acute inflammation. (erythema, pain, tenderness, and edema). They can be associated with recent increased or new motor nerve function impairment/paralysis. During the phase of regression, desquamation can be observed on these patches. Rarely, necrosis and ulceration occur in severe cases.
2. Patients with type 2 reaction (T2R) [Erythema nodosum leprosum (ENL)] (Fig. 2.3).
   Classical history of developing recurrent crops of bright erythematous, tender, slightly raised papules to nodules, (aptly named as erythema nodosum leprosum), which are evanescent, (lasting usually for 2–3 day) in a febrile patient, more so in the evenings would be present. The distribution is bilateral, symmetrical; usually on arms and thighs. While the flexor aspects of forearms and the medial aspects of thighs are favored, but can present on the trunk and face as well. They regress leaving a blue-black pigmentation at their site, which causes occasional desquamation. New crops can keep appearing in chronic ENL. At times, vesicles and bulla develop on them spontaneously that rupture to form ulcers known as erythema/ENL necroticans.

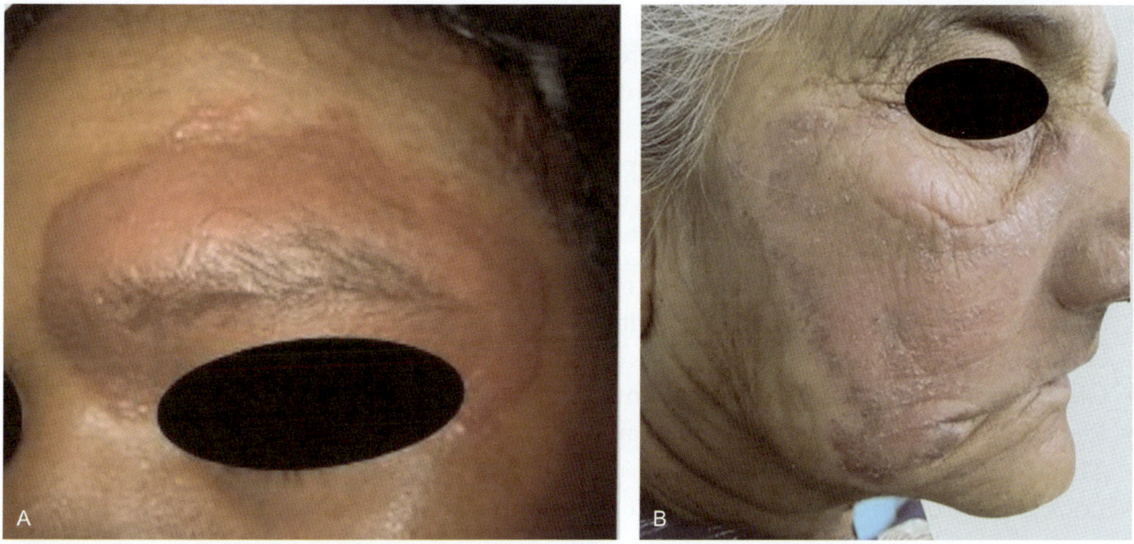

Fig. 2.2: Type 1 reaction: (A) Well-defined, raised outer border of erythematous, tender plaque over left forehead; (B) Erythematous, tender plaque over right face

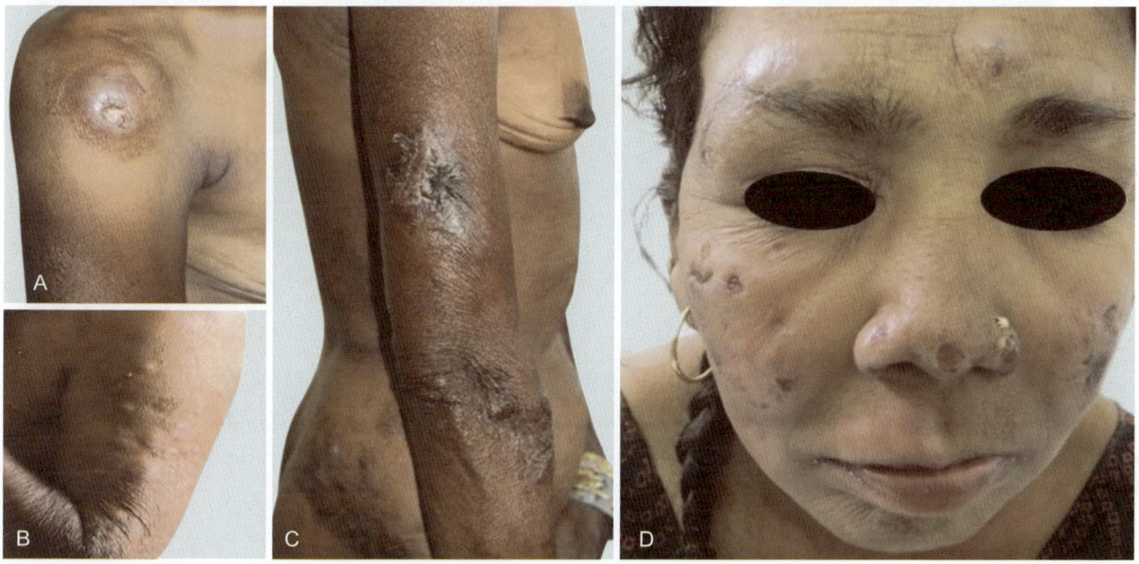

Fig. 2.3: (A and B) Multiple, discrete, erythematous, tender, papules and nodules occurring in crops; (C and D) Necrotic ulcers over ENL lesions (erythema necroticans)

Special Sites for Examination and Attention

Face: Look for following features:

- Erythematous facial patches—indicative of impending T1R.
- Watering of eyes, red eye, lidlag and lagophthalmos—indicative of facial and ophthalmic nerve involvement.

- Diffuse coarse infiltration of the face with papules with thick skin folds, loss of eyebrows and nodularity—Leonine facies in lepromatous leprosy (Fig. 2.4A and B)
- Depressed nasal bridge, due to loss of nasal septal cartilage and inferior nasal spine-advanced lepromatous leprosy
- Mega-lobules of ear in lepromatous leprosy (Fig. 2.4C and D)

Hands and Feet:[6,7] (Fig. 2.5)

- Test for sensations on hands and feet
- Check for trophic changes and loss of muscle mass.
- Note clawing of fingers and toes and inability to extend fingers fully or to bring fingers close together
- Observe for callosities over bony prominences or pressure points.
- Record blisters, fissures and ulcers, if any
- Check for loss of tissue and resorption of fingers tips and toes.
- Look for any other signs and features of disability and deformity.

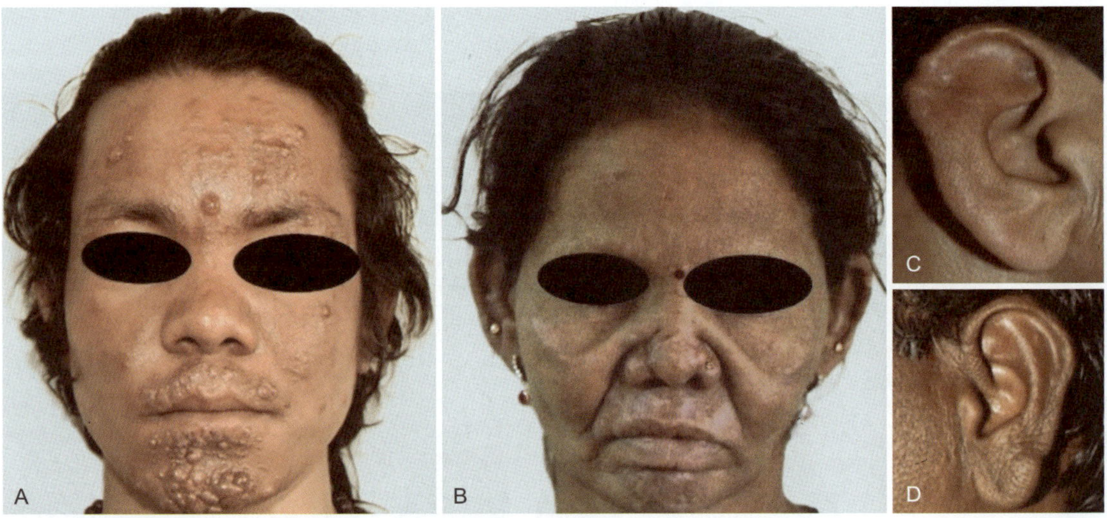

Fig. 2.4: (A and B) Coarse infiltration of face with papulonodular lesions in case of histoid leprosy; (C and D) Infiltrated earlobe

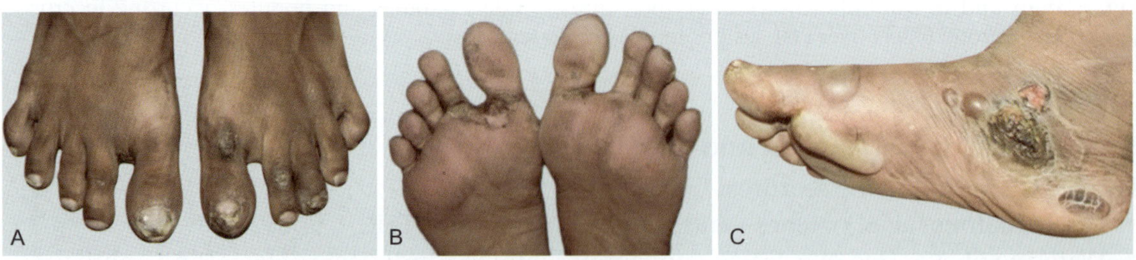

Fig. 2.5: (A and B) Trophic ulcers over bilateral feet; (C) Spontaneous blister over right foot

CONCLUSION

Diagnosis of leprosy and its classification warrants thorough clinical examination of all suspected cases. It is a prerequisite for planning management and administration of appropriate therapy. Findings of initial examination and each follow-up should also be recorded in the pre-formatted leprosy proforma and follow-up sheets. These records, either physical or electronic should always be stored safely for their future use and reference.

REFERENCES

1. World Health Organization. (2009). Microbiology of *M. leprae*. [online] Available from www.who.int/lep/microbiology/en/index.html. [Accessed May, 2014].
2. NLEP Training Manual for Medical Officers, CLD, MoH&FW, Govt of India-2019.
3. Jopling WH, McDougall AC. The disease. In: Jopling WH, McDougall AC (Eds). Handbook of Leprosy,6th Edition: 2020Delhi: CBS Publishers and Distributors; 2020.pp.10-53.
4. Guidelines for the diagnosis, treatment and prevention of leprosy. New Delhi: World Health Organization, Regional Office for South-East Asia; 2018.
5. Singh G, Nagaraja, Prabhu S. Leprosy presenting as macrochelia. Indain J Lepr. 2000;72(1):341-2
6. Indira D, Kaur I, Sharma VK, et al. Palmoplantar lesions in leprosy. Indian J Lepr. 1999;71(2):167-72.
7. Srinivasan H, Dharmendra. Treatment of ulcers in leprosy patients. In: Dharmendra (Ed). Leprosy. Bombay: Kothari Medical Publishing House;1978.pp.599-616.

Chapter

3

Peripheral Nerve Examination

• Shekhar N Pradhan • Anil Patki

INTRODUCTION

Involvement of the nerves is an integral aspect of leprosy. The consequences of nerves damage are responsible for the deformities and disabilities that occur in this disease. Nerve involvement and its inflammation, referred to as 'neuritis' is the major cause of morbidity in leprosy, appreciated clinically as nerve thickening, beading/nodularity or nerve abscess. It results from cell-mediated immune damage, infiltration of nerves with lepra bacilli as well as from reactionary episodes.[1] Sensory component of the nerves is damaged first (the earliest sensation to be lost is temperature, followed by touch and pain), but eventually autonomic as well as motor functions can be deranged.

Damage to the peripheral nerves can lead to sensory loss, motor paralysis and loss of sweating in the areas innervated by the affected nerve. Vibration and proprioception are not affected.

In the various patterns of leprosy, the skin and major peripheral nerves often undergo parallel pathologies. The inflammation is similar, and the same classification system is applied. The severity of the cutaneous and peripheral nervous system abnormalities depends upon whether the patient is 'leaning' toward the lepromatous pole or the tuberculoid pole.[3] Although tuberculoid leprosy patients may have conspicuous alterations in just one specific peripheral nerve trunk, usually in the same segment of the skin lesion, lepromatous leprosy patients often present with variations of thickness and tenderness in many nerves.[4] However, the density of acid-fast bacilli is often a logarithm higher in nerves than in the nearby involved skin.[2] On the whole, clinical examination of the peripheral nerves forms an important aspect of diagnosis and follow-up in patients of leprosy.[5]

In leprosy, the peripheral nerves are affected where they are superficial, cool and subjected to friction and trauma. These 'sites of predilection' are typical for different nerves and usually near the skin surface and where the nerves pass through tough fibro-osseous canals. The swelling of nerves at these sites compromises the blood supply of the nerves causing ischemic damage. The superficial, cool parts of the peripheral nerves are affected because the *Mycobacterium leprae* grows best at an optimum temperature between 27° and 30°C.

IMPORTANCE OF PERIPHERAL NERVE EXAMINATION IN LEPROSY

The palpation of peripheral nerves is a disappearing clinical skill. As presence of thickened peripheral nerve is considered one of the three cardinal signs of leprosy for its diagnosis, it is important that the method and skill of appreciating it by palpation of nerves be learnt. In fact, thickening and/or tenderness of the nerves can be the only diagnostic features of pure neuritic leprosy, a type of leprosy where the skin lesions are absent. This skill can only be honed by repeated practice. In addition, it is also important to supplement it by learning the correct way of sensory testing of suspected areas of skin, with the cotton wool, ballpoint pen and graded nylon filaments.

CLINICAL METHOD OF NERVE EXAMINATION

While examining the peripheral nerves, it is extremely important to be gentle and careful for appreciating any gross structural abnormality. And for that it is important to have an idea of the size and feel of the 'normal' nerves; which can only be obtained by repeated palpation of nerves in normal individuals. Note that the nerve size varies between individuals depending on the age, weight and muscularity of the individual. The normal nerves of a muscular worker may be thicker than of a thin sedentary individual. While palpating the nerves, the features to be noted are thickening, tenderness, nodularity (beaded/abscess) and consistency (soft/firm/fibrosed). Palpation should always be done with pulp and not the tips of the fingers. Once nerve is identified, roll it gently against a firm background (bone or taut muscle) for assessment. And nerves of the both sides should have examined if possible at the same time, for comparison to detect any differences in thickening and tenderness. Box 3.1 illustrates basic necessities before proceeding for peripheral nerve examination.

Box 3.1: How to set up patient before peripheral nerve examination

- Introduce self
- Enquire patients name and what they like to be called
- Explain about the examination
- Wear gloves
- Position the patient in the right way for the nerve to be palpated (Table 3.1)

Table 3.1A: Palpation of major peripheral nerves of upper extremity

Nerve	*Site/bony landmark*	*Patient position*	*Method*
Radial Nerve 1. In the arm	Spiral groove on humerus, Posterior to the deltoid insertion (Fig. 3.1)	Sitting/standing with elbow flexed at 90°. Examiner's hand holds patient's hand in shaking-hand manner	Examiner's fingers of other hand roll the nerve in radial groove
2. At the wrist	Radial cutaneous nerve: Lateral border of radius, just proximal to the wrist; thereafter along the proximal part of extensor policis longus tendon, which stands out prominently on ulnar side of the anatomical snuff box (Fig. 3.2)	Same as above. Patient is asked to extend the thumb to visualize the anatomical snuff box	Examiner's fingers roll the nerve against radius. It can be further traced and rolled from side to side on extensor policis longus tendon and dorsum of hand
Ulnar	Ulnar groove on medial epicondyle of humerus, medial to the point of elbow. (Fig. 3.3A)	Same as above.	Examiner's ring finger locates the nerve in the groove; other fingers palpate the nerve upwards along the medial aspect of arm. (Fig. 3.3B)

(Contd.)

Table 3.1A: Palpation major peripheral nerves of upper extremity *(Contd.)*			
Nerve	***Site/bony landmark***	***Patient position***	***Method***
Median	Proximal to the flexor aspect of wrist joint (proximal to flexor retinaculum), between the tendons of Palmaris longus and flexor carpi radialis	Sitting/standing with elbow flexed at 90°, wrist in supination. Examiner's left hand stabilizes patient's left hand vice versa (Fig. 3.4)	Examiner's fingers palpate and feel for the nerve deep between the tendons. As the nerve is deeply placed, only tenderness can be elicited in almost all cases, when it is involved.

Table 3.1B: Palpation of major peripheral nerves of lower extremity			
Nerve	***Site/bony landmark***	***Patient position***	***Method***
Common Peroneal (Lateral Popliteal)	On the neck of fibula, round the insertion of biceps femoris tendon	Sitting/standing with knees flexed at 90°. Both nerves should be palpated simultaneously with the examiner sitting in front for better comparison	Examiner's thumbs are placed on the tibial tuberosities and the fingers on the lateral side of knees. Fibular head is located and the nerves are palpated just beneath it on the neck of fibula posteriorly and round the insertion of biceps femoris tendon (Fig. 3.5)
Posterior tibial	At the ankle joint, midpoint between the medial malleolus and the tuberosity of calcaneum	Same as above with ankle in the neutral position	Examiner's fingers roll the nerve in the tarsal tunnel below the flexor retinacula (Fig. 3.6)

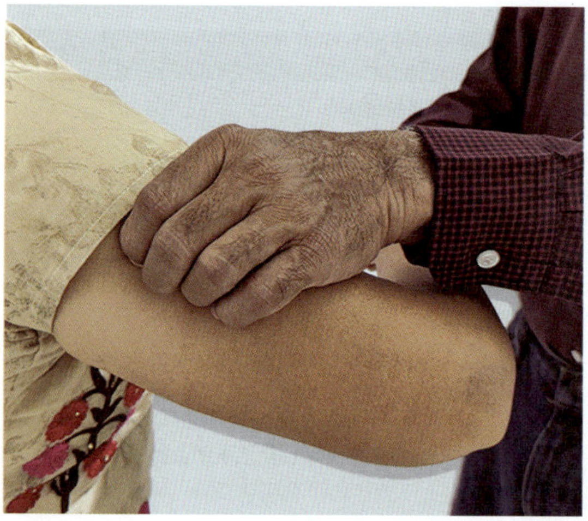

Fig. 3.1: Examination of radial nerve in the arm

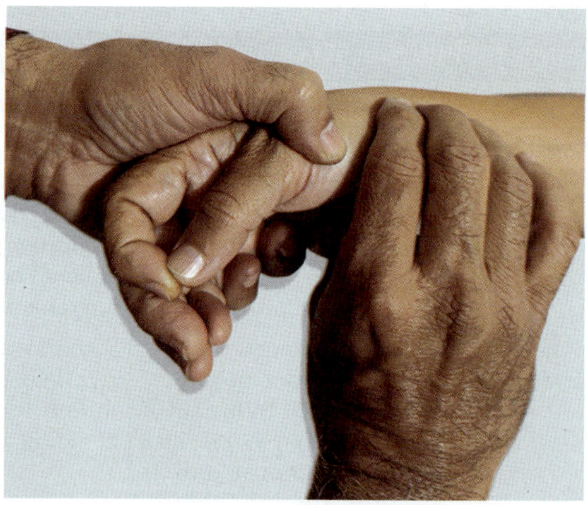

Fig. 3.2: Palpation of cutaneous branch of the radial nerve

Ulnar Nerve

The ulnar nerve is the most commonly involved nerve amongst all the peripheral major nerve trunks. It is subjected to trauma and friction as it traverses through fibro-osseous tunnel at elbow. The ulnar nerve can be palpated in two ways. The examiner holds the right hand of the patient in his left hand and then palpates the right ulnar nerve with the right hand passed medially around the elbow. The ulnar nerve is palpated in the olecranon groove. It is traced above till the mid-arm (Fig. 3.3A).

The patient flexes both the elbows to 70–80° and the examiner examines both the ulnar nerves simultaneously passing the fingers around the lateral sides of elbows. By this method, the two nerves can be palpated simultaneously and the discrepancy in their sizes can be compared (Fig. 3.3B).[7]

Median Nerve

The median nerve is affected just above the wrist joint. When the wrist is flexed against resistance, two tendons viz. flexor carpi radialis and palmaris longus are visible. The median nerve is anatomically placed between and deeper to these tendons. When firmly palpated, while passively flexing the wrist joint, tenderness of the effected nerve can be appreciated. However, it is not possible to assess its thickness as it is placed deep below the flexor retinaculum of the wrist (Fig. 3.4). One should keep it in mind that median nerve is most amenable to imaging by HRUS at this location.

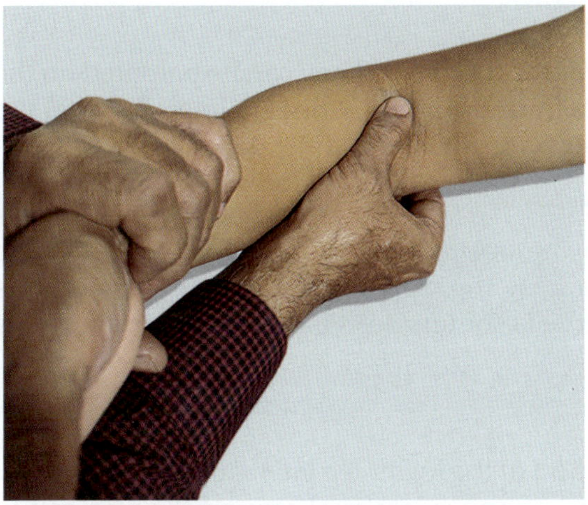

Fig. 3.3A: Examination of ulnar nerve

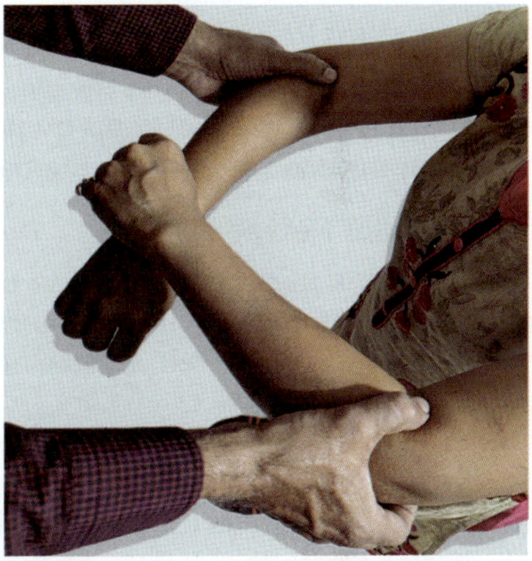

Fig. 3.3B: Examination of ulnar nerve of both hands simultaneously

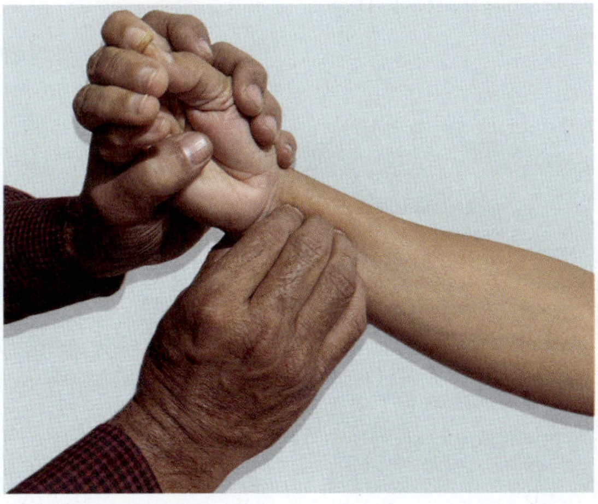

Fig. 3.4: Examination of median nerve at the wrist

Radial Nerve

The radial nerve is the least commonly involved major nerve trunk in the upper limb. It is palpated in the mid-arm just behind the insertion of the deltoid muscle (Fig. 3.1). However, its cutaneous branch which is commonly involved is palpated just above the wrist joint where it lies over the lateral side of the lower end of the radius (Fig. 3.2)

Common Peroneal (Lateral Popliteal) Nerve

These nerves are palpated with the patient sitting on a stool or examination table with the knees bent at right angles. The examiner keeps the thumbs on the patella and passes the fingers lateral to the knee joints to locate the fibular heads. The nerves can be palpated simultaneously where they pass around the neck of the fibulae (Fig. 3.5)

Posterior Tibial Nerve

This nerve is palpated at the ankle joint in between the medial malleolus and the calcaneal tuberosity (Fig. 3.6).

Other Important Nerves Commonly Examined

These nerves run upward from the eyebrows over the forehead. They can be palpated on the forehead just above the eyebrows by passing the thumbs or index fingers laterally from the midline. Supratrochlear nerve is medial to the supraorbital nerve (Fig. 3.7)

Great Auricular Nerve

To examine this nerve, the head is turned to the opposite side in order to stretch the sternocleidomastoid muscle. The nerve runs across the upper third of the muscle. This nerve is better seen than felt. Even a normal nerve is sometimes visible in thin individuals (Fig. 3.8).

Sural Nerve

This nerve is examined on the posterior-lateral aspect of the lower leg lateral to tendo-Achilles. It travels along with the short saphenous vein becoming superficial around the mid-calf to the level of ankle, where it courses between the calcaneus and lateral malleolus. This is the area where it can be best palpated. It is a pure sensory nerve (Fig. 3.9).

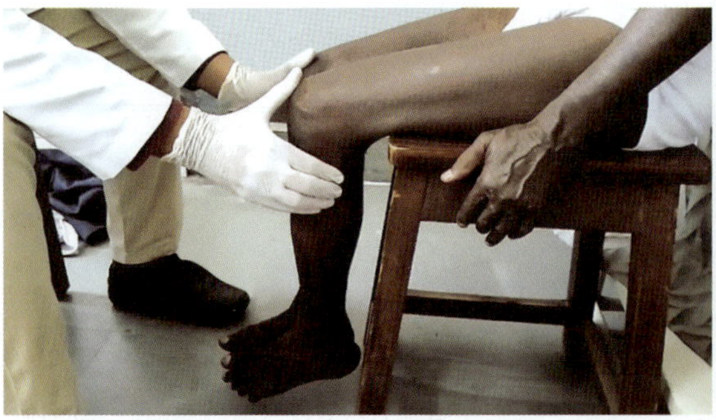

Fig. 3.5: Examination of lateral popliteal nerve

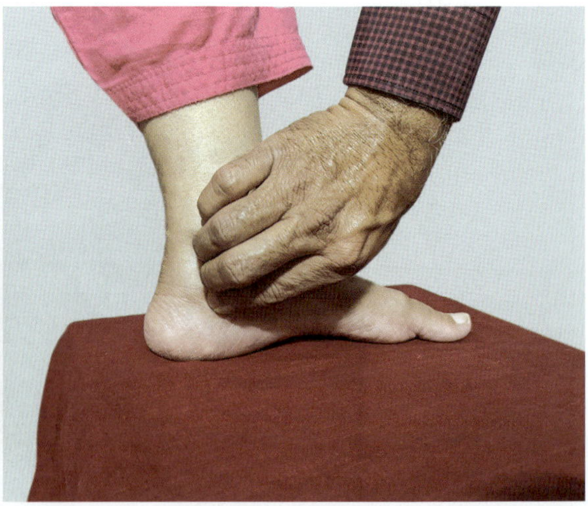

Fig. 3.6: Examination of posterior tibial nerve

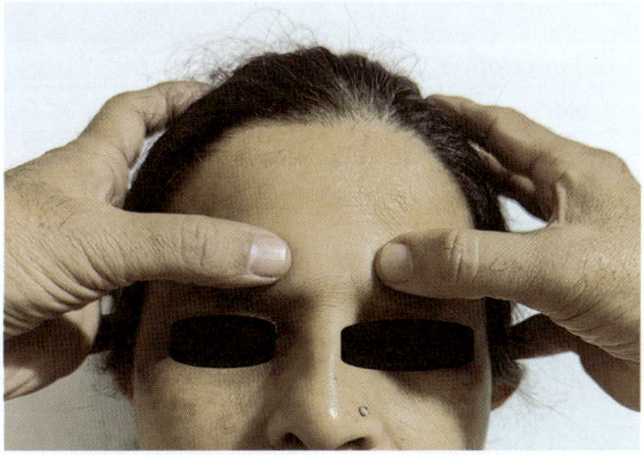

Fig. 3.7: Examination of supraorbital and supratrochlear nerves

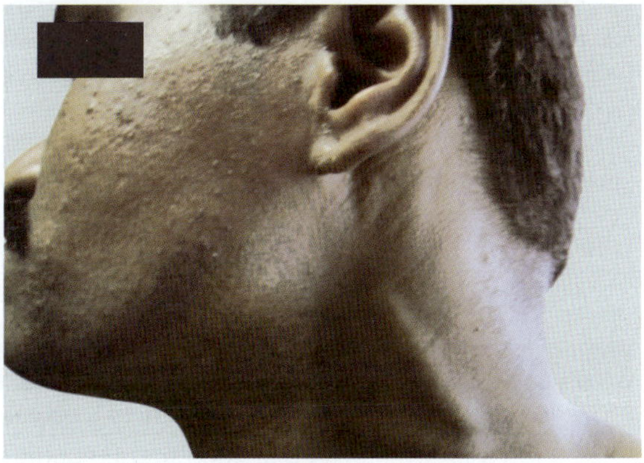

Fig. 3.8: Examination of great auricular nerve

OTHER CUTANEOUS NERVES

The supraclavicular nerves, medial, lateral and posterior cutaneous nerves of the forearm, ulnar cutaneous nerve, superficial peroneal nerve, digital nerves are the common cutaneous nerves which can be seen and/or palpated in patients of leprosy, when they are involved.

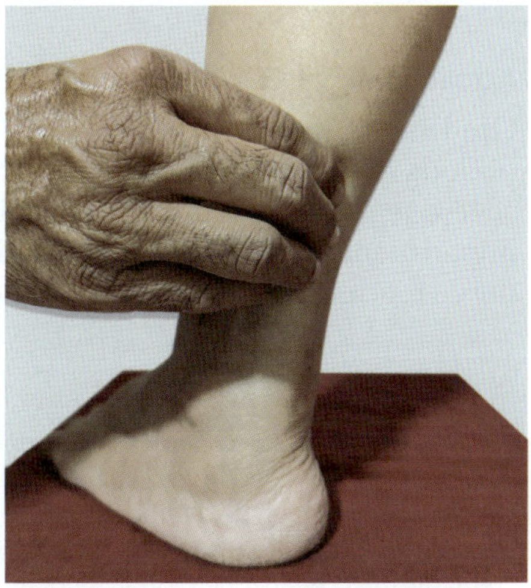

Fig. 3.9: Examination of sural nerve

CLINICAL GRADING OF NERVE THICKNESS AND NERVE TENDERNESS AND ITS APPLICATION

Assessment of nerve thickness and tenderness is subjective in nature. Objective measurement of thickness of nerves can be done with high resolution ultrasonography. A standardized clinical grading of nerve thickness, tenderness and pain are required for (a) systematic recording at the initial and follow-up visit for changes, (b) communication between leprosy workers, and (c) for institution of appropriate therapy and to assess its effect.

Given below is the widely accepted clinical grading of nerve thickness and tenderness.

Grading of nerve thickness: A four-grade scale (0–3) is used to grade nerve thickening. The nerves are palpated at their most superficial locations for at least 5–10 cm of its length to detect beading or nodularity (Table 3.2).

Grading of Nerve Tenderness

A four-grade scale (0–3) is used to grade tenderness. It is elicited by applying mild to firm pressure on the nerve during palpation. To evaluate the grade of tenderness, during palpation, look for patient's response (wincing, expression of distress on face, withdrawing the limb). An experienced examiner can provide a reasonable grading of tenderness. Repeated/overzealous palpation of tender nerves should be avoided (Table 3.3).

Table 3.2: Grading of nerve thickness*		
Grade	***Degree***	***Description***
0	Not thickened	Nerves not thickened and feels normal
1	Mild thickening	Thickened compared to contralateral side
2	Moderate	Thickening is rope like
3	Severe	Nerve thickened and also nodular or beaded

*Normal nerve feels soft to firm, flattish and slightly compressible

Table 3.3 Grading of nerve tenderness		
Grade	***Degree***	***Description: Patient's response***
0	None	Says palpation is not painful even when asked about it
1	Mild	Says palpation is painful only when asked about it
2	Moderate	Indicates palpation is painful by wincing during palpation or says so
3	Severe	On palpation, tries to withdraw the limb; or is clearly distressed by pressure on the nerve

Application of Clinical Grading

Grading of nerve thickness once recorded is usually not prone to changes over short periods of time. However, nerve tenderness is prone to changes over short intervals and severe tenderness indicates acute inflammation of nerve which can lead to nerve function impairment (NFI). Immediate administration of corticosteroid therapy should be done when nerve tenderness is more than or equal to grade 2 along with measures to prevent NFI.

SUMMARY

Palpation of peripheral nerves is an important clinical skill to be learnt to assist the diagnosis of leprosy. It can only be perfected by repeated palpation of peripheral nerves, of both leprosy and non-leprosy affected persons. While high resolution ultrasonography is now available for the objective examination of peripheral nerves in some tertiary centres, the palpation of nerves clinically for their involvement and grading still remains the cornerstone of leprosy diagnosis and management.

REFERENCES

1. Textbook of Dermatology and Sexually Transmitted Diseases with HIV Infections, Sardana K Jan 2019.
2. Atlas and Synopsis of Lever's Histopathology of the Skin, 3rd edition, David E. Elder, Rosalie Elenitsas *et al*, 2013.
3. Dermatology edited by Jean l Bolognia, Joseph l Jorizzo, 2nd Edition 2008.
4. Fitzpatrick's Dermatology Ninth Edition Sewon Kang, Masayuki Magai,Leprosy Claudio Guedes Salgado, Arival Cardoso *et al.*
5. Brycesson ADM, Pflatzgraff RE. Leprosy Third edition, 1990, ELBS, Churchill Livingstone pp57–75.
6. Chen S, Wang Q, Chu T, Zheng M. Inter-observer reliability in assessment of sensation of skin lesion and enlargement of peripheral nerves in leprosy patients. Lepr Rev. 2006;77(4):371–6.
7. Girdhar BK. Methods of nerve examination. In: Kar HK, Kumar B editors, IAL Textbook of Leprosy, 2nd edition 2016, Jaypee Brothers, pp 263–7.

Chapter

4

Cranial Nerve Examination

• Shylaja Someshwar • Pooja Agarwal

INTRODUCTION

In leprosy, a disease with an affinity for nerves, there is sufficient evidence of multiple cranial nerves being affected often. Yet, clinicians seldom gives importance to this part of examination. Nonetheless, it is paramount to examine all the commonly affected cranial nerves in leprosy to rule out their involvement, more so those which exit through bony canals where they can be compressed, especially during a lepra reaction. This can cause a great amount of function loss which may even be irreversible. Furthermore, these nerves supply vital structures of the body, the dysfunction of which results in enormous functional crippling. It is even shown that the manifestations of cranial nerve involvement may resurface even after completion of MDT. In this chapter, we have attempted to fill this lacuna by describing the examination of commonly affected cranial nerves in a simple and practical manner.

CURRENT KNOWLEDGE ON THE INVOLVEMENT OF CRANIAL NERVES IN LEPROSY

In leprosy, cranial nerve involvement is seen in about 10–17% of patients.[1] The infection can reach the nerves via direct exposure or through blood or lymph.[2] While it has been observed that cranial nerve involvement most commonly affects patients suffering from lepromatous leprosy, it has also been shown to occur in other spectra of the disease. Of the cranial nerves involved in leprosy, the commonly involved three cranial nerves are facial, olfactory and the trigeminal nerves.[3] Facial or trigeminal nerve involvement has commonly been reported in borderline tuberculoid (BT) leprosy, while the olfactory nerve involvement has been observed more frequently in borderline lepromatous or lepromatous (BL, LL) leprosy.[4] Auditory, oculomotor, glossopharyngeal, vagus, spinal accessory and hypoglossal nerves are rarely affected[5] and Optic nerve involvement is extremely rare.[6] The most common sign of trigeminal nerve involvement is hypoesthesia and/or anesthesia, of skin supplied by the maxillary division.[7] Multiple cranial nerve involvement in a single patient has been emphasized in many studies. The cranial nerves reported to be involved are I, V, VI, VII, VIII IX, X, and XII.[8–10] MRI evidence of CNS changes in the brain and spinal cord has also been described in leprosy patients.[11] Cranial nerves with their type and designated Roman numerical are summarized in Table 4.1.

Salient Clinical Aspects of Cranial Nerve Involvement

Involvement of olfactory nerve results into hyposmia/anosmia. Olfactory dysfunction has been shown to affect 40% of patients with leprosy.[12] Inability to identify smell of smoke/leakage of cooking gas/other hazardous gases can be a cause of consequences. The quality of

Table 4.1: Cranial nerves overview

Type	*Cranial nerves*	
	Roman Numerical	***Names***
Pure sensory	I	Olfactory
	II	Optic
	VIII	Vestibulocochlear
Pure motor	III	Oculomotor
	IV	Trochlear
	VI	Abducens
	XI	Spinal accessory
	XII	Hypoglossal
Mixed	V	Trigeminal
	VII	Facial
	IX	Glossopharyngeal
	X	Vagus

life gets impaired as the food does not taste good with anosmia. The **optic nerve** involvement though rare, this may manifest as vision loss and visual field defects especially in patients with lepra reaction.

The ocular changes in leprosy are more commonly due to the trigeminal and facial nerve involvement.

Trigeminal and Facial Nerve Involvement

It presents as loss of corneal sensation, in addition to the loss of sensation in area supplied by its sensory branches on face, especially by the maxillary branch. Loss of corneal sensation can lead to injury to corneal epithelium and hinder its healing, which may progress ultimately to ulceration, scarring and perforation.[13]

Leprosy affects the facial nerve in various patterns. Zygomatic branch is preferentially involved due to its superficial location, but hematogenous spread of the lepra bacilli within epineural and perineural vessels may also be seen and could be the reason behind skip lesions and selective involvement of the branches of the facial nerve.[14] The facial nerve supplies muscles of facial expression and of which involvement of orbicularis oculi causes lagophthalmos. Combined involvement of V andVII nerves result in corneal xerosis, exposure keratitis, corneal ulceration, scarring, complicated cataract and blindness. Due to persistent corneal anesthesia, development of new ocular complications even after successful completion of treatment has been shown by many studies[15,16] Patients with lepromatous spectrum of the disease and elderly have increased ocular morbidity.[17]

Facial nerve involvement also affects other muscles of facial expression which manifests as facial asymmetry and Bell's palsy, more often in patients with BT leprosy undergoing type 1 lepra reaction.[5,18] In a patient who presents with bilateral facial palsy, leprosy should always be ruled out. Taste sensation from the anterior 2/3rds is carried by the facial nerve and taste impairment has been observed in about 40% of patients with leprosy.[19]

Involvement of Vestibulocochlear Nerve

It can lead to cochlear type of hearing loss as observed by researchers in a substantial number of patients of leprosy.[8,9] Sensorineural hearing loss is more common in lepromatous leprosy with erythema nodosum leprosum (ENL) reaction.[20]

CRANIAL NERVE EXAMINATION APPROACH

Following prerequisites which should be kept in mind before examining the patient.

W – **W**ash the hands properly/Wear gloves

I – **I**ntroduce yourself politely

P – **P**ermission (informed consent taken from patient after explaining the examination)
Privacy to be maintained
Position of the patient (Seated comfortably in a chair at your eye level).

Examination of Olfactory Nerve

It is an unmyelinated nerve sensory nerve covered with olfactory glia transmitting the smell sensation through olfactory pathway. It may directly get affected by as impairment of the olfactory bulb and olfactory receptors by the lepra bacilli [12] or by primary atrophic rhinitis caused due to mucosal thinning and defects in mucosal innervation with olfactory nerve.

Method of Examination

Enquire the patient for: (a) Any difference in ability to smell, (b) Any recent cold/epistaxis, (c) If they can recognize the smells of the common substances (as these may vary according to the region and subset of patients).

After checking for the patency of the nostrils and explaining the procedure, he is asked to close the eyes. Each nostril is tested separately. Place a familiar scent (non-irritating, non-pungent) like cardamom/soap/asafoetida (*hing*)/clove/peppermint below the nostril and ask him/her to identify the scent. Same procedure is to be repeated on the other side. Test is considered positive when he/she is able to identify the smell on both sides.

Optic Nerve Examination

Optic nerve is responsible for transmitting the special sense of vision. Leprosy can rarely cause visual field defects by damage to any part of the visual pathway and defects in the pupillary light reflex: Direct reflex and consensual reflex (Fig. 4.1).

Method of Examination

Examination of this nerve encompasses

1. *Pupillary reflexes:* Light and accommodation reflexes are tested to check both the optic and oculomotor nerves together (**Afferent: Optic; Efferent: Oculomotor)**
   - *Light reflex:* Light is shone into the patient's eye in a dark room (while keeping a card between the eyes) from the side. The examiner observes for pupillary constriction in the same eye (direct light reflex) and other eye (consensual light reflex). Each pupil constricts briskly if normal. The same procedure is repeated on the other eye. The schematic diagram for pathway of light reflex and possible defects are given in Fig. 4.2
   - *Accommodation reflex:* The examiner keeps his finger near nose of the patient (about 18") and he is asked to focus on it after focussing on a distant object. The reflex comprises of convergence of the eyes along with pupillary constriction.

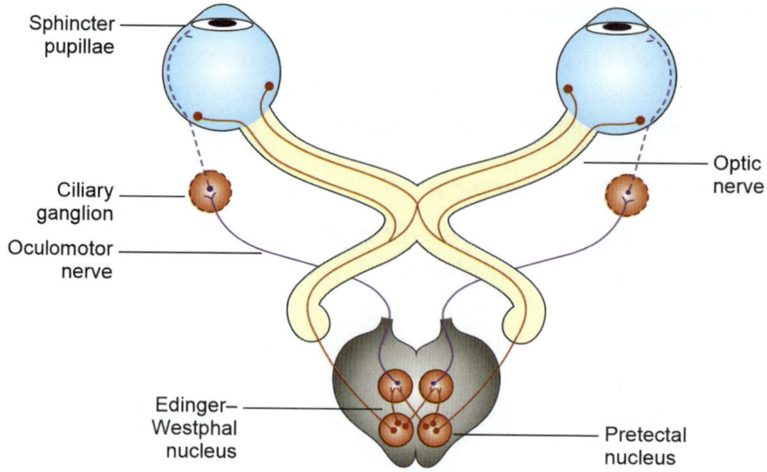

Fig. 4.1: Light reflex pathway

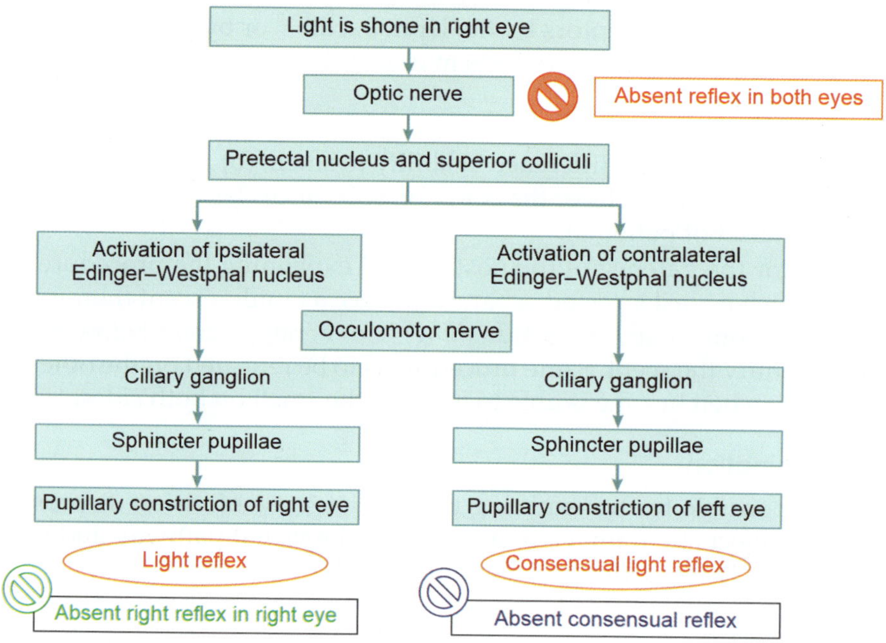

Fig. 4.2: Schematic representation of light reflex pathway

2. *Visual acuity* is the measure of how well the eyes can distinguish shapes and details of objects at a distance. It depends on the intactness of the central retina and the optic nerve. It also depends on the integrity of cornea. It is checked in each eye separately for both near and distant vision. Counting of fingers is simple test to detect gross visual defect for distant vision (start at 1 meter distance. Normal person can count till 6 meter distance). Distant vision can also be checked with the help of standard Snellen's chart. Near vision is checked with the help of Jaeger cards kept at a distance of 1 foot from the patient. In case of severe decrease in acuity, in addition to finger counting, hand movements and light perception are tested to assess the level of blindness.

Oculomotor, Trochlear and Abducens Nerve Examination

All three are mainly motor nerves. They are very rarely involved in leprosy. Oculomotor and trochlear nerves originate in the midbrain whereas abducens originates in the pons and all 3 of them traverse the supraorbital fissure to enter the orbit. Table 4.2 describes their innervations, functions and clinical signs of their damage. Clinical signs of 3rd nerve palsy are illustrated in (Fig. 4.3). The mnemonic LR6 $(SO_4)_3$ helps in remembering the innervation

Table 4.2: III, IVand VI nerves

Cranial nerves	*Innervation*	*Function*	*Clinical signs of damage (Fig. 4.3)*
III	a. Involuntary supply to pupil and lens • Ciliary muscle • Sphincter pupillae	• Controls the shape of lens to focus on closer objects • Constriction of the pupil	• Loss of accommodation • Dilated pupil • Ptosis • "Downward and outward" positioning of the affected eye [due to the unopposed abduction (lateral rectus muscle) (and adduction and downward movement (superior oblique muscle) • diplopia because of misalignment of the eyes
	b. Motor supply • Levator palpebrae superioris • 4 eye muscles (Superior rectus, inferior rectus, medial rectus and inferior oblique)	• Elevates the upper eyelid • Visual tracking and gaze fixation	
IV	Superior oblique muscle	• Forward rotation of the eyeball when the eye is adducted	• Failure to depress the eye during adduction • Diplopia • Difficulty in reading a book/ walking down the stairs • Affected eye is higher and medially deviated because of dominance of inferior oblique
VI	Lateral rectus muscle	• Abducts the eye on the same side	• Inability to abduct the ipsilateral eye • Diplopia and medial strabismus due to the unopposed action of medial rectus

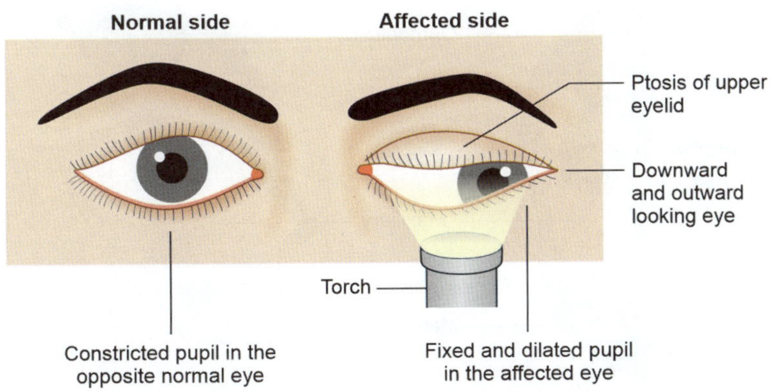

Fig. 4.3: Clinical signs of oculomotor nerve paralysis

by the extraocular muscles. It stands for: LR6: Lateral rectus muscle of eye being supplied by sixth cranial nerve. SO_4: Superior oblique muscle being supplied by fourth cranial nerve. The third (3) cranial nerve innervating the other extraocular muscles.

Method of Examination

The three nerves are additionally tested together for the movements of the eyeball. With the head kept stable, the patient is first asked to look in different directions (approximately corresponding to 12, 2, 4, 6, 8, 10 o'clock positions) on command by following an object kept at about 12" from patient's nose and then moved in the above mentioned directions. Both eyes are observed simultaneously. This can also be observed while doing the visual field mapping. Size of palpebral fissures is additionally observed for any narrowing due to muscle weakness (ptosis) as a result of oculomotor nerve lesion, if any.

Trigeminal Nerve Examination

It provides sensory innervation to the face. After its origin at the junction of pons and the middle cerebellar peduncle, and after its intracranial course, it exits the skull as 3 branches: ophthalmic branch; through superior orbital fissure, maxillary branch through *foramen rotundum* which enters the orbit through infraorbital foramen as infraorbital nerve and mandibular branch through foramen ovale (Fig. 4.4). Details of each branch are described in Table 4.3.

Method of Examination

Sensory examination: The patient is instructed to close his/her eyes and pain, temperature and light touch sensations are examined over forehead and upper side of nose (ophthalmic division), malar region and upper lip (maxillary division) and chin (mandibular division).

- *Corneal reflex:* After explaining the procedure, the patient is asked to fix gaze straight ahead. Then from the side, the lateral margin of cornea is touched lightly with a wisp of cotton. This results in blinking of both eyes. (Afferent—Trigeminal nerve; efferent—Facial nerve) as shown in Fig. 4.5.
- *Blink reflex/orbicularis oculi reflex/glabellar reflex*—The supraorbital ridges are tapped lightly which result in blinking. (Afferent—Trigeminal nerve; efferent—Facial nerve).

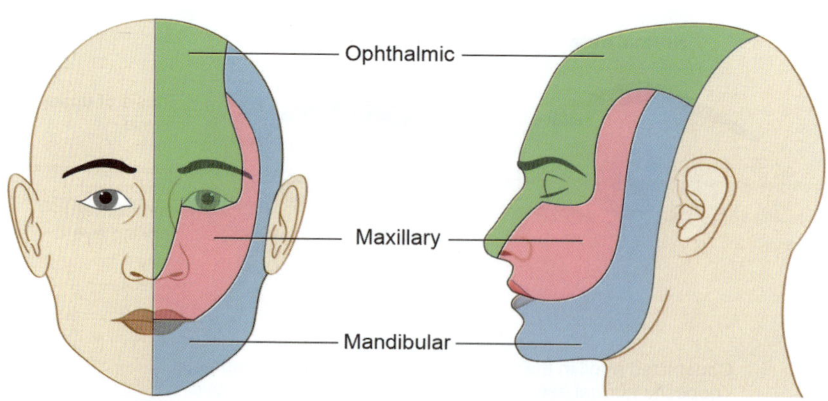

Fig. 4.4: Sensory innervation of trigeminal nerve branches

Table 4.3: Trigeminal nerve					
Branches	***Description***	***Branches***	***Innervation***	***Function***	***Effects of damage***
Ophthalmic	• Smallest • Pure sensory	• Lacrimal • Frontal-2 branches – *Supraorbital* – *Supratrochlear* • Nasociliary	These branches supply • Forehead, scalp • Frontal and ethmoidal sinuses • Cornea • Upper eyelid with its conjunctiva • Dorsum of nose	Sensory	• Loss of sensations of the supplied area • Loss of corneal reflex
• Maxillary	• Second division • Pure sensory	• Gives various branches at various levels	• Lower eyelid with its conjunctiva • Cheeks • Maxillary sinus • Lateral nose and nasal cavity • Upper lip • Upper incisors, canines and molars, with the associated gingiva • Superior palate • Parasympathetic supply—nasal as well as lacrimal glands	Sensory	• Loss of sensations of the supplied area
Mandibular	• 3rd and the largest of the 3 • Mixed nerve with motor and sensory branches	• Sensory supply • Motor supply • Parasympathetic supply	• Mucosa and floor of oral cavity • External ear • Lower lip and chin • General sensation over anterior 2/3 of the tongue (taste sensations by branch of facial nerve) • Lower incisors, canines and molars with the associated gingiva • Muscles of mastication: • Digastric muscle-anterior belly • Mylohyoid muscle • Tensor veli palatini • Tensor tympani • To submandibular, sublingual and parotid glands	• Sensory • Help in mastication of food with various movements of mandible • Normal jaw jerk • Involved in elevation of hyoid bone while swallowing • Elevates soft palate and prevents regurgitation of food into nasopharynx • Dampens sounds like that of chewing by stabilizing malleus bone of middle ear	• Loss of sensations of the supplied area • Difficulty in mastication • loss of jaw jerk

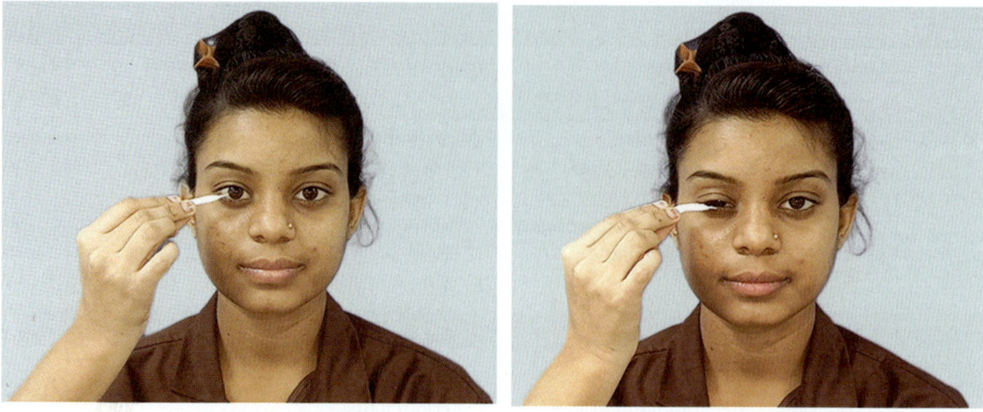

Fig. 4.5: Method of examination to elicit corneal reflex

Facial Nerve Examination

It is a mixed nerve having sensory, motor as well as parasympathetic innervations. It arises from the brainstem and after its intracranial course it comes out of the stylomastoid foramen of the temporal bone and divides into its terminal branches at the posterior edge of the parotid gland. Various branches and functions of facial nerve are described in Table 4.4, the areas supplied by its branches are depicted in Fig. 4.6. The patient is made to sit in good light and is observed for facial symmetry, symmetry of blinking/eye closure and any palsy. *Motor examination*: The patient is asked to raise the eyebrows, close the eyes tightly, frown, puff the cheeks and show the teeth. Any difficulty in doing the actions or asymmetry is noted.

Other cranial nerves are very rarely involved in leprosy and routine testing for their integrity is not needed in leprosy patients.

Table 4.4: VII nerve

Terminal branches	*Functions*		*Effects of damage*
• Temporal • Zygomatic • Buccal • Marginal mandibular • Cervical	• Motor	Posterior belly of the digastric muscle, muscles of facial expression, stylohyoid and stapedius muscles.	Peripheral nerve damage causes: • Ipsilateral paralysis of the muscles of facial expression
	• Sensory	Around the concha	
	• Special sensory	Via chorda tympani—Taste sensation to the anterior 2/3 of tongue	• Taste disturbance in the affected area
	• Parasympathetic	Supplies many glands of head and neck region: Lacrimal glands. Salivary glands: Submandibular and sublingual Nasal, palatine and pharyngeal mucous glands.	• Disturbances in lacrimation and salivation

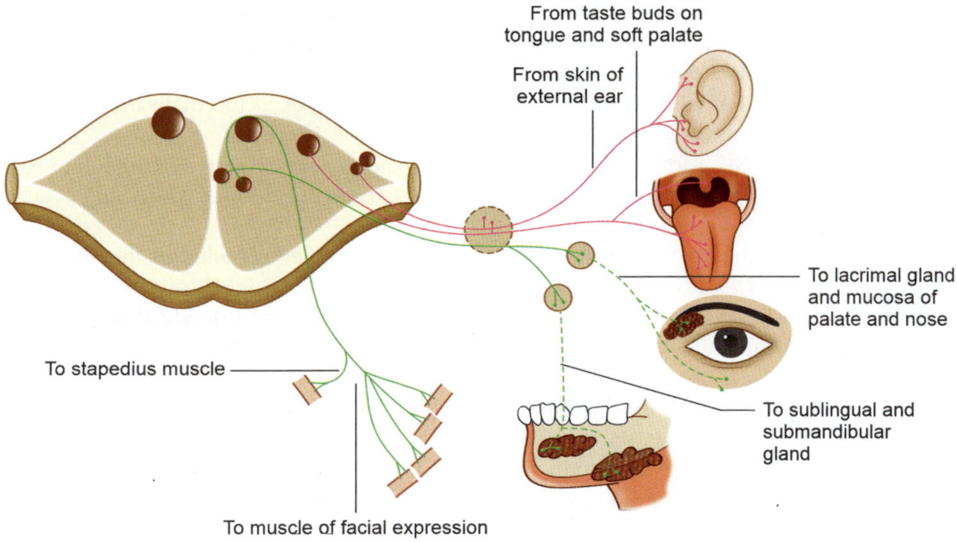

Fig. 4.6: Facial nerve innervation

SUMMARY

In the normal functioning of the human body, cranial nerves play a very essential role, and they can be involved in leprosy. Hence, it should be a routine practice to look for cranial nerve involvement in examining a leprosy patient. Investigations like CT and MRI may sometimes be required for the diagnosis. Patient suspected to have their involvement should be sent for Ophthalmology, ENT and neurology specialist care as needed to tertiary centers.

REFERENCES

1. Kumar S, Alexander M, Gnanamuthu C. Cranial nerve involvement in patients with leprous neuropathy. Neurol India, 2006; 54: 283–5.6
2. Liu TC, Qui JS. Pathological findings on peripheral nerves, lymph nodes and viceral organs of leprosy. Int J Lepr. 1984;52:377–83.
3. Gopinath DV, Thappa DM, Jaishankar TJ. A clinical study of the involvement of cranial nerves in leprosy. Indian J Lepr 2004;76:1–9.
4. Wani AA, Gupta V, Jan N. A clinical study of cranial nerve involvement in leprosy. Egyptian Dermatol Online J, 2009; 5: 3.
5. Gourie-Devi M. Cranial neuropathy in patients with leprosy. Neurology India, 2006;54: 248–9.
6. Arora VK, Dhaliwal U, Singh N, Bhatia A. Tuberculous optic neuritis histologically resembling leprous neuritis. Int J Lepr, 1995; 63: 454–5.
7. Reichart PA, Srisuwan S, Metah D. Lesions of the facial and trigeminal nerve in leprosy. An evaluation of 43 cases. Int J Oral Surg, 1982; 11: 14–20.
8. Dhar MC, Ghosh KC, Basu K, Banerjee G. Polyneuritis cranialis in a case of leprosy. J Assoc Physic India 1999;47:828-30.
9. Paul JT, North-Wilhelm K, Higdon GA, Chesser RS, Hayden DL. Multiple cranial neuropathies associated with leprosy. South Med J 1994;87:937–40.
10. Dhar S, Sharma VK, Kaur S. Facial, glossopharyngeal, vagus and hypoglossal nerve palsy in a case of lepromatous leprosy. Indian J Lepr 1993;65:333–6.
11. Polavarapu K, Preethish-Kumar V, Vengalil S, et al. Brain and Spinal Cord Lesions in Leprosy: A Magnetic Resonance Imaging-Based Study. Am J Trop Med Hyg. 2019;100(4):921–31.

12. Chaturvedi VN, Rathi SS, Raizada RM, Jain SK. Olfaction in leprosy. Indian J Lepr. 1985;57:814–9.
13. Iraha S, Kondo S, Yamaguchi T. et al. Bilateral corneal perforation caused by neurotrophic keratopathy associated with leprosy: a case report. BMC Ophthalmol 2022;22:42
14. Turkof E, Tambwekar S, Kamal S, et al. Leprosy affects facial nerves at the main trunk: neurolysis can possibly avoid transfer procedures. Plast Reconstr Surg 1998;102:1565–73.
15. Lewallen S, Tungpakorn NC, Kim SH, Courtright P. Progression of eye disease in 'cured' leprosy patients: implications for understanding the pathophysiology of ocular disease and for addressing eyecare needs. Br J Ophthalmol 2000; 84(8): 817–21.
16. ffytche TJ. Residual sight-threatening lesions in leprosy patients completing multidrug therapy and sulphone monotherapy. Lepr Rev 1991; 62(1): 35–43.1.
17. Daniel E, Koshy S, Sundar Rao G, Rao PSSS. Ocular complications in newly diagnosed borderline lepromatous and lepromatous leprosy patients: baseline profle of the Indian cohort. Br J Ophthalmol. 2002;86:1336–40.
18. Ramadan W, Mourad B, Fadel W, et al. Clinical, electrophysiologucal and immunopathological study of peripheral nerves in Hansen's disease. Lepr Rev 2001;72:35–49.
19. Soni NK, Chatterji P. Disturbance of taste in leprosy. J Laryngol Otol. 1981;95(07):717–20.
20. Mann SB, Kumar B, Yande R, Kaur S, Kaur I, Mehra YN. Eighth nerve evaluation in leprosy. Indian J Lepr 1987;59:20–5.

Chapter 5

Sensory and Motor Nerve Function Assessment

• *Shashank Bhargava* • *Deepali Tarate*

INTRODUCTION

Mycobacterium leprae attacks the nerve tissue and effects pathological changes which results in the sensory, motor, and autonomic nerve function impairments (NFI). As the peripheral nerves of limbs are involved principally in leprosy, the NFI of these can progress to disabilities and deformities of hands and feet, which often result in social stigma infamously associated with leprosy. Therefore, examination of peripheral nerves in leprosy patients is an important and integral part of clinical examination and a good methodology will aid assessing the extent of their involvement.

SENSORY ASSESSMENT

The different types of sensations based on their receptors are exteroceptive or superficial (touch, pain, temperature) and proprioceptive or deep (joint position, vibration and perception of muscle movement). In leprosy, only the former is altered. The notable changes in sensation are (a) Tactile—hypoesthesia is decreased appreciation and anaesthesia is the total absence of appreciation of touch. (b) Pain—hypoalgesia is decreased appreciation and analgesia is the total appreciation of pain. (c) Temperature for both cold and hot: Thermal hypoesthesia is decreased appreciation and thermal analgesia is the total absence of temperature appreciation.

While the sensory examination in leprosy, as recommended by medical specialists and neurologists, involves evaluation of temperature, touch, pain as mentioned above, testing of all these sensations is not recommended by WHO from programmatic point view of leprosy. WHO and NLEP-India, recommend only testing of cutaneous sensations with the help of tip of light ballpoint pen for leprosy patients,[1] probably because it provides the needed information about loss of sensation sufficient for the diagnosis leprosy, and to assess the protective sensations of hands and feet. However, in this chapter we are providing, in brief, the methods for examination of temperature, touch and pain sensations.

Sensory Examination

It is important that prior explanation of the sensory testing method which is going to be performed is needed to gain the confidence and cooperation of the patient (Box 5.1). Sensory testing should always be performed first on the normal side and later on the suspected area of the contralateral side with diminished sensations. Such testing should ideally be done with patients' eyes closed.

Testing for temperature sensation: Two test tubes filled with water: for cold (5–10°C) and hot (47°C) are to be used. Temperature beyond these ranges should be avoided as they elicit

Box 5.1: Testing the sensation over skin[2]

It is very important to learn the skill of eliciting sensory loss in a skin patch.

- You will need a light ballpoint (with plastic body) without cap.
- Explain to the person what you are going to do and demonstrate it.
- Touch the skin with the tip of the pen lightly and ask the individual to point to the spot touched with his index finger. Do not stroke.
- The pen should be perpendicular to the surface of the skin.
- Repeat this procedure a few times until the patient is familiar and comfortable with the procedure.
- Now ask the patient to close his eyes and repeat the procedure (first on the normal skin, then over the affected area). Only give one stimulus at a time.
- While testing lesions over inaccessible areas (back, buttocks) the patient may be asked to count on each touch.

Do not keep asking the patient whether he feels the touch. You may get misleading results. Vary the pace of testing.

The NLEP Manual recommends testing for sensation only with a ballpoint pen. It does not recommend use of other objects like pin, cotton wool, feather, etc.

painful sensation. With eyes closed, have the patient describe the stimulus. Temperature sensation is the first sensation to be affected/lost in leprosy and is a more sensitive measure of subtle sensory dysfunction than pain testing. Nonetheless, it is seldom practiced in the leprosy program due to the difficulty involved in performing this test.

Testing for touch sensation: Check for the loss of touch sensations over the lesions (permissible limit for mis-reference is 1 cm on face, 2 cm on hands and feet, and 7 cm on back). Check for glove and stocking anesthesia. Also ask and look for signs of previous or current injuries/burns/blisters in the area of suspected sensory loss, especially hands and feet. While leprosy manuals only suggest the use of tip of ballpoint pen, but fine touch conventionally is assessed with a wisp of cotton wool. In addition, a graded set of Semmes Weinstein (SW) monofilaments can also be used, more so for assessing sensations on palms and soles.[2] Identification of the point touched with an error of less than 2 cm by the patient, indicates that the sensation is normal. The sensory nerve distribution of hands and feet are as given in Fig. 5.1A and 5.1B.

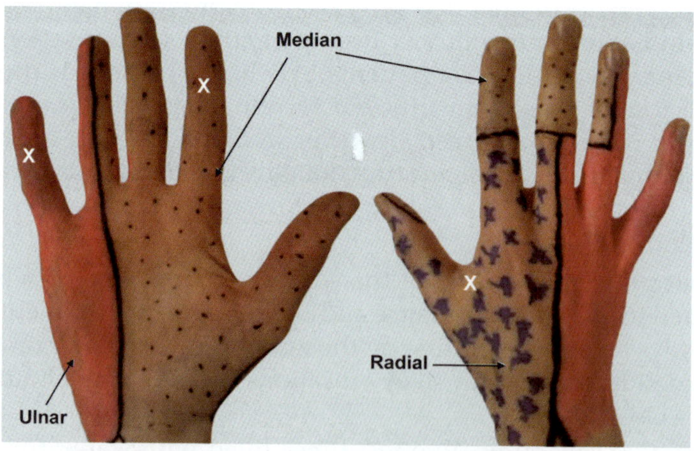

Fig. 5.1A: Sensory nerve distribution of hand

1. Testing with ballpoint pen: When testing, make sure the patient understands what is required by demonstrating the procedure. For the actual test, make sure the patient cannot see the part being tested and ask them to point to the place being touched (Fig. 5.2A).
2. Testing with color-coded Semmes-Weinstein (SW) monofilaments: (Fig. 5.2B and Table 5.1) These monofilaments of six grades, made of nylon 612 and are used to measure both diminishing and returning cutaneous sensations. Testing should be started with the

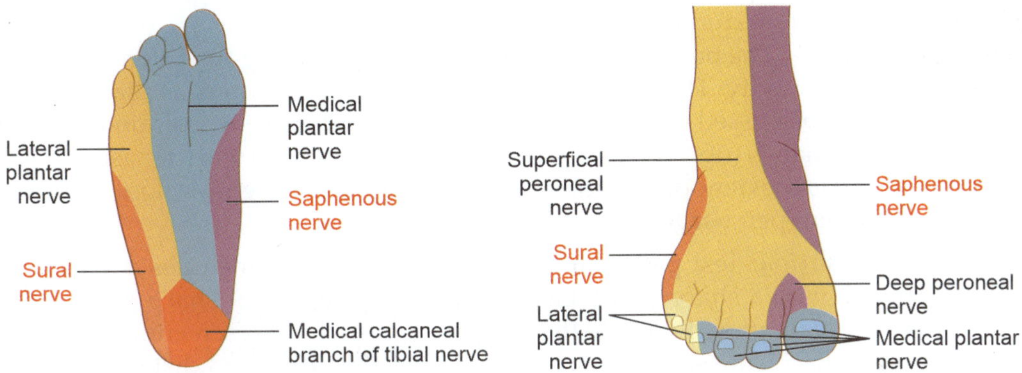

Fig. 5.1B: Sensory nerve distribution of feet

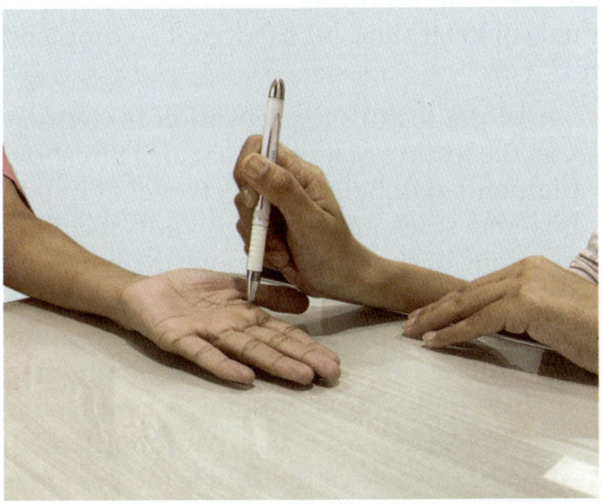

Fig. 5.2A: Testing for sensations with ballpoint pen

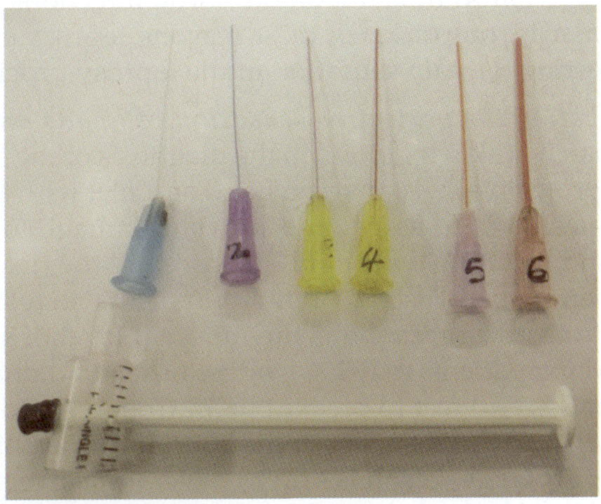

Fig. 5.2B: Semmes-Weinstein monofilaments

Table 5.1: Characteristics of the color-coded set of Semmes-Weinstein (SW) monofilaments[3]		
Filament	***Filament index number****	***Bending force (grams)***
Green	2.83	0.07
Blue	3.61	0.2
Purple	4.31	2
Red	4.56	4
Orange	5.07	10
Pink	6.65	300

finest (the green) filament and built up to the orange one. Testing up to a maximum of three times with each filament, at each site; the lightest filament that is felt is recorded. They test normal, diminished light touch, diminished protective sensation, loss of protective sensation for hands, loss of protective sensation for feet and for deep pressure sensation, in that order. This is quite a time-consuming exercise, and should be done in a quiet room without interruption, which may not be possible everywhere.[3]

If a single nylon monofilament is used, it will bend and give a standardized force, measured as a weight in grams, which makes it more accurate and higher sensitivity than the ballpoint pen. A few studies have shown the comparison for usage of ballpoint pen and monofilaments.[4,5] The ballpoint pen was used instead of 10 g monofilament, having the comparable sensitivity. They mention that absence of sensations as diagnosed with monofilaments can be missed with ballpoint pen, i.e. underdiagnosis. This underdiagnosis was mainly seen in hands (up to 21% patients) and feet (up to 30%) with no visible damage. Paradoxically, the low extent of ballpoint pen overdiagnosis of sensory loss, is a point in favor of the ballpoint pen usage.[6]

Testing for pain sensation: Test pain using a sharp object, which includes a safety pin or a wooden toothpick with a sharp point. Gentle and careful usage of sharp end is advised while them for pain evaluation. Evaluate the same areas tested in the screening examination for tactile sensation. Each side should be compared with the other, and distal and proximal portions of each extremity should be tested. Take care not to puncture the skin and only use clean instruments. These objects should be discarded properly after use, as they have potential to transmit blood-borne infections through small amounts of blood collected on them by pinprick. For these reasons, leprosy manuals of WHO and NLEP do not recommend testing for pain sensation in the leprosy program.[7]

Testing the protective sensation of hands and feet: While testing for sensation on leprosy patch of skin is helpful in the diagnosis of the disease, the testing of level of sensory threshold (protective sensation) on hand and feet with SW filaments will help to detect level of hypo/ anesthesia to assess and prevent damage to palms and soles and thus prevent disability and resulting deformity. However, in the field conditions of the leprosy program, ballpoint pen is used, instead of monofilaments, to test for integrity of sensations on hands and feet. Protective sensation is the minimal level of sensation that is needed to prevent ulceration. Many patients may have nerve function damage but still retain protective sensation in their hands and feet to prevent them from being damaged. A person is said to have a protective sensation of the palm of the hand if the person is able to feel at least a 2 g SW monofilament (purple). A person is said to have protective sensation of the sole of the foot if the person is able to feel at least a 10 g SW monofilament (orange) (Fig. 5.3).

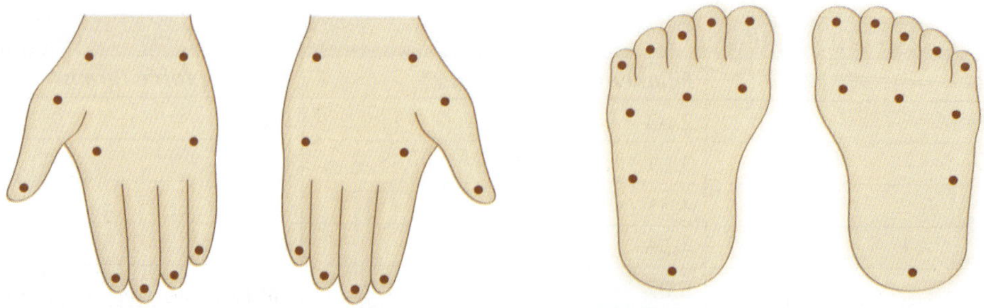

Fig. 5.3: Sensory testing points of hands and feet

Method of testing sensation on the palm or the sole of the foot is similar to what is already explained in Box 5.1. The monofilament is pressed only once at a perpendicular angle and pressed to make a 'C' shaped curve. If a ballpoint pen is used, it is pressed to make a slight dimple on the skin. Detailed score should be recorded on a hand and foot examination card of the patient.

In case of testing with SW monofilaments, the sites are marked with the number specific for the filament used. If no sensation is felt then the site is marked as 0 (zero). If a ball point pen is used, the sensory test site on the patient's record is marked as ✓ if the sensation is felt. If sensation is not felt, *X* is marked to denote that sensation is absent in the particular area.

Motor Examination

Motor NFI is assessed by voluntary muscle testing (VMT) using the modified Medical Research Council (MRC) scale.[3] It has six levels that are easily assessed during clinical examination. Different muscles are tested for each of the motor nerves commonly affected by leprosy (Table 5.2). If the VMT score for any muscle or group of muscles is equal or less than 4 on the MRC scale, it is considered as motor impairment. The modified MRC grading score used for VMT is given in Table 5.3.

Table 5.2A: Method of testing for muscles supplied by specific nerves[2]

Facial nerve	To test for early weakness, ask the patient to close the eyes tightly and try to separate the eyelids with your thumb and index finger, without use of excessive force. Normally, it will not be possible to separate the eyelids. In addition, ask patient to close eyes lightly, as during sleep. Check for lid gap. When present it is indicative of weak orbicularis oculi, which points the need for eye protection during sleep. Record the gap. *See* Chapter 4: Examination, Cranial Nerves for details
Ulnar nerve	Ask patient to abduct the little finger and apply resistance at the base of the little finger ("little finger out, against resistance). Record the strength.
Median nerve	Ask the patient to hold the hand flat in a horizontal position and abduct the thumb (to a point upwards at 90 degrees–*Pen test*). Resistance is applied at the head of the 1st metacarpal toward the index finger. Wrist should be slightly extended.
Radial nerve	Ask patient to extend the wrist ("wrist up"). Apply resistance on the dorsum of the hand.
Lateral popliteal nerve	Ask patient to lift the foot ("foot up"). Apply resistance on the dorsum of foot.

Table 5.2B: Recommendation regarding the frequency of nerve function assessment in leprosy[3]

1	For all leprosy patients	• At the start of MDT • At completion of MDT • Any time when there are complaints suggesting neuritis.
2	Patients at higher risk of developing NFI. e.g. a. MB patients who already have nerve damage. b. Skin patch on the face or near the eye or in the areas supplied by a palpable or visibly enlarged trunk nerve.	• At start of MDT • Every 3 months or if possible every month, while on MDT. • And at the completion of treatment.
3	Patients with reaction	• Monthly while on steroid therapy • Later once in 3 months.

Table 5.3: Voluntary muscle testing (VMT) score

VMT score	*Description of motor power*
Grade 5	Normal power. Full strength in all movements against normal degree of resistance
Grade 4	Full range of movements but less than the normal strength. Movement against gravity present, but not of normal degree
Grade 3	There is full range of movements sufficient to overcome gravity, but not against added resistance
Grade 2	There is some contraction of the muscle, the range of active movement is incomplete, effective neither against gravity nor resistance
Grade 1	Perceptible contraction of muscles(s), but not allowing joint movement
Grade 0	No movement or power representing total paralysis

Peripheral Nerves

Ulnar Nerve

Inspection: Look for wasting or flattening of muscles of hypothenar eminence, i.e. lateral side of palm and little finger. Also guttering over the 1st dorsal interossei

The little finger stays apart from the ring finger on resting the palm, facing upward. Also, there is partial claw due to paralysis of abductor digiti minimi.

Partial clawing of fingers (lumbricals of little and ring finger): Ask patient to flex metacarpiphalangeal (MCP) joint while extending Inter-phalangeal (IP) joint, for 30 seconds. In early ulnar nerve paralysis, the little finger cannot be kept in this position and it will be bent.

Testing for strength of abductor digiti-minimi: Ask patient to abduct the little finger and apply resistance at the base of the little finger (little finger out, against resistance). It will be weak in case of ulnar nerve involvement (Fig. 5.4).

Card test: Failure of adducting fingers (testing interossei)—The examiner places cards between to extended fingers of hand, and asks the patient to hold them firmly between fingers, while the examiner tries to pull it gently away. In a positive test, there is inability to hold the cards firmly and guttering of interosseous spaces.

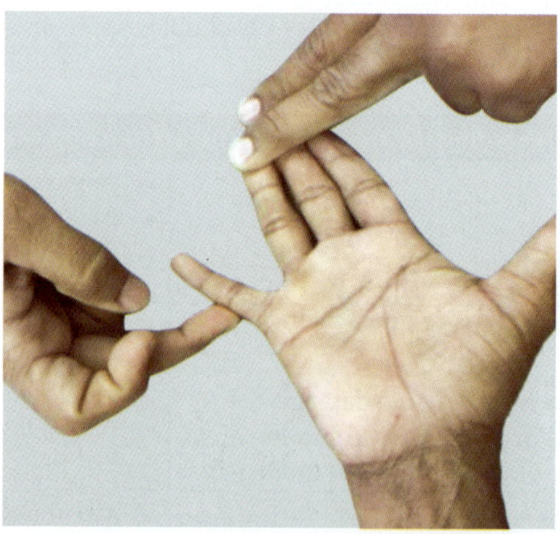

Fig. 5.4: Testing for abductor digiti minimi (ulnar nerve)

Froment's book test: If a book is held between the thumb and index finger, the tip of the thumb flexes because the active flexors of the thumb flexes the finger, as adductors of the thumb supplied by ulnar are paralysed.

Median Nerve

Inspection: Look for wasting or flattening of muscles over thenar eminence, i.e. prominence at the base of the thumb. Look for clawing of all fingers of hand. If the middle and ring finger are involved, it indicates median nerve involvement.

Pen test (for abductor pollicis brevis) elicits ape thumb deformity: Ask the patient to stretch the hand out, with the palm horizontal and facing upwards and fingers including the thumb facing forward. Then ask to lift the thumb upward at 90° away from pam and hold it in that position for at least 30 seconds, touching the pen in that position (Fig. 5.5). The patient is unable to do it if the muscle is affected.

Ask the patient to stabilize the hand and with the thumb parallel to the palm touch the tips of the other fingers firmly-to check for the function of opponens pollicis. Record the strength.

Radial Nerve

Ask the patient to close fist with palm facing down and to extend the wrist against resistance. Inability to extend it against resistance is indicative of weakness and which can progress to wrist drop, indicative of complete paralysis of extensors of wrist.

Common Peroneal Nerve

Inspection: Look for a 'high stepping gait', where the patient has to lift the affected leg high up while walking. Ask to sit on a high stool with legs dangling and lift only the foot without raising the leg. There is foot drop when the dorsiflexors of the foot, extensor hallucis longus and tibialis anterior are affected.

Test dorsiflexors and evertors of foot: Ask the patient to dorsiflex, i.e. extend the foot against resistance. If it is weak, in is indicative of lateral popliteal nerve involvement.

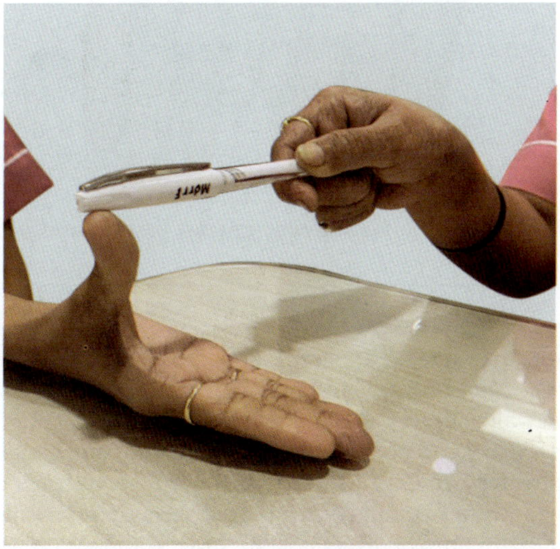

Fig. 5.5: Pen test for median nerve

Facial Nerve

Inspection: Look for signs of facial asymmetry. In case of facial palsy, that side of face is flattened, without any nasolabial fold and the mouth is pulled towards the opposite side by the action of active muscles on that side. Dribbling of saliva of the affected side along with deviation of angle of mouth toward the normal side. In complete facial paralysis, there is difficulty in blowing of cheeks on the affected side.

Check for lagophthalmos. Ask patient to close eyes lightly, as during sleep. Check for lid gap. When present it is indicative of weak orbicularis oculi which indicates the need for eye protection during sleep. A gap of 1 mm may be normal. Look for Bell's phenomenon (rolling up of the eyeball on closing the lid). The affected eye can also show redness due to exposure, as a result of lagophthalmos.

To test for early weakness of eyelids, ask the patient to close the eyes tightly and try to separate the eyelids with your thumb and index finger, without use of excessive force. When there is no motor weakness, it would not be possible.

Assessment of Autonomic Function

A detailed nerve examination should include the signs and symptoms of autonomic dysfunction:

1. Ask the patient regarding decreased or absent sweating over any area of body, especially palms and soles.
2. Examine for presence/absence of sweating. Look for generalized dry skin and/or presence of cracks and fissures over palms/soles (Fig. 5.6).
3. Further, sweating can be elicited by starch iodine test or bromophenol blue test for confirmation.

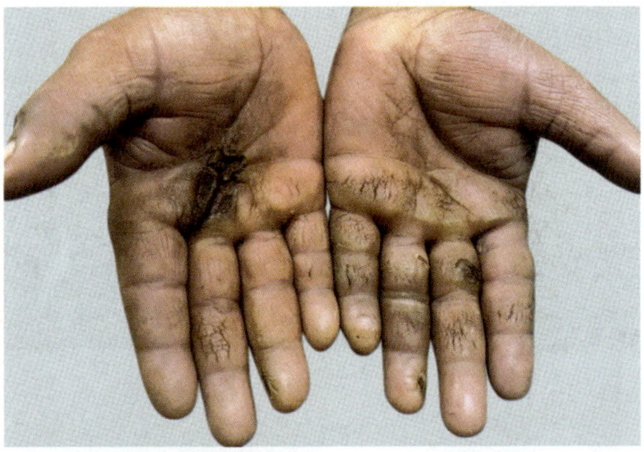

Fig. 5.6: Patient's hands showing cracks, fissures and ulceration

SUMMARY

In leprosy, nerve involvement may not be apparent, hence a detailed examination for nerve function is important in all patients. Also a detailed history often points to the underlying sites and areas for evaluation. The combination of physical palpation for nerve thickening, voluntary muscle testing and use of graded nylon for sensory testing was closely comparable to the nerve conduction studies to confirm neuritis.[8] Silent neuropathy refers to insidious impairment of sensory or motor nerve function without the symptoms of neuritis. Foot drop and claw hand are frequently seen in such cases. Special attention and timely monitoring is required for all patients under treatment, especially in those with lepra reactions, for early identification of neuritis and possible NFI.

REFERENCES

1. NLEP, Training manual for medical officers, CLD, New Delhi-CLTRI, Chengalpattu, MoH & FW, Govt of India, 2019.
2. NLEP, Training Manual for Physiotherapists, CLD, New Delhi–CLTRI, Chengalpattu, MoH &FW, Govt of India, 2020.
3. Leprosy/Hansen Disease: Management of reactions and prevention of disabilities. Technical guidance. New Delhi: World Health Organization, Regional Office for South-East Asia; 2017. Licence: CC BYNC-SA 3.0 IGO.
4. Owen BM, Stratford CJ. Assessment of the methods available for testing sensations in leprosy patients in a rural setting. Lepr Rev, 1995;66:55–62.
5. Koelewijn LF et al. Sensory testing in leprosy: comparison of ballpoint pen and monofilaments. Lepr Rev. 2003; 74:42–52.
6. Brandsma JW. Basic nerve function assessment in leprosy patients. Lepr Rev. 1981;52:161–70.
7. Bigley GK. Sensation. In: Walker HK, Hall WD, Hurst JW, editors. Clinical Methods: The History, Physical, and Laboratory Examinations. 3rd edition. Boston: Butterworths; 1990. Chapter 67.
8. Brandsma JW, Schreuders TAR, Birke JA, et al. Manual muscle strength testing. Intra-and interobserver reliability of the intrinsic muscles of the hand. J Hand Ther 1995;8:185–90.

Chapter

6

Systemic Examination in Leprosy

• Swetalina Pradhan • Usha Khemani

INTRODUCTION

Leprosy is a disease of skin and peripheral nerves predominantly. However, systemic involvement of various internal organs can occur in lepromatous forms of leprosy and due to lepra reactions. Predominantly involved organs are the eye, nose and paranasal sinuses, kidney, reproductive system. Less commonly others organs like liver, spleen, lymph nodes, and bone marrow may also get involved. This chapter describes briefly the details of their involvement and principles of examination.

Eye involvement: It is important always to take help of an ophthalmologist when eye involvement is suspected.

Eyebrows: Madarosis—Loss of lateral one third of eyebrow occurs in lepromatous leprosy as the hair roots are destroyed by cellular infiltration.

Eyelids[1]

- Loss of eyelashes can occur in lepromatous leprosy. Sometimes, dropping of eyelids can occur due to heavy infiltration. Similarly, ectropion of lower eyelid can occur due to tissue weight because of infiltration.
- Lagophthalmos: In tuberculoid leprosy, lagophthalmos is generally unilateral whereas in lepromatous leprosy bilateral lagophthalmos can be seen. Majority of cases lagophthalmos occurs because of type 1 reaction. For checking lagophthalmos ask the patient to close the eye if there is lid gap and eyeball is visible, then patient has lagophthalmos. Always compare the lid gap in both the eyes. To see for weakness of orbicularis oculi ask the patient to close eyes forcefully, then try to open the eye (Fig. 6.1). Look for the presence of spontaneous blink, its frequency and symmetry.

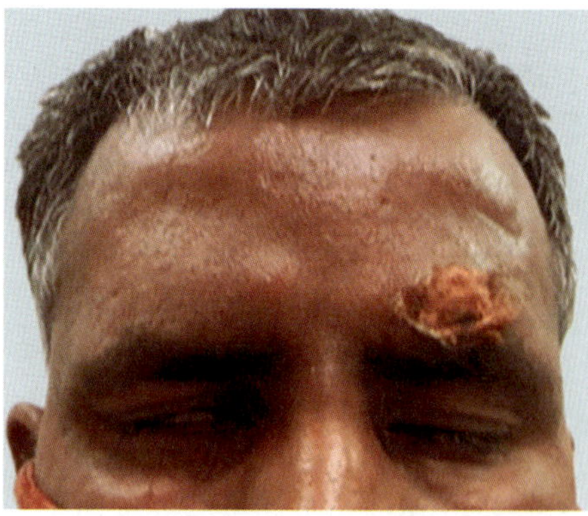

Fig. 6.1: Lagopthalmos on right side due to facial nerve involvement with lid lag

Cornea[1,2]

- Check for any erosion, ulceration or opacity and evidence of exposure—keratitis. Punctate keratitis can be visualized by slit lamp examination.
- Corneal sensation: Corneal reflex is elicited with a sterile wisp of cotton. The examiner approaches the patient from below and side so

that the patient cannot see it. Cornea is touched gently, 2 mm inside the limbus while the patient looks straight (Fig. 6.2). Normally there should be a brisk blinking of the ipsilateral (direct reflex) and contralateral (consensual reflex) eyes. The afferent limb of the reflex is mediated by the ophthalmic branch of the trigeminal nerve, the efferent limb by the facial nerve. With unilateral trigeminal nerve involvement both direct and consensual responses are absent while stimulation of the opposite eye produces normal direct and consensual responses. In case of unilateral facial nerve involvement, direct response is impaired but the consensual reflex will be normal. Beading and opacification of the corneal nerves is seen in lepromatous leprosy patients, which is best visualized by slit lamp broad beam examination.

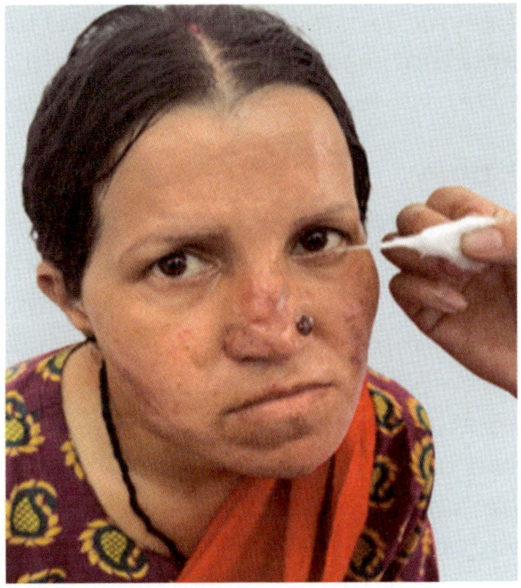

Fig. 6.2: Corneal reflex

Conjunctiva

Conjunctivitis occurs in lepromatous leprosy and type 2 lepra reaction. It presents with conjunctival redness. Rarely, nodules can be found in conjunctiva. Pigmentation of conjunctiva can occur while the patient is on clofazimine.

Visual acuity: Gross visual acuity should be checked in all patients. Check the visual acuity of each eye, using Snellen's chart or by counting at 6 meters. If the patient cannot read the top line of the chart or count fingers at 6 meters, they are visually impaired and have grade 2 disability in that eye.

Intraocular pressure: Secondary glaucoma occurs in type 2 lepra reaction due to uveitis, hence it should be measured periodically in all cases of eye involvement.

Slit lamp examination: It should be done to look for changes in the cornea of its involvement and anterior chamber of eye to observe features of uveitis. It examines the lens for opacities, including secondary cataract.

Nose and Paranasal Sinuses

Common nasal complaints include nasal obstruction, nasal discharge, crusts, hyposmia and rarely epistaxis. The nasal mucosal findings include paleness and granulomatous infiltration. In addition, resorption of anterior nasal spine can occur.[3] Vestibular stenosis and columella retraction can lead to nasal obstruction.

Late features in untreated lepromatous leprosy are; septal perforation, where the cartilaginous wall dividing the nasal cavities develops a hole or perforation. And saddle nose deformity, characterized by the collapse of the bridge of the nose due to the destruction of cartilaginous framework.

The paranasal sinuses (PNS) involvement in leprosy can produce ideal conditions for the growth of bacteria because of the large surface area. All PNS, including the maxillary, ethmoid and frontal sinuses, have been reported to be affected in leprosy. CT scan of PNS has been reported to detect changes in leprosy in the form of mucosal thickening, soft tissue density and fluid levels.[3]

Larynx: Hoarseness of voice due to congestion, infiltration, ulceration, nodulation, thickening and fibrosis can be visualized on laryngoscopy. Paralysis of muscle of larynx, which is very rare, can lead aspiration pneumonia and obstruction.[4,5]

Kidney

Several types of renal lesions including acute and chronic glomerulonephritis, interstitial nephritis, secondary amyloidosis and pyelonephritis have been described on palpation may have firm to hard consistency with tenderness leprosy. Glomerulonephritis has been observed as the most common type of renal lesion in leprosy. Almost all types of glomerulonephritis have been observed in lepromatous leprosy, and they have been thought to have an immunological basis, particularly during reactions. Acute renal failure and renal amyloidosis can occur because of lepra reaction. These will be manifested by proteinuria, microscopic hematuria, granular, hyaline and red blood cell casts; and the biochemical alterations. Chronic kidney disease (CKD) due to amyloidosis has been reported as one of the causes of death in leprosy. Chronic intake of clofazimine can also lead to nephrotoxicity.[6,7] Rarely, interstitial nephritis secondary to higher dose of rifampicin (900–1200 mg) can cause acute kidney injury. Dapsone can induce hemolysis and very rarely intravascular coagulation induced by dapsone can result in acute tubular necrosis.[7]

Reproductive System (Testes and Ovary)

Male reproductive system: In type 2 reaction, testicular swelling and pain can be initial involvement and testes on palpation may have firm to hard consistency with tenderness. In later stages, testes become soft, with reduced volume and finally atrophic leading to oligospermia/azoospermia, resulting in altered hair pattern, gynecomastia and impotency.[8]

Testicular examination: Cup one testicle at a time (best performed during or after a warm bath or shower) and then examine by rolling the testes between thumb and fingers using slight pressure. Palpate the spermatic cord and epididymis and simultaneously feel any change in size or for irregularities. The volume of the testis can be measured using an orchidometer. Cremasteric reflex may be absent because of lower motor neuropathy.[9]

Female reproductive system: As compared to testes, female reproductive organs are less commonly involved. Usually menarche, menstruation and fertility remain unaffected although it may involvement.[10]

CHANGES IN OTHER ORGAN SYSTEMS

Central nervous system: Cranial nerve V and VII are well known to be affected although brain and spinal cord are said to escape the infection. Nonetheless, abnormal conduction of auditory and visual pathways has been documented.[11]

Lymph nodes: In lepromatous leprosy, there can be widespread and generalized lymphadenitis with even visceral nodes being affected.[12] Enlarged lymph nodes do not show any matting or suppuration. Lymphadenopathy can be pronounced during type 2 lepra reactions.

Bone marrow: Leukopenia may occur secondary to infiltration of bacilli and bacilli may even persist in the bone marrow after complete treatment or slit skin smear negative.[13]

Liver and Spleen: Elevation of hepatic enzymes, especially of the aminotransferases, occurs in leprosy mainly during the reactions. Focal infiltration of the liver predominantly by lymphocytes associated with degenerative changes of the hepatocytes can be observed in lepromatous leprosy. Spleen usually is not enlarged, but diffuse infiltration in sinusoids, red and white pulp on microscopy has be documented along with amyloid deposits.[14,15]

Hematology and serology: In lepromatous pole, blood parameters are commonly altered; like low levels of hemoglobin, raised ESR, low serum iron levels and low levels of albumin are often observed. It is important to note that various serology markers can become (false) positive in leprosy, especially during reactions and in lepromatous leprosy. Eg: anticardiolipin, VDRL/RPR, ANA, antispermatozoal antibodies, RA factor, Anti-sDNA, ANCA, APLA, antimitochondrial and anti-beta-2 glycoprotein.[16,17]

REFERENCES

1. Soshamma G, Suryawanshi N. Eye lesions in leprosy. Lepr Rev 1989; 60: 33–8.
2. Ebenezer GL, Daniel E. Pathology of a lepromatous eye. Int J Lepr Other Mycobact Dis. 2000; 68: 23–6.
3. Sharma VK, Bapuraj JR, Mann SB, Kaur I, Kumar B. Computed tomographic study of paranasal sinuses in lepromatous leprosy. Int J Lepr Other Mycobact Dis. 1998 ;66(2):201–7.
4. Sakamoto K. Otorhinolaryngological finding of leprosy. In: makino M, Matsuoka M, Goto M, Hatano K (Eds) Leprosy: Science working towards dignity. Tokyo: Tokai University Press; 2011. Pp209–15.
5. Bretan O, De Souza LB, Lastoria JC. Larygeal lesion in leprosy and the risk of aspiration. Lepra Rev 2007;78;80–1.
6. Da Silva Júnior GB, Daher Ede F. Renal involvement in leprosy: retrospective analysis of 461 cases in Brazil. Braz J Infect Dis. 2006;10(2):107–12.
7. Silva Junior GB, Daher Ede F, Pires Neto Rda J, Pereira ED, Meneses GC, Araújo SM, Barros EJ. Leprosy nephropathy: a review of clinical and histopathological features. Rev Inst Med Trop Sao Paulo. 2015;57(1):15–20.
8. Kumar B, Raina A, Kaur S, Dash RJ, Samuel E, Datta BN. Clinico-pathological study of testicular involvement in leprosy. Lepr India. 1982;54(1):48–55.
9. Testicular cancer screening (PDQ) — Health professional version. National Cancer Institute. https://www.cancer.gov/types/testicular/hp/testicular-screening-pdq. Accessed Dec. 5, 2020.
10. Sarkar R, Pradhan S. Leprosy and women. Int J Womens Dermatol. 2016;2(4):117–21.
11. Mann SB, Kumar B, Yande R, Kaur S, Kaur I, Mehra YN. Eighth nerve evaluation in leprosy. Indian J Lepr. 1987;59(1):20–5.
12. Kar HK, Mohanty HC, Mohanty GN, Nayak UP. Clinico-pathological study of lymph node involvement in leprosy. Lepr India. 1983;55(4):725–38.
13. Sen R, Sehgal PK, Singh U, Yadav MS, Chaudhary SD, Sikka R. Bacillaemia and bone marrow involvement in leprosy. Indian J Lepr. 1989;61(4):445–52.
14. D'Souza GA, Jindal SK, Malik SK, Kumar B, Kaur S. Airway response to aerosol inhalations in leprosy. Indian J Med Res 1988;87:190–3.
15. Powell CS, Swan LL. Leprosy: pathologic changes observed in fifty consecutive necropsies. Am J Pathol. 1955;31(6):1131–47.
16. Karat AB, Rao PS. Haematological profile in leprosy. Part I--general findings. Lepr India. 1977;49(2):187–96.
17. Pradhan V, Badakere SS, Shankar Kumar U. Increased incidence of cytoplasmic ANCA (cANCA) and other autoantibodies in leprosy patients from western India. Lepr Rev. 2004;75(1):50–6.

Section 2

Diagnosis and Investigations

Chapter 7

Preparation and Interpretation of Slit Skin Smear

• Biswanath Behera • Patnaik Satyadarshi

INTRODUCTION

Slit skin smear (SSS) test, also called skin smear (SS) test is an integral part of leprosy work-up. It is a simple and minimally invasive test which can be performed on an outpatient basis.[1] It helps demonstrate AFB which is one of the confirmatory criteria for the diagnosis of leprosy. Often it supports the clinical diagnosis of leprosy when in doubt, as sole dependency on the clinical features to diagnose and classify leprosy can sometimes be inconclusive. The 100% specificity of SSS makes it the gold standard diagnostic technique. However, the sensitivity can vary between 20–50%, based on the expertise of the laboratory worker.[2] There is a concern among leprosy experts of declining skill and accessibility of SSS due to the lack of dedicated laboratories and trained technicians. This chapter will provide a broad overview of the various aspects of SSS that will enable the clinician to confirm the diagnosis in a suspected case and facilitate instituting appropriate therapy depending on the bacillary load.[3]

DEFINITION

Slit-skin smear (SSS) is an outpatient laboratory procedure and a cytodiagnostic technique, wherein collection of tissue fluid from dermis is obtained from a tiny cut in the suspected skin with a surgical blade. The thus obtained tissue smear is stained, and examined under a microscope to detect AFB.

Role of SSS in Leprosy: The role of SSS in the management of leprosy is manifold and is mentioned in Box 7.1.

Box 7.1: Uses of slit skin smear in leprosy

i. To confirm the presence of AFB in skin of suspected leprosy patient
ii. To assist in classifying leprosy into subtypes of Ridley-Jopling classification
iii. To decide the therapy, paucibacillary (PB) or multibacillary (MB) multidrug therapy (MDT)
iv. To assess the response to therapy, and to record bacillary index (BI) of SSS during follow-up
v. To suspect relapse of leprosy/drug resistance in leprosy.

The reduction in leprosy cases, less exposure to the leprosy patients and reduction and lack of adequate training, have in general reduced severely the expertise in performing and interpreting the skin smears.

Tools needed: The various tools needed to perform a SSS are enumerated in Box 7.2.

Box 7.2: Tools needed for preparation of slit skin smear

Equipment

- Sterile gloves
- Cotton swabs and surgical spirit
- Spirit lamp
- Clean glass slides
- Dressing (first aid) strips
- Scalpel handle with blade number 15
- Sterile gauze pieces and blotting paper
- Tincture benzoin
- Safe disposal bin for used blades and cotton balls and Gauze.

Stains

- Freshly prepared 1% carbol fuchsin solution
- 1% Acid-alcohol solution
- 0.2% Methylene blue solution

Others:

Sink with running water, Clock or a watch, Pipette, staining rack, tissue paper

PREPARATION OF SSS

Sites for SSS

A SSS should be done for all the suspected or diagnosed cases of leprosy before the commencement of anti-leprosy therapy. The smear should be collected from the suspected lesions, especially from the active-looking edge. In addition, a smear should be ideally done from regions with a high bacillary load, such as ear lobes, forehead, chin, buttocks, extensor aspect of the forearms, fingers, and knees.

There are differences in opinion regarding the selection and number of skin smear sites. The original recommendation was for smears to be taken from 6 "routine sites" (both earlobes, elbows, and knees) as well as several typical lesions from the patient. However, as per WHO 1988 recommendations, they were revised to three sites; one earlobe and two active lesions, to be chosen for SSS.[4] For cases with solitary lesions, two smears from the diagonally opposite active edge should be taken.[5] Some recommend four skin smears from the following sites: right earlobe, forehead, chin, and left buttock in males or left upper thigh in females. In addition, skin smear from the active lesion can be included.[6] However, ILEP manual of 2003 recommends only two sites for skin smear, one form ear lobe and other from active skin lesion. In general skin smears from lepromatous leprosy without identifiable skin lesions, earlobes, eyebrow, nodules and infiltrated skin, and even skin over extensors of fingers, are considered preferred sites for skin smear. However, a single skin smear done accurately is enough to demonstrate AFB and reach a leprosy diagnosis. For follow-up, ideally the smear should be repeated from the same sites. To detect relapse, smears from the prior site and new lesions should be done.[7]

Steps in the Preparation of SSS

i. The glass slide should be cleaned and made air dry. Record ID number of patient at one corner of the slide, on the same side where smears to be taken.

ii. The skin from where the smear is to be taken should be cleansed using 70% alcohol and dried.
iii. A skin fold is made and held between the thumb and index finger to exsanguinate it. This pressure is maintained till the skin smear is collected and smeared. To maintain adequate and uniform pressure, a chalazion clamp, curved artery and sponge-holding forceps have also been used to exsanguinate the earlobes.[7, 8]
iv. A scalpel with Bard Parker blade number 15 is used to make a thin cut of length 5 mm and depth 2–3 mm without causing bleeding. Following this, the blade is turned at 90 degrees, and the incised area is scarped to collect the dermal tissue and tissue fluid. Bleeding, if any, should be wiped using a sterile gauge piece so that the smear is free from blood. The skin cut is sealed with a tincture of benzoin.
v. The collected sample is placed on the cleaned glass slide and spread evenly to make a smear of size 5–7 mm. The smear should be moderately thick and should have uniform visible opacity.
vi. The sample for the next site is taken using the second blade or after cleaning and sterilizing the same blade by passing over a flame of spirit lamp. A total of 3–4 smears can be made in a single slide.

The steps in modified Ziehl-Neelsen (ZN) staining method are described in Flowchart 7.1.[8, 9]

Flowchart 7.1: Steps in Modified Ziehl-Neelsen (ZN) staining method

Fixing of smear: Fix the smears by passing the slide, with the smears upward slowly through the flame of a spirit burner, 3 times. Do not overheat. The slide should not be too hot to touch. Put the slide in a slide box and send to the laboratory with the skin smear request form.

Before staring the staining, register the slide in the lab register. Put the slide on the staining rack with stained side up and start the staining procedure as mentioned below,

Just before use, filter the 1% carbol fuchsin solution through ordinary filter paper.

Staining

Cover the slide with freshly prepared 1% carbol fuchsin (basic fuchsin, phenol crystals, 95% ethanol and water) and leave it for 20 minutes

Or

The slide with carbol fuchsin can be gently heated so that fumes come out without causing boiling. Repeat it three times during a period of 5 minutes. The stored carbol fuchsin should be filtered before using for staining.

Decolorizing

The slide is washed in running water and decolorized with either 5% sulfuric acid (H_2SO_4) or 1% hydrochloric acid (HCl) in 70% absolute alcohol for 3–5 seconds.

Counter Staining

The slide is washed again in running water and counterstained with 0.2% methylene blue (10% KOH, methylene blue, 95% ethanol and water) and kept for 1 minute and washed in running water

The slide is dried by keeping inclined over a blotting paper on its narrow edge

Possible Offshoots/variations

The sensitivity of detecting *M. leprae* increases by adding auramine-rhodamine staining of the slit skin smear, especially in PB patients.[10]

Examination of Skin Smears

A microscope with a 10x eyepiece and 10x and 100x objectives is needed. Start the examination using the 10x objective. Put the slide under the microscope with the smears and the ID number upward. First focus the smear using the 10x objective for the overall integrity of the smear. Then, put a drop of immersion oil on the smear and switch to the 100x objective. Adjust the objective so that it would touch the immersion oil. Open the diaphragm completely and raise the condenser to its highest position. Focus precisely with the fine adjustment screw. Look for AFB, which appear as fine red short lines or as clumps against a blue background.

Solid-staining bacilli are characterized by uniform staining, parallel sides, and blunt round ends, and the length is five times the width (Fig. 7.1). These represent live bacilli. Fragmented bacilli are highlighted by the interruption of the acid-fast staining at one or more points. (Fig. 7.2). Granular bacilli are typified by round granules arranged in a line or clump and represent dead bacilli. Both fragmented and granular bacilli are considered dead bacilli. Globi represents clumps containing hundreds of bacilli and is seen in lepromatous leprosy (Fig. 7.3).

Ridley's logarithmic scale is used to calculate the total number of bacilli (both living and dead), also called the **Bacteriological index (BI).** The following parameters of the acid-fast bacilli are examined: number per oil immersion field (x100), and their structure (solid, fragmented and granular). [11]

- Zero: No bacilli noted after searching for 100 microscopic fields
- 1+: 1–10 bacilli in 100 microscopic fields
- 2+: 1–10 bacilli in 10 microscopic fields
- 3+: 1–10 bacilli in one average microscopic field
- 4+: 10–100 bacilli in one average microscopic field (Fig. 7.4)
- 5+: 100–1000 bacilli in one average microscopic field
- 6+: over 1000 bacilli in one average microscopic field or presence of globi.

Calculate the BI for each smear separately and record it. In the case of variation in the number of bacilli in each site, the highest BI observed may be considered as BI of the patient. Some studies/manuals suggest to calculate BI by adding the values from each site divided by the number of sites. It should be discouraged.

Morphological Index

Morphological index (MI) may be defined as the average of the percentages of morphologically normal forms (solid rods) of *M. leprae* found in smears taken by a standard procedure and stained and examined by a standard technique. In practice, it is defined as the percentage solid staining bacilli out of 200 bacilli examined. MI indicates the proportion of bacilli that are presumably viable and capable of multiplying.

False-negative Results

The following can be responsible for a false-negative SSS report:

i. Superficial skin cut
ii. Uneven spreading the material on the glass slide and smear admixed with blood
iii. Failure to fix the specimen immediately can lead to degeneration of bacilli
iv. An uneven light source can can lead to reduction in visualisation of solid staining bacilli.

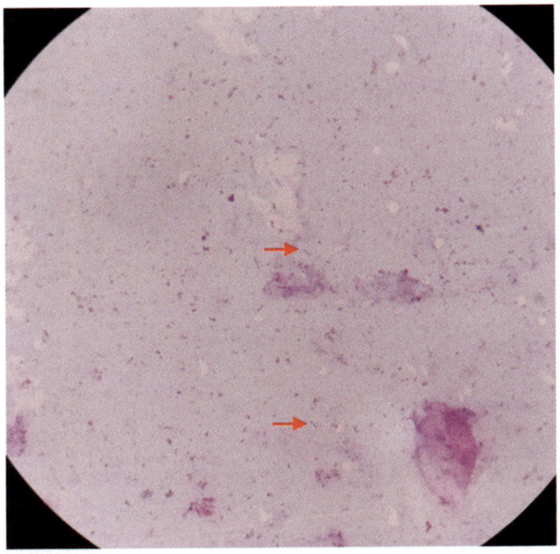

Fig. 7.1: Solid-staining bacilli (arrows)

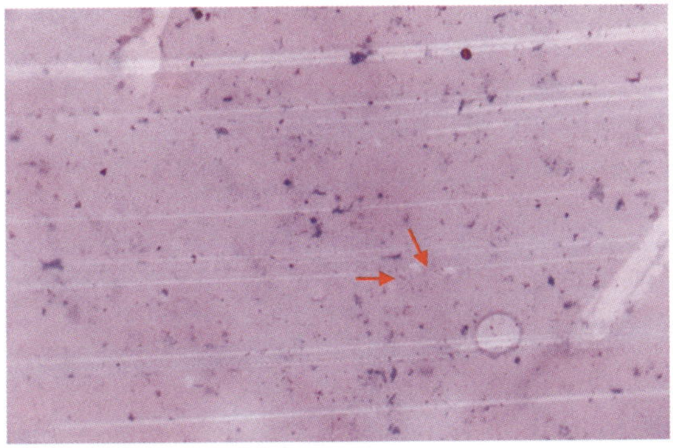

Fig. 7.2: Fragmented bacilli (arrows)

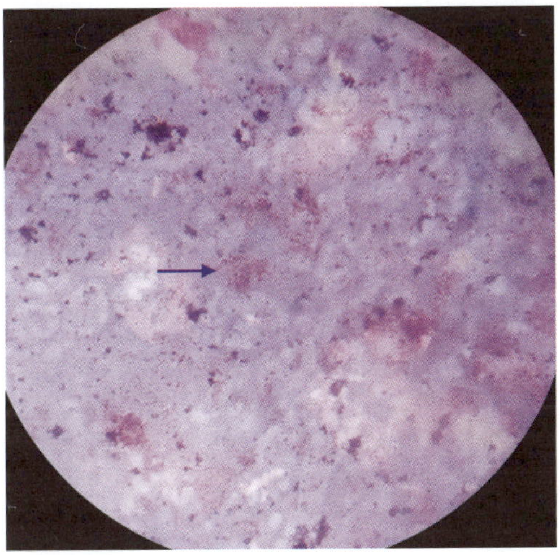

Fig. 7.3: Globi consisting of clumps of bacilli (arrow)

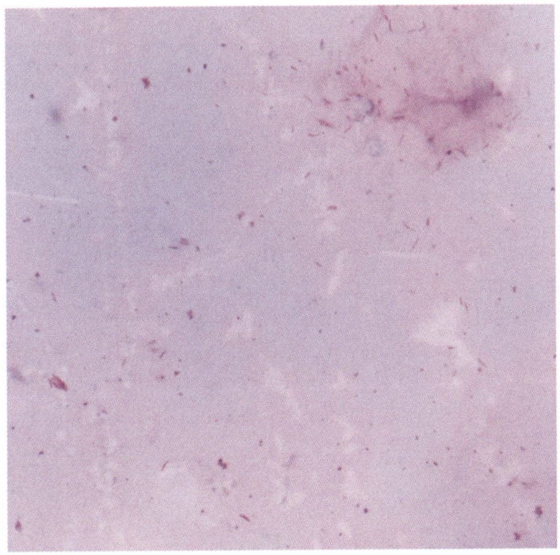

Fig. 7.4: Bacteriological index 4, 10–100 acid-fast bacilli per average oil immersion field. Note the presence of solid-staining, fragmented and granular bacilli

SUMMARY

Skin smear taking and its examination is a simple outpatient test to confirm smear-positive multibacillary leprosy in a suspected case. It also helps diagnose multibacillary relapse in a patient who has previously been treated. Moreover, SSS findings can solve the ambiguity between relapse and reactions. It can be used as a prognostic marker. In addition, skin smear can also be used as an substrate to perform PCR and other molecular tests to detect *M. leprae* in both PB and MB cases.[12] As the percentage of MB cases are increasing over past decade, there is a need to re-introduce slit skin smear as a programmatic measure across India.

REFERENCES

1. Training Manual for Medical Officers 2019. NLEP, Govt of India.
2. Report of the International Leprosy Association Technical Forum. 25–28 February 2002. Paris, France. Lepr Rev. 2002;73 Suppl:S3–61.

3. Demsiss W, Van Henten S, Takarinda KC, Kamau EM, Abdela SG. Slit-skin smear for the classification of leprosy; are we wasting time and resources? J Infect Dev Ctries. 2022 ;16(8.1):3S–7S.
4. WHO Expert Committee on Leprosy (1988). A guide to leprosy control. World Health Organization, 6th Technical Report Series No. 768, 1988.
5. World Health Organization (1992). A guide to end leprosy control. WHO, Geneva, 2 edition, 1988; reprint 1992.
6. Chacko CJ. Microbiology. A Manual of Leprosy, 4th edition. Thangaraj RH (ed). New Delhi: The leprosy Mission; 1985. pp.43–60.
7. Mahajan VK. Slit-skin smear in leprosy: lest we forget it! Indian J Lepr. 2013 ;85(4):177–83.
8. Gupta A, Sharma YK. The use of chalazion clamps to create adequate sustained pressure for slit skin smear. J Am Acad Dermatol. 2016 ; 74(1): e15.
9. Deshmukh KM, Sharma YK, Kumar A. The use of forceps for creating sustained pressure for slit skin smear. J Am Acad Dermatol. 2020 ;82(3):e77–e78.
10. Bhatia VN, Cherian E, Harikrishnan S. Auramine staining in detecting small number of bacilli in skin smears. Indian J Lepr. 1988; 60(1):13–6.
11. Gautam M, Jaiswal A. Forgetting the cardinal sign is a cardinal sin: Slit-skin smear. Indian J Paediatr Dermatol. 2019;20:341–4.
12. Azevedo MC, Ramuno NM, Fachin LR, Tassa M, Rosa PS, Belone AF, et al. qPCR detection of *Mycobacterium leprae* in biopsies and slit skin smear of different leprosy clinical forms. Braz J Infect Dis. 2017;21(1):71–8.

Chapter

8

Skin and Nerve Biopsy

• *Sujai Suneetha* • *Ankit Bharti*

INTRODUCTION

Early diagnosis of leprosy is important in preventing the complications and sequelae of the disease. Clinical diagnosis is based on a thorough examination of skin lesions: palpation of peripheral nerves, sensory testing (ST), and voluntary muscle tests (VMT), all of which aid in the definitive diagnosis of leprosy. Laboratory diagnostic tests include slit skin smears (SSS) which is discussed in the previous chapter; skin biopsy and nerve biopsy are the focus of this section.

INDICATIONS FOR SKIN AND NERVE BIOPSY

- **Diagnosis of leprosy:** Leprosy is diagnosed on the basis of the identification of the characteristic clinical and histopathological changes in the skin and nerves.[1,2] A skin and/or nerve biopsy helps in the accurate diagnosis of leprosy, particularly in suspected cases where a clinical diagnosis is still in doubt.
- **Classification of leprosy:** The classification of leprosy is important for an improved understanding of the disease and also for therapeutic purposes. As leprosy presents as a clinical spectrum, a skin biopsy helps in the exact typing of the disease. The histopathology of the skin biopsy generally gives adequate information about the type of leprosy. On the other hand, the role of a nerve biopsy in the classification of leprosy is not well documented. It should be noted, however, that in most of the cases the lesions in the nerves have a higher bacillary index than the cutaneous lesions, and that the pathological changes in the nerve persist even after the skin lesions have resolved.[3–5]
- **Diagnosis or confirmation of lepra reactions:** The normal course of leprosy is usually interrupted by acute acerbations of the disease which are referred to as 'Lepra reactions'. Reactions are important in that they can lead to nerve damage and disability. A skin biopsy is useful in diagnosing reactions early or in confirming the clinical suspicion of a reaction.[2] This can help in early treatment interventions that can circumvent irreversible nerve function impairment (NFI).
- **Follow-up and prognosis:** Histopathology provides a prognostic indicator in patients under treatment and gives an idea of the progression or regression of the disease.[6] It is very useful in research studies, especially where response to an intervention needs to be assessed. It is ideal to perform biopsy, at tertiary care centers or wherever facilities are available, at the time of diagnosis (start of MDT) and at RFT (12 months in MB patients and 6 months in PB patients) and later during follow-up, to assess the improvement. A comparison is made between the granuloma fraction (GF–the extent of dermal involvement by the inflammation or granuloma) at baseline and at completion of therapy

to determine the degree of histological resolution of the disease. Persisting or increasing histological activity in the follow-up biopsy may indicate that the patient needs further treatment or closer follow up during the post-RFT period of surveillance.

- **Detection of relapse:** The reappearance of leprosy after completion of a full course of MDT is termed a relapse. Relapse may present as new skin lesions, new nerve pain/enlargement, or new sensorimotor symptoms. A biopsy of the suspected skin lesions or the cutaneous nerve can yield a definitive diagnosis of relapse. It can be compared with the biopsy done at baseline and more importantly at end of treatment/RFT to confirm a relapse.

SKIN BIOPSY

Indications

As mentioned above a skin biopsy is useful in the accurate diagnosis, correct classification, identification of lepra reactions, as a prognostic tool during follow up of patients on treatment, and to diagnose relapse. Before taking a biopsy a basic set of steps need to be followed to decide on the site, type of biopsy, method and ideal size of the biopsy.

Site of Biopsy

For best results it is important to choose a representative site for the biopsy. In general, the edge of an active skin lesion is the best site to take a skin biopsy. In treatment naïve cases of MB leprosy with a BI of ~ 2+ at any site, the type of skin lesions to choose are—large papules, nodules, plaques, patches or areas of heavy skin infiltration, as they yield the best results. The active lesions present on any part of the body can be biopsied but universally the extensor aspects of the trunk and limbs are considered the most appropriate sites for a skin biopsy. Although the involvement of the earlobes is very common in MB leprosy, it is rarely chosen as a site for a skin biopsy but is a preferred site for slit skin smears. A skin smear test site from a skin lesion with the highest BI can also be an ideal site to biopsy.

In PB leprosy, biopsy should be taken from the most active skin lesion among the 1–5 skin lesions present, with the clinically active lesions being preferred. When the selected lesion is annular, the biopsy should be preferably taken from the active raised rim, close to the outer edge. In the same way, for a plaque or a macule, it is desirable to take the biopsy from just inside the edge of the lesion. If there is only one skin lesion except on face, two biopsies may be done from its active edge at sites diametrically opposite to one another.

In patients on treatment requiring a follow-up biopsy, a site close to the baseline biopsy should be chosen for a proper comparison and assessment of response to treatment. In RFT cases that have responded to therapy the biopsy should be taken from sites earlier found to be smear positive. In the suspected drug-resistant cases relapse lesions tend to be extensively disseminated and in uncommon sites; it is important to choose lesions that are clinically active.

Size of the Biopsy

The size of the biopsy can be based on the clinical picture. In well-established and clear leprosy lesions a 4–6 mm punch biopsy is adequate. For lesions on the face and in case of children a 3 mm punch can be used to ensure minimum scarring. In early lesions with doubtful sensorimotor changes it is advisable to do a larger biopsy of up to 1 cm size and this can be an elliptical incision biopsy with adequate depth containing both dermis and subcutis. The depth of the biopsy while using a punch should also be deep enough to include sufficient deep dermis and subcutaneous tissue.

Procedure

The two basic methods of performing a skin biopsy—punch biopsy and incision biopsy are described below.

Instruments: A sterile tray containing a draping cloth, cotton, spirit, betadine, 2% lignocaine, 2 ml disposable syringe, 4 mm and 3 mm punch and biopsy fixative (10% formalin or alternative). In case of an incisional biopsy the additional items needed will be a scalpel handle, 14 no. scalpel blade, non-toothed forceps, curved or straight scissors, curved needle, thread, and needle holder.

Preparation of the site: Clean the site chosen for the biopsy and surrounding area with spirit and betadine. Drape the lesion with a sterile towel with a window to highlight the area to be biopsied. Infiltrate a local anesthetic 2% lignocaine intradermally (Fig. 8.1A) into the area surrounding the site chosen.

PUNCH BIOPSY

Depending on the site a punch can be chosen. Preparation of the site and infiltration of the anaesthetic is as mentioned above. The sterile punch is placed perpendicularly on the site chosen (Fig. 8.1B) and turned in a circular fashion while applying pressure to obtain a clean cut in the skin. Ensure that the desired depth has been achieved and withdraw the punch. Gently lift the biopsy using the non-toothed forceps and cut it below at the level of the subcutaneous fat (Fig. 8.1C). Gently dab it on a piece of filter paper to remove excessive blood and place it immediately in the fixative, seal, label and send it to the lab for further processing. For a minute or two, pressure at the biopsy site is maintained to stop any bleeding. To minimize scarring a single suture using sterile cotton/silk thread may be given (Fig. 8.1D), after which a light dressing is applied.

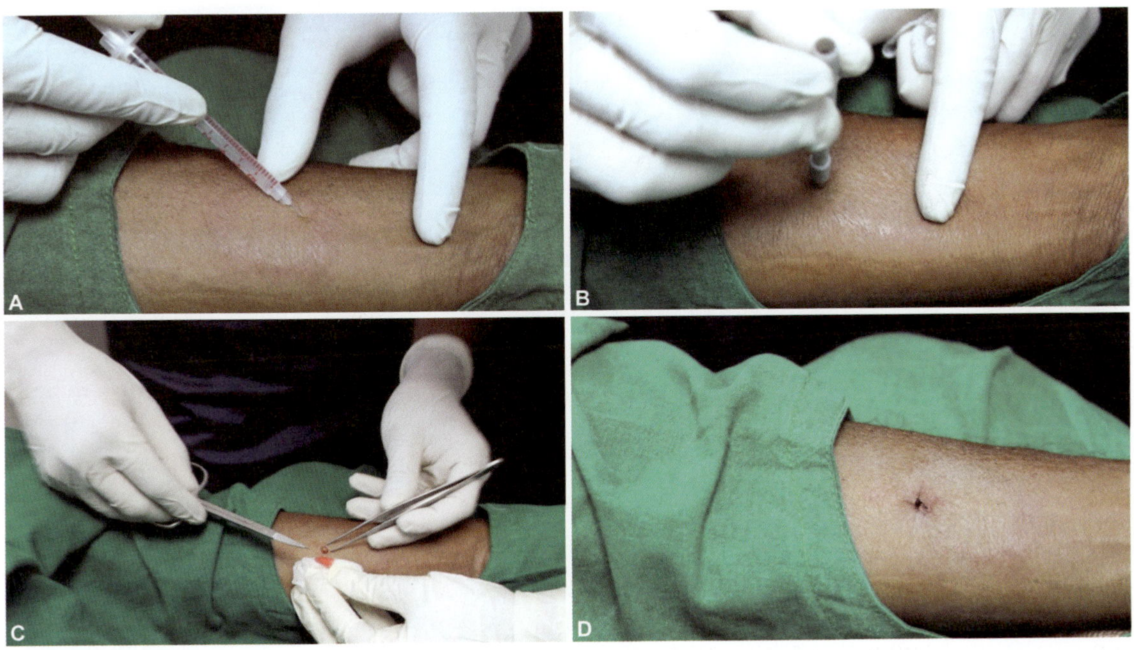

Fig. 8.1: Punch biopsy: (A) Injection of local anesthetic 2% lignocaine; (B) A biopsy punch is placed perpendicularly on the margin of the skin lesion and pressed downward in a circular motion to the depth of the subcutaneous tissue; (C) A cylindrical punched out tissue is gently extracted using a plain forceps taking care not to crush the tissue; (D) Closure with a simple suture

INCISIONAL BIOPSY

A few minutes after infiltration of the local anaesthetic (Fig. 8.2A) an elliptical incision is made with a 14 or 22 No. scalpel blade (Fig. 8.2B) on either side of the site chosen. Ensure that the incision is a clean cut and that it has achieved the desired depth (Fig. 8.2C). Slowly and delicately lift the sample using a non-tooth forceps without damaging the tissue and excise it below while ensuring that the dermis and subcutaneous fat both have been included. Once the biopsy is harvested the edges of the skin incision are brought together and one or two sutures are given using a fine needle and thread (Fig. 8.2D). Close and careful approximation of the two edges will ensure that there is minimal scarring.

The biopsy is gently dabbed on a piece of blotting or filter paper to remove the excessive blood and to prevent it from curling and it is immediately placed in the fixative to preserve the morphology of the tissue. Preparation of different fixatives is given in Box 8.1. Delay in transferring the specimen can lead to autolysis of the tissue, rendering it inappropriate for study. The bottle is properly labeled, sealed and sent to the lab for further processing.

Limitations/Precautions: An accurate histological diagnosis of leprosy is dependent on the choice of lesion biopsied. Often if the lesion chosen is not representative of the overall clinical picture there is poor clinico-histopathological correlation. The presence of inflammation or granuloma is also dependent on the biopsy sectioning, hence it is important to include only the active lesion while preforming biopsy.

Assessment/Interpretation: The skin biopsies are routinely processed; 4–5 microns thin sections cut and stained with haematoxylin and eosin (H and E stain) to study morphology and Fite-Faraco stain to identify lepra bacilli. Morphological study includes the location and type of cells composing the granuloma, the absence or presence of subepidermal free zone,

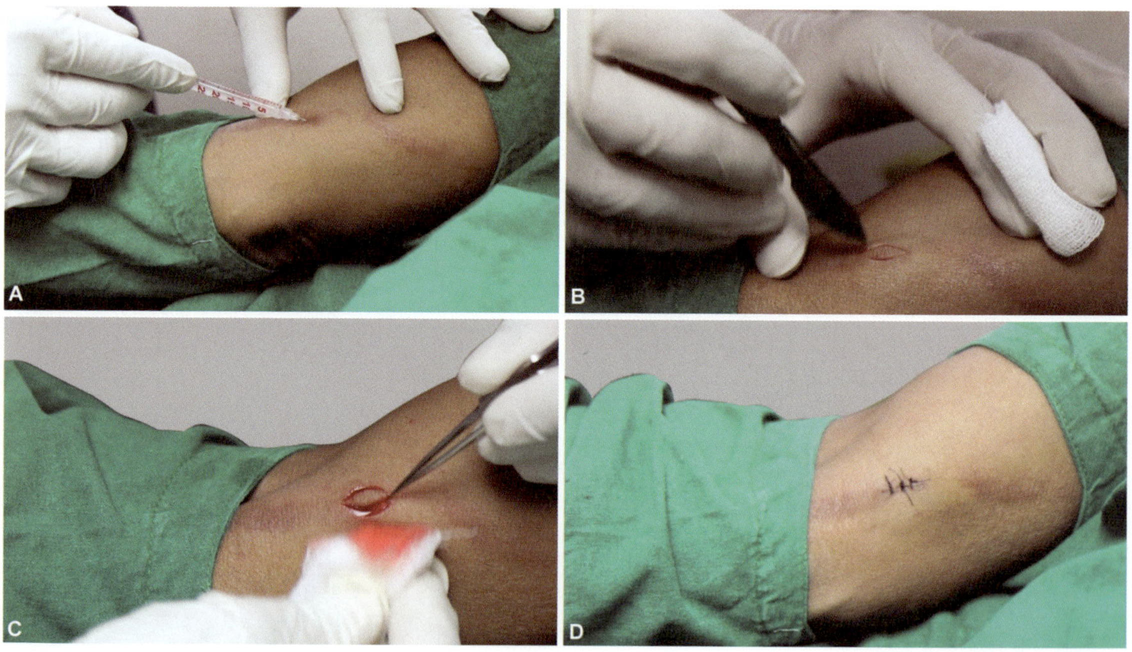

Fig. 8.2: Incisional Biopsy: (A) Injection of local anesthetic using 2% lignocaine; (B) An elliptical incision is made using a scalpel blade within the margin of the lesion; (C) A clean incision is a made to the level of the subcutaneous fat and the biopsy gently lifted out using a plain forceps taking care not to crush the tissue; (D) Approximation of the edges and simple sutures for closure

Box 8.1: Preparation of different fixatives

a. Preparation of 10% formalin
b. Procedure for modified Fite Faraco staining

Preparation of Fixative

a. Preparation of 10% Formalin

Formaldehyde (37–40%)	–100 ml
Distilled water	–900 ml

Procedure: Pipette 100 ml of concentrated formalin (37–40%) into a measuring jar. Then add 900 ml of distilled water to it to make up 1000 ml or 1 liter of 10% formalin.

b. Procedure for modified Fite Faraco staining

Modified Fite–Faraco (Ziehl–Neelsen) stain for demonstrating *M. leprae* in tissue sections

Procedure

1. Deparaffinize sections with xylol and liquid paraffin mixture (2 parts of xylol and 1 part of liquid paraffin). Two changes of 12 min each.
2. Drain, wipe excess of oil and blot to opacity. The residual oil helps to prevent shrinkage and injury to sections. It also prevents removal of acid-fast material from the organisms.
3. If the tissue is fixed with fixatives containing mercuric chloride, do the additional two steps:
   a. Treat the section with Lugol's iodine for 5 min and wash in water.
   b. Bleach the sections with 5% hypo (sodium thiosulfate) for 5 min and wash in water for 5 min.
4. Stain with Ziehl–Neelsen carbol fuchsin solution for 30 min at room temperature.
5. Wash in tap water until all the excess stain runs out.
6. Decolorize slides individually with 5% sulfuric acid for 10 min.
7. Wash in tap water for 10 min.
8. Counterstain with Harris' hematoxylin for 15 sec.
9. Wash in running water for 5 min.
10. Blot and dry.
11. Dip in xylol.
12. Mount in gum dammar or DPX mounting medium.

Adapted from: Suneetha S. Histopathological Techniques. In: Handbook of CMAI Medical Laboratory Technology. Editor, Carman RH. 2nd Ed. 1993: 508–41.

involvement and destruction of skin appendages and nerves in the dermis and the presence of AFB. Histology helps in the classification into the 5 conventional Ridley-Joplin (RJ) groups, TT, BT, BB, BL and LL. The fraction of the dermis occupied by granuloma is known as the granuloma fraction (GF) which is determined by observing the section under low power objective and is expressed as a percentage.[7,8]

The bacillary index of skin biopsies is graded as 'bacterial index of granuloma' or 'BIG' on a similar logarithmic scale of $0–6^+$ similar to the scoring of BI in skin smears. The grading is based on the number of bacilli in the areas of inflammatory infiltrate or granuloma and not on the entire section that includes the uninvolved dermis or subcutaneous tissue.

NERVE BIOPSY

Indications

Due to the morbidity related with the procedure, the decision to do a nerve biopsy is made only when all other less invasive methods have been exhausted. Complete patient history and physical examination are required to be performed, including the identification of nerves affected and functional status.

A nerve biopsy is an important diagnostic test for the diagnosis of pure neural leprosy (PNL). Nerve histology in PNL reveals specific histological features of leprosy and helps in clinching a diagnosis of leprosy. In addition, a nerve biopsy can help in the early detection of acute neuritis that requires urgent intervention to prevent permanent NFI (Flowchart 8.1).

Sites for Nerve Biopsy

The nerves that are usually biopsied in leprosy are:

1. Sural nerve
2. Radial cutaneous nerve (RCN) or superficial branch of radial nerve
3. Ulnar cutaneous nerve (UCN) or dorsal cutaneous branch of ulnar nerve
4. Musculocutaneous nerve (MCN) or superficial peroneal nerve of dorsum of foot.

Other cutaneous nerves that can be biopsied in special situations where the above nerves are not clinically enlarged or are distant from the leprosy lesions are:

1. Nerve feeding a skin patch, e.g. in tuberculoid spectrum
2. Great auricular nerve
3. Supraorbital branch of 5th cranial, nerve
4. Supraclavicular nerve
5. Cutaneous nerve of thigh

Procedure

Ideally a nerve biopsy should be performed by a neurosurgeon, neurologist, surgeon, or a dermatologist who is well trained in nerve biopsy. The procedure described below is for a sural nerve biopsy which is the most frequently biopsied nerve in leprosy.

Flowchart 8.1: Steps describing the investigation for a case of pure neuritic leprosy

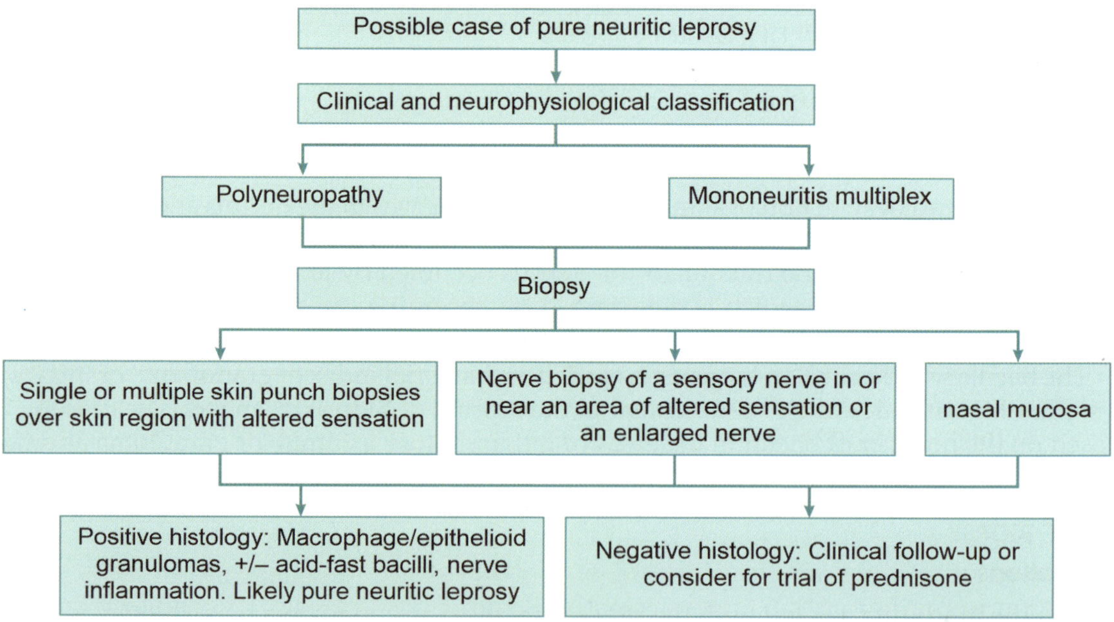

(*Adapted from* Wilder-Smith E. Diagnosis of pure neuritic leprosy. Neurol J Southeast Asia. 2002;7(1):61–3.)

Instruments: A sterile tray containing a draping cloth, scalpel handle, 14 no. scalpel blade, non-toothed forceps, curved or straight scissors, curved needle, thread, needle holder, cotton, spirit, betadine, 2% lignocaine, 2 ml disposable syringe, and biopsy fixative (10% formalin or alternative).

Cleaning the site: The patient is positioned in a prone position to access conveniently the posterior/lateral part of the leg. The area is cleaned with spirit and betadine. Usually, the procedure is initiated by marking out the sural nerve at the posterior border of fibula in the part between the Achilles tendon approximately 5–7 cm proximal to the lateral malleolus (Fig. 8.3A). A modified approach also exists at proximal calf to minimalize complications.[9]

There are two ways of doing a nerve biopsy: One is a complete nerve biopsy and another is a fascicular biopsy. A biopsy of the whole nerve is indicated if the pathology may not involve all of the fascicles, which can happen in leprosy, and when patient's symptoms are severe. Similarly, if the patient's symptoms are minimal and the pathology may be localized in the fascicles, then a fascicular biopsy should be performed.[10]

Complete nerve biopsy: Make a 3–5 cm vertical incision in the skin in the area marked out for the nerve (Fig. 8.3B); the lesser saphenous vein is identified; and the vein is retracted superficially to expose the sural nerve. The nerve is dissected from the surrounding tissue (Fig. 8.3C); two untied sutures are inserted into the two ends of the nerve; the nerve is transected above and below these sutures (Fig. 8.3D); and the nerve is extracted (Fig. 8.3E) using these sutures as a sling to avoid nerve compression. The biopsy is placed on a small piece of filter paper wherein the biopsy sticks to the paper and this prevents contraction and curling of the nerve (Fig. 8.3F). The biopsy can be placed with the filter paper in the fixative.

Fascicular biopsy: For a fascicular biopsy, the nerve is visualized, dissected out, and a sliver of the nerve is partially transected using a similar technique as above, avoiding the compression of the nerve during harvesting. As mentioned above the nerve is placed on filter paper and transferred to the fixative. The steps for fascicular nerve biopsy are detailed in Flowchart 8.2.

During a fascicular biopsy, after the harvest the surgeon can attempt a repair by carefully matching nerve patterns and executing an end-to-end repair of remaining structures under a microscope.[11] Many products, including collagen-based conduits and nerve-wraps, are available in an attempt to reduce morbidity and risks of neuroma formation after the procedure.[12]

Limitations and complications: The most frequently affected nerves in leprosy comprise the posterior tibial, common peroneal, ulnar and median nerves which are mixed peripheral nerves carrying motor and sensory fibers. Proof of a leprosy etiology is often sought in the affected peripheral nerves. However, these peripheral nerves should not be biopsied as it can cause iatrogenic sensory loss and paralysis. Given this situation cutaneous nerves are biopsied with the view that they reflect the changes in the trunk nerves. This may be challenging as nerve biopsy is limited by sampling errors and low sensitivity as the biopsy may not always include the involved fascicles. Additionally, a nerve biopsy may produce permanent sensory deficit in the area of distribution. Overall. the sensitivity of nerve biopsy for leprosy varies across studies from 33 to 75%.

In a study with 50 cases of sural nerve biopsy performed, the biopsy changed the diagnosis in 14% of cases, and altered management in 60% of cases[13] with 33% of the cases reporting a rise in pain 6 months after the nerve biopsy. However, another study described complete resolution in post-surgical pain following both fascicular and whole nerve biopsy.[14] This study also described that the key complaints 5 years after both whole and fascicular biopsy

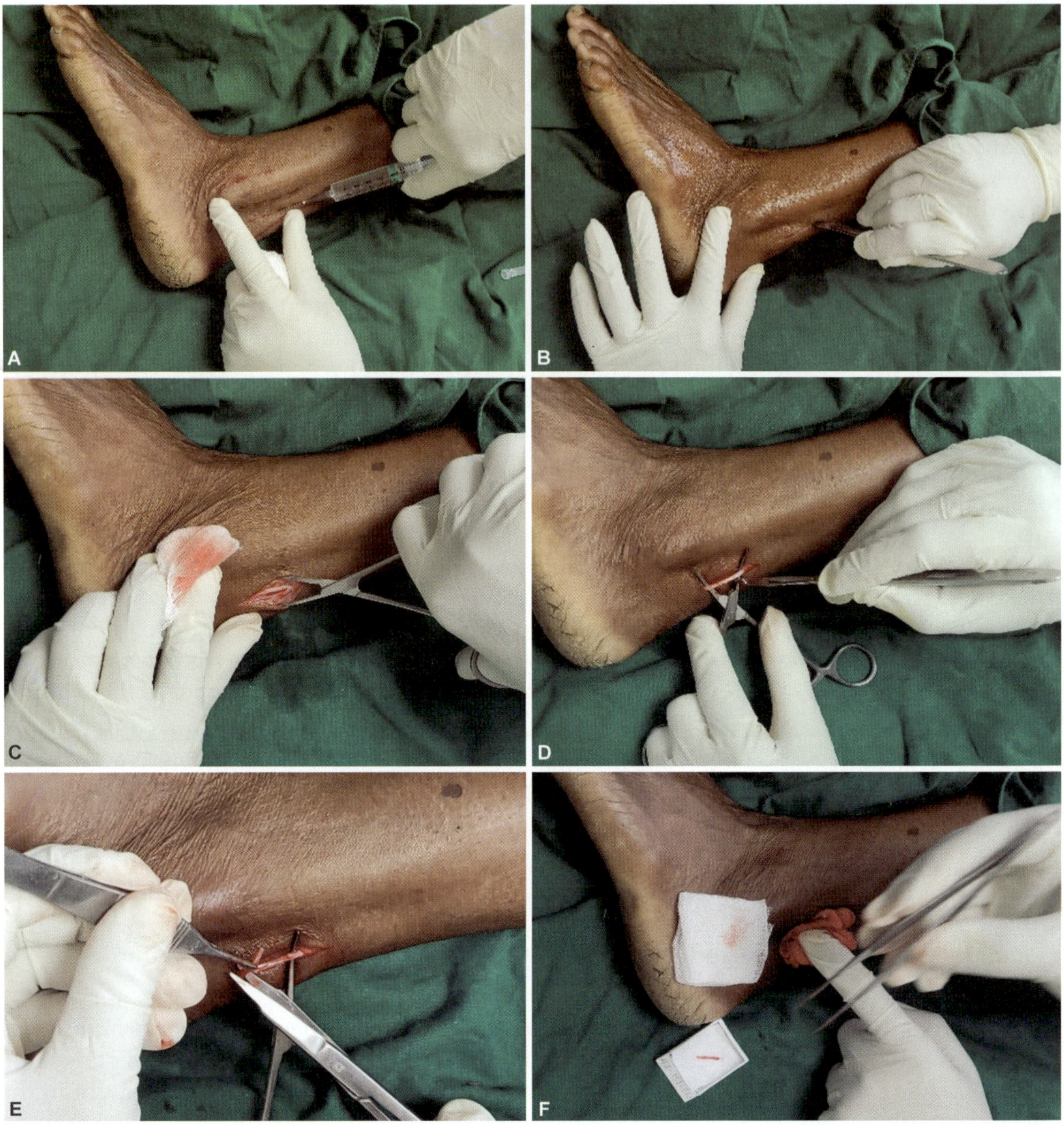

Fig. 8.3: Nerve biopsy: Local anesthesia using infiltration of biopsy site with 2% lignocaine; (B) A transverse skin incision of 4 cm at the location of the nerve; (C) Blunt dissection using plain forceps and curved hemostatic forceps to isolate the sural vein and locate the sural nerve which is seen as a silvery structure; (D) Partial nerve extraction: The nerve is incised longitudinally ensuring that a few fascicles are included and a sliver of the nerve is gently cut and extracted; (E) Removal of the sliver of the nerve using a scissor ensuring a length of 2–3 cm of the nerve and allowing the remaining half of the nerve intact; (F) The nerve tissue is placed on a filter paper or blotting paper to avoid curling onto itself and then immediately place it in the fixative solution.

was tactile induced dysesthesias located to the sural nerve distributional area. Hypoesthesia in the sural nerve distribution happened in 18.4% of patients who underwent a whole nerve biopsy.[15] Sensation loss did not differ based on whether patients had a fascicular or whole nerve biopsy.

Flowchart 8.2: Steps of nerve biopsy

- Decide on the nerve to biopsy and markout the location of the nerve

↓

- Tubeculoid specturm
- Pure neuritic leprosy

↓

- Clean the site with spirit and betadine (keep for 30 seconds) and clean with spirit
- Local infiltration with 2% lignocaine

↓

- Cover the surrounding area with the surgical towel (wait for 5 minutes)

↓

- Put a longitudinal incision of 3–5 cm at the location of the nerve
- Blunt dissection below to subcutis level to find nerve

↓

- Silver shiny cord like if nodular thickening present; prefer nodular lesion for biopsy

↓

- Put a longitudinal small nick and divide the nerve into fascicles, strip apart a fascicle from the nerve bundle and cut 2 cm long nerve twig

↓

- Put the excised tissue on blotting paper or filer paper to keep longitudinal orientation preserved and immediately store it in 10% buffered formalin.

Assessment/Interpretation

Nerve histology in leprosy exhibits a spectrum which includes TT where there is extensive destruction by granuloma, even caseation; BT neuritis where epithelioid granuloma predominate; BL where macrophages and lymphocytes predominate; and LL where bacilli are abundant in the Schwann cell cytoplasm and substance of nerve but the lymphocytic response is limited.[16] Segmental necrotizing granulomatous neuritis (SNGN) is the term used to denote rarely observed extensive destruction of nerve tissue by granuloma along with caseous necrosis in tuberculoid leprosy.

Nerve biopsy also helps in diagnosing early changes of neuritis, by features which include a sudden influx of lymphocytes accompanied by tissue oedema, which cause damage to nerve fascicles. When a specific histological pattern or acid-fast bacilli (AFB) are not observed in the nerve biopsy, the value of other nonspecific histological alterations should be considered along with pertinent clinical, nerve ultrasound, electroneuromyographical and laboratory data, such as—the detection of *Mycobacterium leprae* DNA by PCR and elevated PGL1 antibody levels—to support a probable diagnosis of neural leprosy.[17]

Use of special stains: Leprosy is a demyelinating neuropathy and hence use of special stains for myelin are valuable when available in determining the degree of demyelination which may be graded as mild, moderate or severe/extensive. Solochrome cyanine stain is a versatile stain for myelin wherein myelin stains a brilliant blue.[18] Other myelin stains include luxol-fast blue (LFB) stain, osmium tetroxide stain, Kulchitsky Pal (K Pal) stain and fluoro-myelin stain.[19]

Silver stains are useful in delineating the axons and can be used to study the integrity of the axons. Glees stain for axons in paraffin-embedded tissues is a time tested and dependable silver staining method.[20] Bodian silver stain uses silver (and copper and gold chloride) to stain neuronal cell bodies and axons dark brown. Axonal loss may be graded as mild, moderate and severe based on the degree of disruption of the axons. Other axonal stains include Bielschowsky's silver stain. Silver stains are a bit finicky and need care and finesse while performing to prevent staining artefacts.

CONCLUSION

Histopathology of the skin is a valuable tool in the precise diagnosis, classification, and follow-up of leprosy patients. It can be easily performed in the out-patient and a basic understanding of the histological features and its interpretation can improve the quality of care offered to leprosy patients. A nerve biopsy is invaluable in clinching the diagnosis, especially in PNL and should be considered when the clinician is in a diagnostic dilemma. The Fite Faraco stain is a versatile staining method to demonstrate the causative organism and could be a game changer in the diagnosis and grouping of patients for therapeutic purposes.

While the Ridley-Jopling classification is widely accepted, its histological component mentions only features in the skin with the presumption that there may be no noteworthy difference in the classification in the nerve. Still, discrepancies have been brought out, as many nerve biopsies show histological grading lower than the skin with a higher bacillary load. This highlights the values of both skin and nerve biopsy in leprosy.

REFERENCES

1. Beneson AS. Control of communicable disease in man, Fifteenth Edition. American Public Health Association, Washington, 1990:243–7.
2. Lockwood DN, Lucas SB, Desikan KV, Ebenezer G, Suneetha S, Nicholls P. The histological diagnosis of leprosy type 1 reactions: identification of key variables and an analysis of the process of histological diagnosis. J Clin Pathol. 2008;61(5):595–600.
3. Antia NH, Pandya NU. Qualitative histology and quantitative bacteriology in various tissues of leprosy patients. Lepr Rev, 1976;47:175–83.
4. Srinivasan H, Rao KS, Iyer CAS. Discrepancy in the histopathological features of leprosy lesions in the skin and peripheral nerve. Lepr India, 1982;54:275–86.
5. Haimanot RT, Mshana RN, McDougall AC, Andersen JG. Sural nerve biopsy in leprosy patients after varying period of treatment: Histopathological and bacteriological finding in light microscopy. Int J Lepr, 1984;52:163–70.
6. Brundha MP. A Comparative Study: The Role of Skin and Nerve Biopsy in Hansen's Disease. Journal of Pharmaceutical Sciences and Research. 2015 1;7(10):837.
7. Ridley DS. Skin biopsy in leprosy. Basel Documenta Geigy, 1985;59.
8. Charles K Job, Joyce Ponnaiya. Laboratory diagnosis.1st ed. In: IAL Textbook of Leprosy, Eds. Hemanta Kumar Kar, Bhushan Kumar. New Delhi: Jaypee Publishers; 2010; 177–87.
9. Ducic I, West JA modified approach to sural nerve biopsy: minimizing complications. Ann Plast Surg. 2009;62(2):220–2.
10. Bevilacqua NJ, Rogers LC, Malik RA, Armstrong DG. Technique of the sural nerve biopsy. J Foot Ankle Surg. 2007;46(2):139–42.
11. Schoeller T, Huemer GM, Shafighi M, Gurunluoglu R, Wechselberger G, Piza-Katzer H. Microsurgical repair of the sural nerve after nerve biopsy to avoid associated sensory morbidity: a preliminary report. Neurosurgery. 2004;54(4):897–900; 900-1.

12. Saeki M, Tanaka K, Imatani J, Okamoto H, Watanabe K, Nakamura T, Gotani H, Ohi H, Nakamura R, Hirata H. Efficacy and safety of novel collagen conduits filled with collagen filaments to treat patients with peripheral nerve injury: A multicenter, controlled, open-label clinical trial. Injury. 2018;49(4):766–74.
13. Gabriel CM, Howard R, Kinsella N, Lucas S, McColl I, Saldanha G, Hall SM, Hughes RA. Prospective study of the usefulness of sural nerve biopsy. J Neurol Neurosurg Psychiatry. 2000;69(4):442–6.
14. Pollock M, Nukada H, Taylor P, Donaldson I, Carroll G. Comparison between fascicular and whole sural nerve biopsy. Ann Neurol. 1983;13(1):65–8.
15. Luigetti M, Di Paolantonio A, Bisogni G, Romano A, Conte A, Barbato F, Del Grande A, Madia F, Rossini PM, Lauretti L, Sabatelli M. Sural nerve biopsy in peripheral neuropathies: 30-year experience from a single center. Neurol Sci. 2020;41(2):341–6.
16. Suneetha S, Arunthathi S, Kurian N, Chacko CJ. Histological changes in the nerve, skin and nasal mucosa of patients with primary neuritic leprosy. Acta Leprol 2000-2001;12:11–8.
17. Antunes SL, Chimelli L, Jardim MR, Vital RT, Nery JA, Corte-Real S, Hacker MA, Sarno EN. Histopathological examination of nerve samples from pure neural leprosy patients: obtaining maximum information to improve diagnostic efficiency. Mem Inst Oswaldo Cruz. 2012;107(2):246–53.
18. Page KM. A stain for myelin using solochrome cyanin. J Med Lab Technol. 1965;22(4):224–5.
19. García-García ÓD, Weiss T, Chato-Astrain J, Raimondo S, Carriel V. Staining Methods for Normal and Regenerative Myelin in the Nervous System. Methods Mol Biol. 2023;2566:187–203.
20. Marsland TA, Glees P, Erikson LB. Modification of the Glees silver impregnation for paraffin sections. J Neuropathol Exp Neurol. 1954;13(4):587–91.

Chapter 9

Electrophysiological Tests (Nerve Conduction Studies and Others)

• *Chirag Desai* • *Neelam Kumari Bhatt*

INTRODUCTION

Electromyography (EMG) and simultaneous study of nerve conduction are the principle electrophysiological tests. These tests are mainly used by neurologists but their knowledge is important to leprosy practitioners when dealing with pure neuritic leprosy and special scenarios where patient is referred to dermatologist by neurologists to confirm the diagnosis of leprosy as they usually come with these reports to the dermatologist and often asks about the interpretation of the same.

Nerve involvement is one of the cardinal features of the leprosy, and it can present in various patterns according to the classification of the leprosy in form of motor, sensory and autonomic symptoms with resultant loss of function and ensuing deformities, if not identified and managed early. If only one trunk is involved as in case of tuberculoid form of the disease it results in the mononeuritis and in other forms multiple nerves can be effected asymmetrically or symmetrically, resulting into progressive sensory motor polyneuropathy.

DEFINITIONS

Electromyography (EMG): It is a study of electrical activity occurring in muscle during voluntary contraction, or in denervated muscles at rest, recorded with needle electrodes inserted percutaneously into the belly of the muscle, or with surface electrodes.

NCV: Nerve conduction velocity (NCV) is the study of conduction of nerve impulse along the peripheral nerve.[1] The speed of conduction of afferent impulses (sensory nerve conduction velocity) and efferent impulses (motor nerve conduction velocity) is assessed. For nerve conduction study, suitable muscle along with its nerve supply is required.

Latency: This term denotes duration between the stimulus and the onset of the response which includes nerve conduction time and neuromuscular transmission time in motor nerve studies. Two types of latency: Proximal latency (proximal stimulation point to the first deflection from baseline) and distal latency (distal stimulation point to the first deflection from baseline) need to be studied.

Amplitude: This term denotes summation of all activity of the axons within a nerve trunk. It depends on the number of axons conducting impulses from the stimulus point to the muscle, number of functioning motor endplates and muscle volume. Amplitude is measured from the baseline to the negative peak.[2]

Conduction velocity (CV) is derived by using following formula

$$\text{CV (m/s)} = \frac{\text{Distance (millimeters)}}{\text{Proximal latency–distal latency (milliseconds)}}$$

Hence, calculated motor conduction velocity reflects the conduction in the motor axons.[3]

Testing methods and Tools/facilities needed

Tools for NCV study

- NCV machine
- Electrodes—Active or recording electrode
  Reference electrode
  Ground electrode (metal plate)

Tools for EMG study

- EMG machine
- Electrodes—twin core needle electrode

Procedure: Most commonly nerve conduction studies are performed in nerves such as ulnar, median, peroneal and tibial nerves (Tables 9.1 and 9.2)

Stimulating electrodes are generally two metal electrodes which are placed 1.5–3.0 cm apart. Electrodes which deliver mild electrical impulse is applied over the skin above the nerve being tested are called stimulating electrodes. These are generally two metal electrodes which are placed 1.5–3.0 cm apart. Conventionally monopolar needle electrodes which has advantages like requirement of smaller stimulus intensity, more selective stimulation of nerves and stimulation of nerves that lie deep anatomically have been used (Flowchart 9.1).

INTERPRETATION OF THE NERVE CONDUCTION STUDIES

1. Reduction in CMAP or SNAP amplitudes suggests ***axonal degeneration.***
   a. Amplitude can be considered as one of the important indicators of abnormal nerve conduction but further studies are recommended.

Table 9.1: Parameters for nerve conduction study

Nerve conduction study	*Nerves to be tested*	*Parameters analysis*
• Upper limb and lower limbs	• Ulnar nerve • Median nerve, Common Peroneal nerve • Tibial nerve	• Velocity, latency and amplitude

Table 9.2: General principle of nerve conduction study (NCS)

Response	*Active or recording electrode*	*Reference electrode*	*Ground electrode (metal plate)*
Motor	Over muscle or nerve segment to be studied	Distal to the muscle, on a nearby bone or tendon	Body prominence between the stimulating electrodes and recording electrodes.
Sensory	Over muscle or nerve segment to be studied	Distal to and on the nerve segment being studied	Body prominence between the stimulating electrodes and recording electrodes.

Flowchart 9.1: Difference between motor and sensory action potential

Nerve conduction study

Motor: Compound muscle action potential (CMAP)
- Measures CMAP upon stimulating the supplying nerve to muscle
- Place Active/recording electrode(E1) over motor point of muscle
- For example, for testing ulnar nerve CMAP, E1 to be placed over skin surface of abductor digiti minimi
- E2 (reference electrode) to be placed on nearby tendon or bone

Sensory: Sensory nerve action potential (SNAP)
– Can be recorded by two ways:
(1) Anti-dromically: Reference electrode is placed distal to the recording electrode
(2) Orthodromically: Reference electrode is placed proximal to the recording electrode.
Recording and reference electrodes are usually surface electrodes with spring ring, disc or bar which are used for sensory responses.

2. Slowing of CV and prolonged distal latency suggests ***demyelination.***
   a. A study of sensory conduction velocity (SCV) in normal subjects compared to leprosy patients showed slowing of conduction velocity in all nerves of leprosy patients, without any difference between lepromatous and tuberculoid cases. The same study also concluded that the SCV in radial cutaneous nerve is reliable as an early diagnostic tool for leprosy.[4] The slowing of nerve conduction in leprosy is due to demyelination of nerve rather than axonal damage.[5] This results from slowing in velocity of nerve conduction of fast conducting fibers than the slow conducting fibers.[6] In affected nerve, a functional blockade of nerve impulse conduction almost always precedes visible pathological changes.[7] Electrophysiological studies of affected nerves in leprosy have shown marked slowing of conduction.[8] In leprosy cases, clinically normal nerves on routine examination showed a significant slowing of motor nerve conduction velocities. Such patients may progress to clinical nerve damage when a certain quantum of nerve fibers are damaged. In general, the affected nerves of leprosy show more pronounced changes in sensory nerve conduction with reduction in nerve conduction velocity, along with changes in amplitude and latency.
3. Presence of mixed patterns/both of above suggests ***primary demyelination and secondary axonal loss.*** The most common pattern of peripheral neuropathy in leprosy is sensory-motor axonal type, hence NCV may show presence of mixed pattern. A study showed that tuberculoid cases showed more segmental demyelination while lepromatous cases showed mixed axonal and demyelinating changes, and it correlates well with clinical and histopathological findings. [9]
4. Loss of CMAP amplitude at the site of nerve block and normal CMAP amplitudes above and below the blocked segment suggests ***focal nerve conduction block.***

Applications of NCS in Leprosy[10]

1. **To look for subclinical neuropathy:** In leprosy nerve damage is quite advanced by the time it is clinically evident. This complication can be prevented to a great extent if it is detected early (preclinical phase) by nerve conduction studies. Detection of subclinical neuritis should prompt addition of steroids to ongoing MDT for prevention of nerve function impairment.

2. **Neuritis management:** To plan management of neuritis it is ideal to have baseline and follow up NCV studies of the patient.
   a. For patient with new onset/recent neuritis: If EMG worsens and NCV drops, it is a sign of failure of medical and surgical therapies.
   b. For Long-standing neuritis: Surgery is contraindicated if there is clinically complete sensory-motor deficits with abnormal EMG/NCV.[11] It should be only attempted if EMG shows some intact motor units with signs of regeneration. Surgery is worthwhile, only when NCV is more than 25–30 m/s.
3. **Medical management monitoring:** By monitoring improvement in NCV at regular intervals: A follow-up study[8] observed no significant improvement in the sensory conduction in both the multibacillary (MB) and paucibacillary (PB) groups of nerves at the first 6-monthly follow-up, while motor conduction showed a significant improvement in the nerves of MB patients. This is because damage in sensory fibers is earlier than motor fibers resulting in a greater reduction of sensory conduction velocity when compared to motor, while more significant amplitude changes occur in motor fibers. It is also helpful to study the drug efficacy in leprosy reactions using motor NCV.
4. **Diagnosis of peripheral neuropathy induced by thalidomide:** Peripheral neuropathy in leprosy cases may be due to disease *per se* or due to treatment of type 2 lepra reaction by thalidomide, which can be differentiated by NCS. On electrophysiological testing, thalidomide-induced neuropathy show reduction in SNAP amplitude with relative conservation of nerve conduction velocities.
5. In pure neuritic leprosy cases with clinically suspected peripheral neuropathy, to detect the type and the extent of nerve involvement, NCS is recommended for early diagnosis of NFI so that early treatment can be initiated as to prevent disabilities.

Electrophysiological Study by EMG

EMG records motor unit potentials by recording the electrical activity from a portion of a muscle. Each muscle is tested separately by EMG.[12] Needle EMG is commonly used method in leprosy patients in which twin core needle electrode is inserted into the muscle being tested. The electrical potentials in the tested muscle are observed at three points on an oscilloscope. (1) During the insertion of needle, (2) During muscle at rest, (3) During full muscle contraction (Tables 9.3 and 9.4).

LEPROSY NEURITIS

Disease of ventral horn cell, nerve root or peripheral nerve resulting in damaged nerve supply to muscle, leads to muscle denervation. EMG findings of such muscles are known as 'chronic partial denervation' and such pattern is observed in leprosy. It is important to note that EMG changes are more severe in MB patients as compared to PB patients. In manifest muscle paralysis, sensory amplitude and latencies changes were more severe than motor amplitude and latencies.[13]

Application of Electrophysiological Studies in Leprosy

- *Correlation with other method of sensory testing:* They along with warm detection thermal tests (WDT) helps early detection of leprous neuropathy.[14]
- *Difference between sensory and motor nerve conduction study*: The changes are more severe in sensory latencies and amplitude when presents along with muscle paralyses.[15]

Table 9.3: Muscles usually examined in leprosy for testing nerve functions

Nerve	*Muscle to be tested*
Median	Abductor pollicis brevis
Ulnar	Abductor digiti minimi
Lateral popliteal	Extensor digitorum brevis

Table 9.4 Normal vs abnormal EMG pattern:

Normal EMG	*Abnormal EMG (In neuropathies)*	*Abnormal EMG (In myopathies)*
Complete electric silence at rest, individual motor unit potentials, complete interference pattern	Fibrillation, fasciculation, giant motor unit potentials, incomplete interference, reduced recruitment pattern	Low amplitude and short duration of motor unit potentials, reduced interference pattern

- *Comparison with traditional nerve examination to detect nerve thickening*: Even non-thickened nerves may show insidious deterioration in function on electrophysiological tests signifying they are more sensitive than clinical nerve palpation in early detection of nerve function impairment.[16]

  The combination of clinical palpation for nerve thickening and SW graded nylon filament sensory testing along with VMT: It is very useful, reliable and often comparable to measurement of nerve conduction in detecting nerve function impairment in leprosy. Use of this combination in field conditions increases the clinical detection sensitivity of neuropathy by two-fold as compare to detection by only physical palpation of nerve thickening.[17]

CONCLUSION

Electrophysiological tests reflect the manifest nerve damage and help characterise its type. It does not reflect the cause of neuropathy. This is more useful in diagnosis of peripheral nerve disorders, particularly those due to local compressive lesions such as carpel tunnel syndrome and in the clinical assessment of nerve plexus or radicular disease. When used in combination with peripheral nerve clinical palpation, assessment of sensory function by SW monofilament they give better idea if the cause of peripheral neuropathy is leprosy. They are not much helpful when used in isolation.

REFERENCES

1. Marahatta S, Bhattarai S, Paudel BH. Nerve conduction study in leprosy: a hearty need or a customary practice? Lepr Rev. 2016;87:201–10.
2. Soysal A, Atay T, Ozu T, Arpaci B. Electrophysiological Evaluation of Peripheral and Autonomic Involvement in Leprosy. Can. J. Neurol. Sci. 2004; 31(3): 357–62.
3. Indu Krishnan MU, Sobhanakumari K, Jose P, Amitha NP, Irimpan KJ. High resolution ultrasound, nerve conduction study, and other non-invasive investigations in leprosy. J Skin Sex Transm Dis 2021;3:136–42.
4. Sebille A. Respective importance of different nerve conduction velocities in leprosy. J Neurol Sci. 1978;38(1):89–95.
5. Shetty VP, Mehta LN, Antia HN, et al. Teased fibre study of early nerve lesions in leprosy and in contacts, with electrophysiological correlates. J Neurol Neurosurg Psychiatry. 1977;40(7):708–11.
6. Marquees W, Barreira AA. Normal median nerve near potential. Braz J Med Biol Res. 1997;30:1431–5.
7. Hackett ER, Shipley DE, Livengood R. Motor nerve conduction velocity studies of ulnar nerve in patients with leprosy. Int J Lepr. 1968;36(3):282–7.

8. Samant G, Shetty VP, Uplekar MW, et al. Clinical and electrophysiological evaluation of nerve function impairment, following cessation of multidrug therapy in leprosy. Lepr Rev. 1999;70(1):10–20.
9. Celine MI, Jaleel A, Palakkal S, Vasanthi B, *et al*. A clinicopathological and electrophysiological study of nerve involvement in leprosy in a tertiary care centre in South India. Lepr Rev. 2021;92:225–35.
10. Gupta P, Mainra A, Dhanta A. Nerve conduction studies in leprosy a review. IOSR J Dent Med Sci 2018;17:27–32.
11. Carayon A, Rigal J. Value of electrophysiological investigation for therapeutic indications in leprous neuritis. Med Trop (Mars) 1972;32:9–21.
12. Ramdan W, Mourad B, Fadel W, et al. Clinical, electrophysiological, and immunopathological study of peripheral nerves in Hansen's disease. Lepr Rev. 2001;72(1):35–49.
13. Husain S, Malaviya GN. Early nerve damage in leprosy: an electrophysiological study of ulnar and median nerves in patients with and without clinical neural deficits. Neurol India. 2007;55(1):22–6.
14. Van Brakel WH, Nicholls PG, Wilder-Smith EP, *et al*. Early diagnosis of neuropathy in leprosy-comparing diagnostic tests in a large prospective study (the INFIR Cohort Study). PLoS Negl Trop Dis. 2008;2(4):1–12.
15. Husain S, Malaviya GN. Early nerve damage in leprosy: an electrophysiological study of ulnar and median nerves in patients with and without clinical neural deficits. Neurol India. 2007;55(1):22–6.
16. Rao SP, Bharambe MS. Electro-neuro physiological studies in early tuberculoid leprosy. Indian J Lepr. 1993;65(2):181–187.
17. Suneetha SK, Rao NP, Jain S. Structure, Electrophysiological and Ultrasonographic Studies of Peripheral Nerve. In: IAL Textbook of Leprosy, 2nd edn, (Kumar B, KarHK eds), Jaypee Brothers Medical Publishers Pvt Ltd, New Delhi, 2016;p.157.

Chapter 10

Ultrasonography and Imaging Techniques in Leprosy: Value and Applications

• Sujai Suneetha • Ranugha PSS

INTRODUCTION

Polyneuropathies are frequent neurological disorders causing significant morbidity. Symptoms are usually similar though underlying etiologies are different. Hence, early diagnosis of neuropathies due to treatable causes is important but often difficult. Nerve conduction studies are essential for etiological classification, but their use is limited.[1] Usually, there is a lag phase between the onset of nerve degeneration and clinically evident dysfunction. Hence, tests which can detect peripheral neuropathy at subclinical stages are essential. Magnetic resonance imaging (MRI) has been shown to visualize some early alterations in peripheral nerve morphology before clinical signs are seen.[2] However, its sensitivity and specificity are low.[3] High resolution ultrasound (HRUS) has emerged over the last few decades as a diagnostic tool with the potential to significantly enhance the accuracy of testing for common mononeuropathies by adding morphological information regarding nerve and surrounding structures.[4]

ULTRASOUND IN LEPROSY

High-resolution ultrasonography (HRUS) is a noninvasive technology and has been used over the last two decades to measure peripheral nerve thickening in leprosy. Nerve thickening with sensorimotor impairment is one of the cardinal signs of leprosy. Early identification of nerve enlargement and/or neuritis and initiation of therapy is important to prevent disabilities. However, palpation of nerves in leprosy is highly subjective with wide inter- and intraobserver variability. Nerve HRUS is an important tool for the 'objective' assessment of nerve involvement in leprosy.[5] Moreover, while HRUS is very helpful for nerves which are not easily palpable clinically, e.g. median nerve at the wrist, it has shown higher sensitivity and specificity for ulnar and common peroneal nerves.[6]

Indications[7]

- Identify/confirm nerve enlargement in all types of leprosy
- Confirmation of pure neuritic leprosy (PNL) when skin lesions are absent and SSS is negative.
- Early detection of neuritis
- Diagnosis of leprosy nerve abscess

Advantages[1,7]

- Easy to perform
- Cost-effective

- Noninvasive technique (a nerve biopsy can be avoided in pure neuritic leprosy)
- Difficult to palpate nerves like median nerve can be objectively assessed
- Can be used for detection of neuritis, to detect new nerve enlargements or relapse and to monitor response to treatment

Procedure

Knowledge regarding the normal sonographic appearence of the nerve and its size, echo-intensity, nerve and fascicle anatomy, vascularity, elastography and morphology of surrounding tissue is essential before scanning nerve of a leprosy patient.

a. Equipment, high-resolution probe and nerves usually tested

HRUS with broadband frequency of at least 12 MHz (15–18 MHz is preferable) with a linear array transducer should be used for imaging all the peripheral nerves.

While any superficial nerve can be imaged, in leprosy commonly the following nerves are tested bilaterally:

1. Ulnar nerve (UN) at the elbow and proximal to the medial epicondyle
2. Median nerve (MN) at the wrist and forearm
3. Lateral popliteal (LP) nerve at the head of fibula, and
4. Posterior tibial (PT) nerve at the ankle and proximal to the medial malleolus.

The size and echo-density of the above nerves should be measured using HRUS to determine the length of abnormality.[8]

b. Parameters assessed

i. **Size and cross-sectional area (CSA)**

The nerve's transverse section should be visualized and measurement done at the point where thickness of nerve is maximum. The nerve CSA is measured from the area within the inner margin of the hyperechoic rim.[8]

In a recent meta-analysis, 5.9 mm^2, 8.3 mm^2, 8.4 mm^2 and 10 mm^2 was the mean pooled CSA of ulnar (at elbow), median (at wrist), lateral popliteal (at head of fibula) and tibial (at malleolus) nerves, respectively among healthy adults. They did not find any correlation between CSA and age, weight and height of the individual. They concluded that influence of age, height, and weight need not be considered in clinical practice.[9,10]

ii. **Echotexture**

The epineurium and perineurium of healthy nerve are seen as hyperechoic areas and the nerve bundle as hypoechoic area. Nerves can be hyperechoic (particularly fascicles) due to scar tissue, fibrosis or axonal damage. Inflammation or oedema can cause hypoechogenicity of nerves.[1] Quantitative analysis of the nerve by software tools (gray-scale analysis and fraction of black) is being used as a common method, though qualitative description of echo signal may be more suitable for daily routine.[11]

Nerves' echo density is studied on imaging and graded as: mild—some hypoechogenicity, moderate—obvious hypoechogenicity, and severe—absence of any fascicular pattern.[8]

iii. **Vascularity by color Doppler**

Blood flow signals within a nerve are visualized using color Doppler (CD). Weak signals from slow velocity vessels are identified by adjusting the settings accordingly. 1 kHz is the PRF (pulse repetition frequency) and band filter is set at 50 Hz. If blood flow signals are observed using CD in the perineural plexus or intrafascicular vessels, it is indicative of nerve hypervascularity. When nerve pain or tenderness are absent on clinical examination, HRUS might be able to demonstrate early hemodynamic changes in the nerve which is going into reaction. Identification of this should alert the dermatologist to start corticosteroid therapy. HRUS is also useful as a follow-up tool to assess the response to steroid therapy by appreciating a reduction in the blood flow.[8]

Analysis and interpretation of HRUS image findings should be based on:[8]

1. Measurement of the maximum cross-sectional area of the nerve
2. Length of nerve enlargement
3. Analysis of nerve echotexture
4. Identification of nerve compression within osteofibrous tunnels
5. Detection of endo and epineural color flow signals.

Limitations

- The HRUS data should be evaluated/correlated in the context of clinical examination and NCS, which remain key components of examination of peripheral nervous system.
- HRUS requires a long learning curve and is dependent on the intra- and interrater reliability and on the examiners experience
- The validity of the findings depend on the frequency and resolution of the probe used.
- In order to make a correct diagnosis, knowledge about nerve HRUS as well as anatomy of musculoskeletal and nervous system is a must.
- HRUS is less useful in deeper layers at present, and data on contrast enhanced nerve is lacking
- There is a lack of standard protocols for HRUS examination of nerves and paucity of data from large studies in Indian and Asian populations on nerve parameters of normal individuals.

OTHER IMAGING TECHNIQUES

MR neurography (MRN): Magnetic Resonance neurography (MRN) or MRI of peripheral nerves is an advanced technique where the high contrast resolution, multiplanar imaging capabilities, and noninvasive nature enables excellent visualization of the peripheral nerves. MRI enables study of the nerve throughout its course, evaluate it for changes in morphology, internal characteristics (signal intensity), compare it with the contralateral side, and simultaneously evaluate adjacent bones and soft tissues. Its limitations, however, include its high cost, the longer time needed to perform the test, the operator dependence and limited availability as compared to HRUS. Contraindications include patients with pacemakers, cochlear implants and those who are claustrophobic. A possible approach could be to use HRUS for preliminary imaging and if the results are inadequate or inconclusive then go for an MRI.[12] In leprosy MRI may also be useful to the surgeon to localize a nerve abscess for nerve decompression.

Ultrasound elastography: US elastography, a recent technique is used to evaluate biological tissue stiffness. Strain elastography (SE) and shear wave elastography (SWE) are the two commonly used methods. At present, knowledge regarding the relationship between the severity of peripheral neuropathy and the stiffness of peripheral nerves in leprosy is lacking. Whether elastography changes occur before nerve function anomalies become detectable on NCS is not known. Hence, the role of US elastography in leprosy has to be studied further.[3]

Diffusion tensor imaging (DTI) tractography: DTI is an MRI technique that uses anisotropic diffusion to estimate the axonal organization of nerve tissue. It is a quantitative method that could provide useful information for the diagnosis and follow-up of nerve lesions, entrapments, and regeneration. It is also useful to study details of myelin discontinuity, demyelination, and remyelination.[13]

REFERENCES

1. Kramer M, Grimm A, Winter N, Dörner M, Grundmann-Hauser K, Stahl JH, Wittlinger J, Kegele J, Kronlage C, Willikens S. Nerve Ultrasound as Helpful Tool in Polyneuropathies. Diagnostics (Basel). 2021;11(2):211.
2. Martinoli C, Derchi, L, Bertolotto M. et al. US and MR imaging of peripheral nerves in leprosy. Skeletal Radiol 2000;29,142–50.
3. Zakrzewski J, Zakrzewska K, Pluta K, Nowak O, Miłoszewska-Paluch A. Ultrasound elastography in the evaluation of peripheral neuropathies: a systematic review of the literature. Pol J Radiol. 2019;84:e581–91.
4. Jain S, Visser LH, Praveen TL, Rao PN, Surekha T, Ellanti R et al. High resolution sonography: a new technique to detect nerve damage in leprosy. PLoS Negl Trop Dis 2009; 3(8): e498.
5. Maymone MBC, Laughter M, Venkatesh S, Dacso MM, Rao PN, Stryjewska BM. Hugh J, Dellavalle RP, Dunnick CA (2020). Leprosy: Clinical Aspects and Diagnostic Techniques. Journal of the American Academy of Dermatology, S0190962220304746. doi:10.1016/j.jaad.2019.12.080.
6. Frade MA, Nogueira-Barbosa MH, Lugao HB, Furini RB, Marques Junior W, Foss NT. New sonographic 666 measures of peripheral nerves: a tool for the diagnosis of peripheral nerve involvement in leprosy. Mem Inst 667 Oswaldo Cruz 2013;108
7. Suneetha SK, Rao PN. High-Resolution Ultrasonography in Leprosy: Value and Applications. Indian Dermatol Online J. 2021;12(4):497–9.
8. Jain S, Visser LH., Suneetha S. Imaging techniques in leprosy clinics, Clinics in Dermatology. Clin Dermatol. 2016;34(1):70–8.
9. Fisse AL, Katsanos AH, Gold R, Pitarokoili K, Krogias C. Cross-sectional area reference values for peripheral nerve ultrasound in adults: a systematic review and meta-analysis—Part I: Upper extremity nerves. Eur J Neurol. 2021; 28: 1684–91.
10. Fisse AL, Katsanos AH, Gold R, Krogias C, Pitarokoili K. Cross-sectional area reference values for peripheral nerve ultrasound in adults: A systematic review and meta-analysis-Part II: Lower extremity nerves. Eur J Neurol. 2021;28(7):2313–8.
11. Baute Penry, V.; Cartwright, M.S. Neuromuscular Ultrasound for Peripheral Neuropathies. Semin. Neurol. 2019;39:542–8.
12. Upadhyaya V, Choudur HN. Imaging in peripheral neuropathy: Ultrasound and MRI. Indian J Musculoscelet Radiol 2021;3(1):14–23.
13. Colonna MR, Tallarida G, Stagnod 'Alcontres F, Noto S, Parodi A, Tagliafico A. Diffusion tensor imaging tractography in pure neuritic leprosy: First experience report and review of the literature. Case Rep Neurol Med 2016;2016:2767856.

Chapter

11

Serological Diagnosis of Leprosy

• Itu Singh • Utpal Sengupta

INTRODUCTION

Diagnosis of leprosy is mainly based on clinical evaluation of the patients for the cardinal signs of leprosy, i.e. presence of hypopigmented or erythematous anesthetic patches, enlarged nerves, and the presence of acid-fast bacilli (AFB) in slit skin smears. However, it is problematic to diagnose the disease in the absence of cardinal signs or due to inability to elicit these signs, especially in regions where prevalence is very low. In such situations, laboratory tests based on serological, molecular, histopathological techniques will support, strengthen, and confirm the diagnosis.

Diagnosis of leprosy is usually confirmed by histopathological examination of tissue sections obtained from the margins of active lesion. Molecular techniques to detect genes of *M. leprae* in the lesions could also be used to diagnose early leprosy. Serological tests in leprosy are mainly used for determining exposure with *M. leprae* because antigen stays for long time after subsidence of clinical or subclinical infection.

DEFINITION

In serodiagnosis, the serum of the suspect is used to detect antibody response due to *M. leprae* specific antigen in the host. Serodiagnostic test has limited value for diagnosis of active leprosy as the antigens and associated response persists for long time even after subsidence of clinical or subclinical infection. Hence, this test is mainly used to determine exposure level.

CURRENT AVAILABLE KNOWLEDGE ON THE SUBJECT

i. *Phenolic glycolipid–1 based Serology:* Phenolic glycolipid-1 (PGL-1) is a *M. leprae* specific lipid antigen present on the cell wall of *M. leprae*. PGL-1 as a whole or its terminal sugars [Natural disaccharide (ND)/natural trisaccharide (NT)] have been extensively used for serodiagnostic tests. PGL-1 based enzyme-linked immunosorbent assay (ELISA) test is used for detection of IgM antibodies in patients against PGL-1. This test is mainly useful for diagnosis of BL/LL (90–95% positivity) cases however, it has limited value in diagnosing TT/BT patients (25–60%). Specific B cell epitopes of PGL-1 were identified as sugar molecules, ND/NT were synthesized and conjugated with bovine serum albumin (BSA) as ND-O-BSA/NT-O-BSA. These glyco-conjugates were found to have better specificity in diagnosis than their whole molecule PGL-1.[1] IgM antibody level against ND-O-BSA/NT-O-BSA was found to be positively correlated with bacterial index (BI) of the patient. There are different immunochromatographic techniques like lateral flow (ML flow test), dipstick and particle agglutination test using PGL-1/ND-O-BSA have been developed to use in field conditions. The results are visible in ML flow test within 10 minutes, and it showed 91% agreement with that of ND-O-BSA ELISA.[2]

It was reported that >50% of school children from hyperendemic areas of leprosy have positive anti-PGL-1 responses.[3] Presence of anti-PGL-1 antibodies were considered to be a risk factor for development of disease,[4] nonetheless, other studies have shown that majority of individuals having positive antibodies never developed the leprosy disease.[5] In Indian scenario, especially in endemic regions the benefits of PGL–1/ND-O-BSA/NT-O-BSA ELISA is yet to be determined at present.

ii. *35 kDa Antigen-based serology:* Competitive inhibition ELISA for 35 kDa antigen of *M. leprae* using monoclonal antibody (MLO4) was standardized by Sinha et al. for detection of antibodies in leprosy patients.[6] It was observed that with the help of this assay 40% of PB gave positive reaction.[6] Antibody level against 35 kDa antigen was found to be correlated with treatment in leprosy patients.[7] Purified 35 kDa protein was used for direct ELISA, and it was observed to be highly specific (97.5%) and sensitive (90%). This protein was purified from the sonicate of *M. Smegmatis* and transformed in pW19.[8]

iii. *Major membrane protein-II based serology:* Serodiagnostic value of *M. leprae* derived major membrane protein-II (MMP-II) was evaluated by Maeda et al.[9] Percent positivity of MB cases was reported as 82.4% while for PB cases showed 39% positivity. However, it cross reacted with sera of TB patients with 16.4% positivity.

iv. *18 kDa antigen-based serology:* 18 kDa antigen was found to have T cell epitopes, but its serological reactivity has not been worked out satisfactorily.[10]

v. Early secretary antigen target–6 (ESAT–6) and culture filtrate protein-10 (CFP–10): M. leprae ESAT–6 (ML0049) was used in antigen-based ELISA and its' sensitivity was observed to be 82.4% in MB and 19.4% in PB cases and specificity was 100%.[11]

CFP-10 was evaluated in direct ELISA test in leprosy patients, it was observed to be comparable with PGL-1.[12]

vi. Leprosy IDRI diagnostic–1 (LID–1): M. leprae proteins ML0405 and ML2331 were used to form a fusion construct named leprosy IDRI diagnostic 1 (LID-1).[13] It was found to have the diagnostic potential. ELISA test for detection of antibodies response against LID-1 were found to be positive in 95% of MB cases. However, in PB cases positivity varied between 20 and 40%.[13] Recently, in a study which detected antibody levels using all the three antigens PGL-1, LID-1, and NDO-LID, found that the antibody levels declined significantly after a full course of MDT.[14]

Basic details of testing methods

A. Serology-based testing methods–

i. *Phenolic glycolipid-1 based ELISA test.*

ii. *ND-O-BSA-based ELISA test.*

Reagents required for ELISA

1. Antigen
2. Primary antibody
3. Enzyme-linked secondary antibody
4. Phosphate-buffered saline (PBS)
5. O-Phenylenediamine
6. Tween–20
7. Bovine serum albumin (BSA)

B. Existing SOPs/guidelines of relevance

Basic Protocol

i. Type of sample: Blood.
ii. Blood collection: 5 ml of venous blood is aseptically collected from patients.
iii. Serum separation: Blood is stored at room temperature for 2 hours. Then serum is separated by centrifugation. It will be stored at-20°C till further use.
iv. ELISA for ND-O-BSA is done as described in Table 11.1.
v. Cutoff value is calculated by taking mean value of healthy controls ± 2 Standard deviation (Cutoff value = Mean ± 2SD).
vi. Data are analyzed.

Personnel required: Lab technician, for the collection of blood. Immunologist to process the sample, perform ELISA and data analysis and reporting the results.

ELISA tests targeting different antigens in PB and MB leprosy patients and its usefulness is mentioned in Table 11.2.

Table 11.1: How to perform ELISA test (Fig. 11.1)

ND-O-BSA-based ELISA test
(i) Coat a 96 well micro-titer plate with 100 µl per well of diluted ND-O-BSA (Stock conc. 1 mg/ml) at final concentration of 1 µg/ml dissolved in 0.05 M carbonate–bicarbonate buffer (pH 9.6) and incubate overnight at 37°C.
(ii) Wash plates with PBS (pH 7.4), two minutes washing cycle for three times (300 µl/well).
(iii) Block the plates with 2% BSA in PBS (200 µl/well) and incubate at 37°C for 1 hour.
(iv) Repeat step 2.
(v) Add diluted serum sample (100 µl/well) and incubate at 37°C for 2 hours. [Dilution factor 1:100 in 1% BSA in PBS-Tween 20 (0.05%]
(vi) Repeat step 2 with PBS-Tween 20 (0.05%) [PBST]
(vii) Add antihuman IgM (100 µl/well) diluted in 1% BSA in PBS-Tween 20 (0.05%) [dilution factor 1:4000] and incubate at 37°C for 1 hour.
(viii) Repeat step 6.
(ix) Add substrate solution (100 µl/well) of O-Phenylenediamine (OPD) dissolved in D/W at final conc. of 0.5 mg/ml added with 0.5% H_2O_2 and incubated for 20 min in dark at RT.
(x) Add stop solution 3N HCl/2N H_2SO_4 (50 µl/well).
(xi) Determine OD at 492 nm.
***Tools and facilities needed (Figs 11.2 to 11.4)**: 1. ELISA Reader. 2. Micro-pipettes (2–20 µl, 20–200 µl, 100–1000 µl) 3. Multi-channel pipette (20–300 µl). 4. Micro-titer plate. 5. Deep freezers. 6. Incubator 37°C 7. Refrigerator. 8. Electronic weighing balance 9. Desktop 10. Software for data analysis*

Table 11.2: ELISA tests targeting different antigens in PB and MB leprosy patients and its usefulness

Serological marker	*PB cases (% positivity)*	*MB cases (% positivity)*	*Sensitivity and specificity (%)*
PGL-1	0–40	70–95	91
ML flow test	40	97	97 and 90
35 kDa	46.7	98.5	98.4 and 100
LID	20–40	95	95

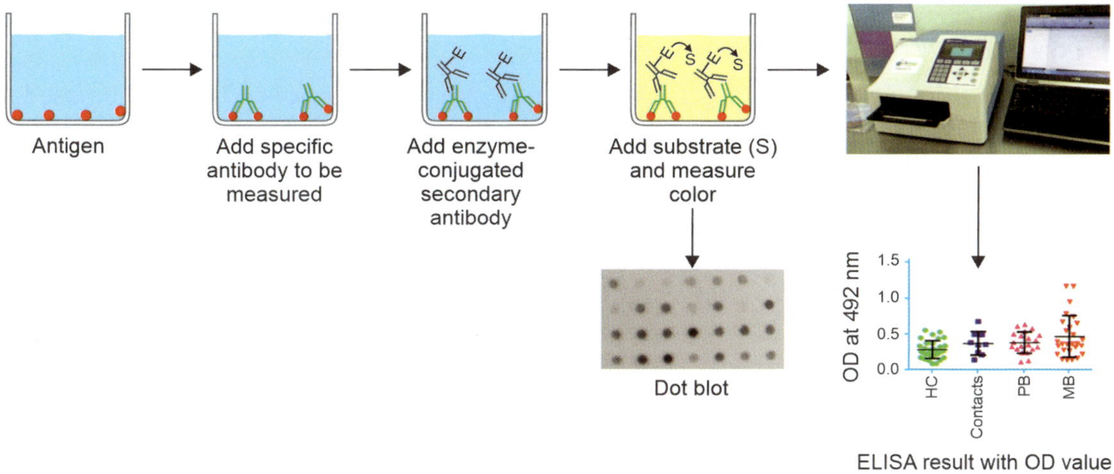

Fig. 11.1: Basic principle of ELISA

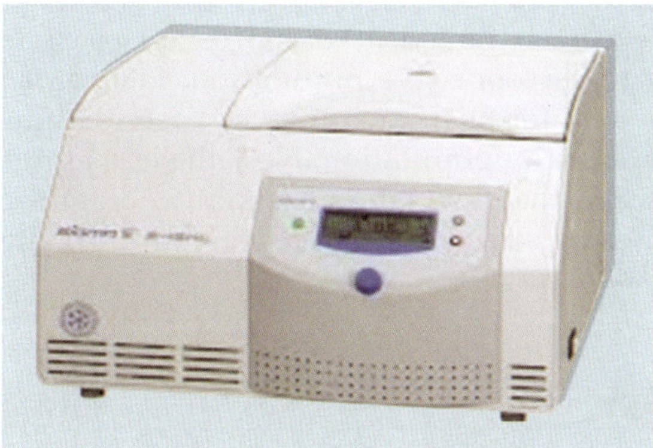

Fig. 11.2: Cooling centrifuge

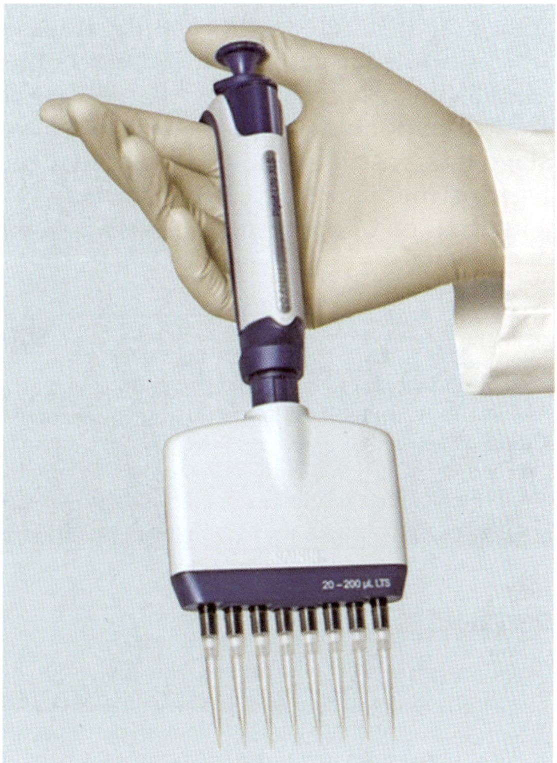

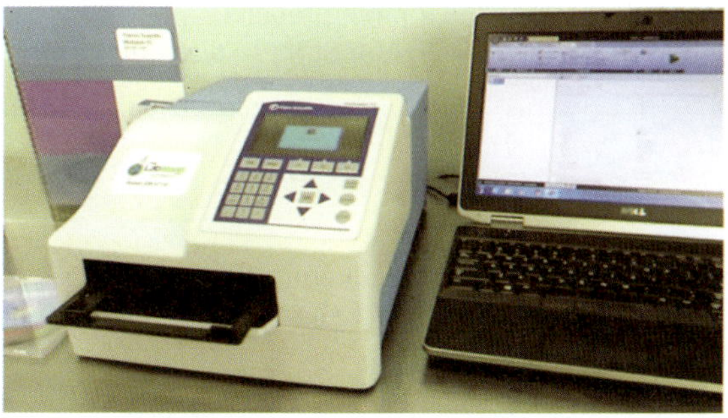

Fig. 11.4: ELISA reader

Fig. 11.3: Multi-channel pipette

C. Management options and variations

ELISA is used to measure antibody level against a particular antigen of *M. leprae*. However, measurement of CMI by cytokines (both pro and anti-inflammatory) as well as humoral immunity to *M. leprae* can be a valuable additional tool for the diagnosis as well as classification of leprosy, which can further lead to timely treatment and reduce disability.

Practical problems: None of the serological diagnostic tests mentioned here can be used as a gold standard method to diagnose leprosy. Using the cardinal signs of leprosy the disease can be diagnosed efficiently by an experienced clinician. While the serological tests described can be used to diagnose MB cases efficiently, where usually cardinal signs of leprosy are present, however, in PB or early cases of leprosy cannot be diagnosed perfectly by any of the serological test available, where cardinal signs are mostly absent or ill-defined. Hence, there is an urgent need to develop a specific and sensitive serological test for the diagnosis of all types of early leprosy cases.

SCOPE FOR FURTHER RESEARCH

As already mentioned, serological tests can diagnose MB cases efficiently, but these are unable to diagnose early or PB cases with good accuracy. Study on use of antibody assay against LID-1 has been carried out in Philippines, Brazil, and Japan for predicting potentially household contacts at a higher risk of developing leprosy.[15] Establishment of such a predictive test for a long incubating disease such as leprosy requires a long-term double blinded cohort study. It was observed that majority of leprosy cases came from sero-negative population as compared to sero-positive population. Hence, for establishment of any standardized diagnostic test for such a chronic disease requires controlled double blinded screening of normal healthy population. Nonetheless, at this stage it is possible that in a suspected case when the clinician is hesitant to diagnose leprosy, these serological tests specially targeting specific antigens can support the confirmation of the case as leprosy.

SUMMARY

Establishment of a gold standard method is urgently needed for definite diagnosis of early cases of leprosy. All the above-mentioned serological methods may help detect up to 60% of early leprosy cases. Efforts are needed to search and develop new and novel biomarkers or antigens which will mainly support the diagnosis of subclinical infection/early leprosy cases. In addition, guidelines are needed for interpretation and relevance of serological test results in contacts of leprosy who might come positive with any of these tests but do not develop cardinal signs and symptoms of the disease.

REFERENCES

1. Gigg J, Gigg R, Payne S et al. The allyl group for protection in carbohydrate chemistry. 17. Synthesis of propyl O-(3,6-di-O-methyl-beta-D-glucopyranosyl)-(1 4)-O-(2,3-di-O-methyl-alpha-L-rhamnopyranosyl)-(1–2)-3-O-methyl-alpha-L-rhamnopyranoside: the oligosaccharide portion of the major serologically active glycolipid from *Mycobacterium leprae*. Chem Phys Lipids. 1985;38:299–307.
2. Buhrer-Sekula S, Smits HL, Gussenhoven GC, et al. Simple and fast lateral flow test for classification of leprosy patients and identification of contacts with high risk of developing leprosy. J Clin Microbiol. 2003;41:1991–5.
3. Barreto JG, Guimaraes LS, Frade MA, Rosa PS, Salgado CG. High rates of undiagnosed leprosy and subclinical infection amongst school children in the Amazon Region. Mem Inst Oswaldo Cruz. 2012; 107(Suppl 1):60–7.
4. Beers, vSM., Hatta M, Klatser PR. Seroprevalence rates of antibodies to phenolic glycolipid-I among school children as an indicator of leprosy endemicity. Int J Lepr Other Mycobact Dis. 1999; 67:243–9.

5. Spencer JS, Kim HJ, Wheat WH, et al. Analysis of antibody responses to *Mycobacterium leprae* phenolic glycolipid I, lipoarabinomannan, and recombinant proteins to define disease subtype-specific antigenic profiles in leprosy. Clin Vaccine Immunol. 2011;18:260–7.
6. Sinha S, Sengupta U, Ramu G, et al. A serological test for leprosy based on competitive inhibition of monoclonal antibody binding to the MY2a determinant of *Mycobacterium leprae*. Trans Royal Soc Trop Med Hyg. 1983;77:869–71.
7. Chaturvedi V, Sinha S, Girdhar BK, *et al*. Association of mycobacterial-specific and *Mycobacterium leprae* specific antibody levels with clinical activity in tuberculoid leprosy: a comparative study of three serological enzyme-immunoassays. Lepr Rev. 1991;62:122–33.
8. Triccas JA, Roche PW, Britton WJ. Specific serological diagnosis of leprosy with a recombinant *Mycobacterium leprae* protein purified from a rapidly growing mycobacterial host. J Clin Microbiol. 1998;36:2363–5.
9. Maeda Y, Mukai T, Kai M, et al. Evaluation of major membrane protein-II as a tool for serodiagnosis of leprosy. FEMS Microbiol Lett. 2007;272:202–5.
10. Dockrell HM, Stoker NG, Lee SP, et al. T-cell recognition of the 18-kilodalton antigen of *Mycobacterium leprae*. Infect Immun. 1989;57:1979–83.
11. Geluk A, van Meijgaarden KE, Franken KL, Subronto YW, Wieles B, Arend SM, Sampaio EP, d Boer T, Faber WR, Naafs B, Ottenhoff TH. Identification and characterization of the ESAT-6 homologue of *Mycobacterium leprae* and T-cell cross-reactivity with *Mycobacterium tuberculosis*. Infect Immun. 2002; 70:2544–8.
12. Geluk A, van Meijgaarden KE, Franken KL, Wieles B, Arend SM, Faber WR, Naafs B, Ottenhoff TH. Immunological crossreactivity of the *Mycobacterium leprae* CFP-10 with its homologue in *Mycobacterium tuberculosis*. Scand J Immunol 2004;59:66–70.
13. Duthie MS, Hay MN, Morales CZ, Carter L, Mohamath R, Ito L, Oyafuso LK, Manini MI, Balagon MV, Tan EV, Saunderson PR, Reed SG, Carter D. Rational design and evaluation of a multiepitope chimeric fusion protein with the potential for leprosy diagnosis. Clin Vaccine Immunol 2010;17:298–303.
14. Hungria EM, Bührer-Sékula S, Oliveira RM, Aderaldo LC, Pontes MAA, Cruz R, et al. *Mycobacterium leprae*- specific antibodies in multibacillary patients decrease during and after treatment with either regular 12 doses MDT or the uniform 6 doses MDT. Front Immunol 2018;9:915.
15. Leturiondo AL, Noronha AB, do Nascimento MOO, Ferreira CO, Rodrigues FDC, Moraes MO, Talhari C. Performance of serological tests PGL1 and NDO-LID in the diagnosis of leprosy in a reference center in Brazil. BMC Infect Dis. 2019;19(1):22.

Chapter

12

Molecular Diagnosis of Leprosy

• Mallika Lavania • Ravindra P Turankar

INTRODUCTION

Mycobacterium leprae is the causative organism of leprosy, and till date cannot be grown on any artificial media. Diagnosis of leprosy is therefore still based on the clinical signs and symptoms of the disease. Leprosy presents a challenge as conventionally, the definitive diagnosis is based on the demonstration of AFB in slit skin smears and/or tissue sections with the disease characteristics on histopathology. This is not always feasible and testing for AFB in slit skin smears (SSS) has been done away with in the programme. With the whole genome sequencing of *M. leprae* and development and use of molecular methods, definitive diagnosis of leprosy is achievable. In the recent past, molecular tests and serological tests/techniques for diagnosis of leprosy have been developed. Serological diagnosis has been described in the preceding chapter but, it was observed that, these tests are less sensitive and specific and do not distinguish active disease from latent disease.

Deciphering the structure and functionality of the *Mycobacterium leprae* genome have led to the creation of specialized PCR-based specific gene amplification assays for leprosy diagnosis, antimicrobial resistance (AMR) testing, understanding the transmission dynamics and also for household contact screening and monitoring. Current literature search suggests, that molecular diagnostic methods, such as RLEP PCR, real-time PCR (RT PCR), quantitative PCR (qPCR), and LAMP assays, would be the preferred method/techniques due to their high sensitivity and specificity, for early and definitive diagnosis of leprosy.

As in other diseases as well, these molecular methods have been tested and found advantageous for specific and rapid DNA detection of causative agent, and are being used as a point-of-care (POC) technology in field situations. These techniques ensure rapid and specific diagnosis of diseases including TB in program settings. Similar methods can be applied for detection of *M. leprae* as well and would help in early diagnosis, and treatment of leprosy. While the term 'molecular' is a broad one, this chapter will be focusing on *M. leprae* specific nucleic acid-based techniques and review relevant recent technological advances in the molecular biology of *M. leprae*.

CURRENT KNOWLEDGE

Molecular detection of *M. leprae* using *M. leprae* specific probes and application by PCR technology, have been investigated by several scientists worldwide. These are being used to improve early definitive diagnosis. These molecular tests use *M. leprae* specific probes which are amplified by polymerase chain reaction (PCR). Besides the conventional use of

PCR for *M. leprae* DNA and RNA probes, other advances include real-time PCR (RT PCR), quantitative PCR and LAMP-based rapid testing systems. They have been found to be helpful in early diagnosis, and identifying *M. leprae* viability, monitoring treatment, assessing drug resistance, and to some extent leprosy transmission pathways. These PCR-based tests have also been found to be useful to diagnose challenging cases, such as pure neuritic leprosy (PNL), indeterminate leprosy, paucibacillary leprosy (PB) and patients with unusual clinical symptoms. Additionally, *M. leprae* DNA was also found in various samples of the household contacts of active leprosy patients. Although a positive result is not sufficient to certify active disease, careful follow-up and quantification as seen by real-time PCR can lead to early definitive diagnosis. Furthermore, if bacillary load increases during follow-up, the results can/will also alert and signal a greater risk of contracting the disease, thereby alerting the doctors/epidemiologists/health workers, to monitor these contacts more closely at frequent regular intervals. Detection of mutation in the gene region can help in detecting drug resistance and used as a tool for surveillance of AMR activity.

TESTING TOOLS AND METHODS

In the past several years (20–30 years), definitive identification of *M. leprae* has been made possible through the development of versatile methods for the extraction, amplification, and identification of *M. leprae* DNA (later also *M. leprae* RNA) from clinical specimens. There are still, some limitations on the number of organisms which can be identified from clinical specimens. The molecular advances in technology have been utilized, so that even 1–10 organisms DNA/RNA can be detected and this has helped in developing rapid detection tools for various diseases including TB and leprosy.[1–3] Several specific gene sequences of *M. leprae* have been identified. These include, specific sequences/genes encoding the 36-kDa antigen, 18-kDa antigen, 65-kDa antigen, antigen complex 85, 16S rRNA, and the repetitive sequence RLEP (*M. leprae* specific repetitive element). Based on these advances gene probes have been designed for direct demonstration and amplification of *M. leprae* specific sequences in different specimens, like slit skin smears (SSS), nasal smears, biopsy specimens, tissue sections, blood, urine etc. The different types of gene probes [DNA, RNA targeting probes] used and described for the detection of *M. leprae* is mentioned below.[4]

Types of Probes

- **DNA targeting probes:** Specific *M. leprae* DNA-targeting probes have been shown to have a detection sensitivity of up to 10^4–10^5 organisms. These can be used in the cases where the bacterial load is low like paucibacillary disease and also neural leprosy. RLEP PCR or specific *M. leprae* repetitive sequence PCR is more sensitive due to the presence of multiple copies in the *M. leprae* genomic DNA. Amplification and real-time detection and quantification of these probes is achieved by real-time 'RT' PCR to increase the sensitivity of the assay and led to detection of even 1–10 organisms/specimen tested.
- **RNA targeting probes:** After cell death RNAs degrade quicker than DNA and are therefore related to live organisms. Their detection and additionally quantitation corresponds better with the presence of live bacteria and/or active disease. It is known that messenger RNA (mRNA) has the most limited half-life and in this way could be an ideal marker of viability. However, tests focusing on mRNA have not been very fruitful due to the extremely short half-life and difficulties of purification and identification of mRNA. Ribosomal RNA (rRNA) is another specific sequence particle which is available as a few duplicate numbers (2,000–5,000) per live mycobacterial cell. Microdensitometric scanning has been used to

establish an assay for the quantitative detection of these signals and it has been found to be helpful for both identifying relapses and tracking the progress of treatment. These rRNA-based probes can be utilized for the detection of viable *Mycobacterium leprae* from the clinical specimens.[5] Among these 16S RNA has been used by several investigators for detection of live *M. leprae* in clinical patient samples, in patients having reactions, and also in the environment, in close proximity to active patients.[5–7]

Suitable Specimens Commonly Used for Detecting M. leprae Specific Sequences

Skin biopsy: Leprosy molecular diagnosis can be carried out in fresh skin biopsies, frozen skin biopsies, paraffin embedded in 70% ethanol and nerve biopsies. However, usually in samples fixed in formalin and 70% ethanol,[8] impurities from the fixation process are more likely to contain inhibitors for PCR and the sequences may not be properly amplified in such fixed tissue samples.

Slit skin smears/scrapings (SSS): There have been reports and evidence supporting the PCR testing of *M. leprae* from fresh slit skin smears/scrapings as an alternative to biopsy. These specimens can improve the diagnosis with a higher degree of sensitivity and specificity. The tests can also be carried out on stained slit skin smears glass slides.[6] The advantage of slit skin smear scrapping is that, it is easy to perform even in field conditions as well as easy and simple to transport from the place of collection to testing center. This can be done either by an individual and/or courier. This is done easily-after heat fixation, the sample is put in 70% ethanol and/or in RNA-Ladder solution. Moreover, the probes can be directly applied to stored SSS specimens as well. The skin-smear specimen exhibits similar recovery rates like that of skin biopsy.

Nasal swabs: It is now established that untreated actively infected individuals, transmit the infection through airborne droplets from the mouth and nose particularly untreated multibacillary (MB) patients. In order to screen possible contacts and control the spread of leprosy, *M. leprae* specific PCR can be done from nasal secretions/swabs.[4, 9] However, it is crucial to distinguish between healthy and subclinical carriers.

Blood: The diagnosis of leprosy can be done from blood by identifying and demonstration of *M. leprae* specific sequence from blood also. This has mostly been carried out in household contacts as well as in posttreatment patients. It may be noted that, and DNA sequence PCR positivity might persist for an extended period. It has been observed that some contacts of multibacillary index individuals who have been shown to be *M. leprae* PCR positive are more likely to develop leprosy. These contacts, need careful clinical examination, and more frequent and careful follow-up.

Urine: The testing of *M. leprae* antigens in urine was demonstrated earlier in established patients of leprosy.[10] Diagnosis of leprosy was made by amplifying 151-bp PCR fragment, (PCR-pra), and has been shown to be positive in paucibacillary (PB), smear negative cases.[9] Its sensitivity however, still has to be established in early diagnosis of leprosy.

Molecular Tests Based on PCR Technology

Conventional PCR: Conventional PCR is widely used in most laboratories. Different sequences such as genes encoding the 36-kDa antigen,[1] 18-kDa antigen,[2] 65-kDa antigen r X,[3] antigen complex 85, 16S rDNA and rRNA[5–7, 9] and the repetitive sequences RLEP,[4, 9,11,12] targets have been used as for PCR amplification and identification. This has been proven to be useful in the early definitive diagnosis of leprosy, understanding the possible leprosy transmission pathways, assessment of *M. leprae* viability, monitoring household contacts, monitoring antileprosy drug therapy and molecular detection of drug resistance in leprosy.[13] In conventional PCR, the amplified DNA product, or amplicon, is detected in an end-point analysis (shown in Flowchart 12.1). The sensitivity of these conventional PCR varied between 50 and 93% and its specificity between 90 and 100%.

The results of the test can be made available quickly (within 24 hours), and only the specific probes as well as laboratory requirements for undertaking PCR are required.

Multiplex PCR: To increase the sensitivity of a single sequence fragment PCR, multiplex PCR (M PCR) methods have been developed and are in use. In multiplex PCR, more than one target sequence is amplified at the same time and results collated together for greater sensitivity. Using multiplex PCR in PB cases (BI-negative cases) the percent positivity significantly increased up to 80.3%[4] and 93.3%. Multiplex PCR includes two and more targets. RLEP, 16S RNA and *sod*A were the common sequences used in these PCRs. Multiplex PCR test has also been used in household contacts of both MB and PB cases, to detect early disease occurrence.[14,15]

Real-time PCR (RT PCR): The steps of RT-PCR are the same as conventional PCR, with the additional first step of reverse transcription. Here, complementary DNA (cDNA) is produced first using reverse transcriptase (RT). The cDNA, thus formed, is then used as a template for the standard amplification process by PCR. This is more sensitive than ordinary PCR methods described above, but more sophisticated instruments are required to undertake it. The enhanced DNA or cDNA (reciprocal DNA) is quantitated as it gathers in the experiment. In addition, analyses using real-time PCR showed that total DNA content estimated at the molecular level could be correlated to bacterial load, which can be useful to determine a molecular bacteriological index.[16] The results of the molecular bacteriological index can be monitored over time to monitor the progression/regression of the disease.[13] Similarly, the increase in molecular bacteriological index in contacts during follow-up can alert the clinicians for a more detailed clinical examination and a more closer and frequent follow-up. It is very helpful in differentiating leprosy from diseases that cause similar symptoms, thus ensuring a correct definitive diagnosis. Slit Skin Smears, histopathology specimens, nasal specimens, etc. can be used in this method.[17]

Flowchart 12.1: Detection of *M. leprae* DNA/RNA by conventional PCR

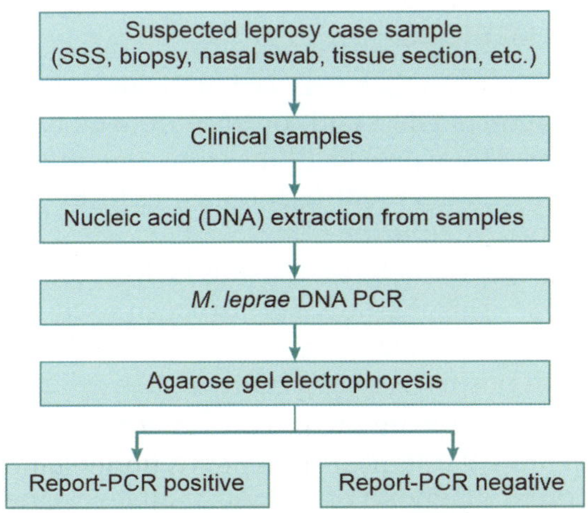

Quantitative real-time PCR assay (qPCR): This is a more sensitive faster with which detailed real-time results can be obtained that can be used to quantify nucleic acids[18] continuously, after every intensification cycle.[19] The accumulation of amplification product is measured as the reaction progresses, in real time, with product quantification after each cycle. A probe is usually used for quantitative detection of *M. leprae* nucleic acids in clinical samples. It quantifies and measures the products generated during each cycle of PCR process. This has been used by different research groups across the globe by targeting various sequences such as RLEP, 16SrRNA, *soda*, *exs*A and Ag 85B genes for the differential diagnosis of leprosy.[9] The effective sensitivity of qPCR shifted from 51 to 91% and specificity from 46 to 100%. It requires specialized instruments and care. It can be undertaken in specialized laboratories. Several of such laboratories have come up in recent past. The clinical samples can also be outsourced to some of these laboratories and get the result at a price. qPCR has a much wider dynamic range of analysis than conventional, end-point PCR .

***In situ* PCR:** This is a simple PCR done in tissue samples and the sequence can be identified and localized in these tissue samples. It can be undertaken on fresh tissue samples as well as old sections utilizing proper probes/stains for identification of target.

Loop-mediated isothermal amplification assay (LAMP assay): Isothermal amplification techniques are favored over traditional PCR methods as they are sensitive as conventional PCR, faster than the real time PCR analysis and is also applicable at peripheral field-based healthcare level. LAMP assay is a rapid, accurate nucleic acid based (NAAT) point of-care (POC) diagnostic test. This technique employs a *Bacillus stearothermophilus* (*Bst*), derived DNA polymerase and a set of four to six primers (two inner and two outer primers). To speed up the reaction and augment sensitivity, a pair of loop-primers that recognize six distinct sequences of the target DNA are usually used. This makes them highly specific to the target. DNA amplification can be completed in a single step by incubating the mixture of primers with polymerase and template it into a reaction buffer using a simple water bath. The results can be obtained using easy and simple eye identification of amplicons. This is also simple and suitable to be applied to skin specimens[19–21] and have been used for early definitive diagnosis of leprosy. Among a range of gene targets, used with this technology, the *M. leprae* specific repetitive element RLEP is regarded as highly sensitive and specific for diagnostic applications. The light amplicons are read/noted, utilizing identification frameworks of fluorometry. LAMP tests were developed by using RLEP or 16S rRNA gene region for detecting *M. leprae*.[19–21]

SUMMARY OF MOLECULAR METHODS

PCR using RLEP region of *M. leprae* is a very sensitive and specific molecular method for amplification and identification of DNA and/or RNA from all types of clinical samples. The reported positivity rate was 73% using RLEP-based conventional PCR in patients with a bacillary index of zero, Further, PCR identification using RLEP of pure neuritic leprosy has also been reported to be sensitive up to 50–70%.[9,12,22,23]

Multiplex PCR as an alternative method of using PCR technology employing more than one gene specific to *M. leprae*. This method has also been used for detection of *M. leprae* in all types of clinical cases as well as in HHCs.[4,24] It has reported that by employing multiplex PCR in PB cases, the percent positivity significantly increased up to 93.3%.[14]

Molecular viability determination by real-time PCR of 16S RNA is a well-known method used for the identification of viable *M. leprae* from various clinical samples.[4,6,9] LAMP assays are useful POC tools for rapid diagnosis of leprosy at all levels including field settings.

SCOPE FOR FURTHER RESEARCH

Observing and examination of the family contacts of leprosy patients helps in early disease detection and diagnosis. Contacts could be screened even at CHC/PHC level using RLEP PCR which is easy to perform and can be undertaken in these centres specially after the facilities were upgraded due to COVID-19 infection. LAMP test using RLEP is equally sensitive POC technology and can be implemented. These can also easily be done in all medical colleges and tertiary care hospitals with their infrastructure, laboratories, personnel and equipment. Furthermore, AMR activities can be taken up by NLEP and State Health Systems to survey, detect and treat MDR cases early, at these peripheral centers as well as tertiary care centers.

Overall, field investigations have demonstrated that DNA as well as RNA based PCR assays can be 100% specific, and >70% sensitive. Also, since demonstrating *M. leprae* is crucial in SSS/tissue sample for the confirmatory diagnosis of early leprosy, the use of PCR technique to enhance the confirmation of diagnosis in difficult cases is strongly recommended. In difficult to diagnose cases, such as Indeterminate and neuritic leprosy, or patients with unusual clinical presentations, qPCR can be used to reach the correct diagnosis and administer appropriate treatment. This can be easily done in all state and private medical colleges and central institutions. This will help in early diagnosis, proper and close follow up of contacts, giving adequate treatment, help in prevent disabilities, helping to break the transmission chain, and early diagnosis of AMR.

FOR FURTHER READING

Detailed information about methodology of various types of sample collection for PCR probes, extraction of DNA from clinical samples, various primers for mRNA PCR tests and qRT-PCR methodology can be downloaded from this open access article by the authors of this chapter (10.1016/j.ijmyco.2014.11.062).

REFERENCES

1. Sharma RK, Katoch K, Shivannavar CT, Sharma VD, Natrajan M, Bhatia AS, Saxena N, Katoch VM. Detection of *M. leprae* by gene amplification; combined ethidium-bromide staining and probe hybridization. Int J Lepr Other Mycobact Dis. 1996;64:409–16.
2. Kampirapap K, Singtham N, Klatser PR, Wiriyawipart S. DNA amplification for detection of leprosy and assessment of efficacy of leprosy chemotherapy. Int J Lepr Other Mycobact Dis 1998;66:16–21.
3. Scollard DM, Gillis TP, Williams DL. Polymerase chain reaction assay for the detection and identification of *Mycobacterium leprae* in patients in the United States. Am J Clin Pathol 1998;109:642–6.
4. Turankar RP, Pandey S, Lavania M, Singh I, Nigam A, Darlong J, Darlong F, Sengupta U. Comparative evaluation of PCR amplification of RLEP, 16S rRNA, rpoT and Sod A gene targets for detection of *M. leprae* DNA from clinical and environmental samples. Int J Mycobacteriol. 2015;4:54–9.
5. Katoch VM, Kanaujia GV, Shivannavar CT, Katoch K, Sharma VD, Patil MA. Progress in developing ribosomal RNA and rRNA gene (s) based probes for diagnosis and epidemiology of infectious diseases especially leprosy. Sushil Kumar, Sen AK, Dutta GP Sharma RN (Eds.), Tropical Diseases-Molecular Biology and Control Strategies. 1994:581–7A.
6. Katoch VM. Molecular techniques for leprosy: present applications and future perspectives. Indian J Lepr. 1999;71:45–59.
7. Lavania M, Katoch K, Katoch VM, Gupta AK, Chauhan DS, Sharma R, Gandhi R, Chauhan V, Bansal G, Sachan P, Sachan S, Yadav VS, Jadhav R. Detection of viable *Mycobacterium leprae* in soil samples: insights into possible sources of transmission of leprosy. Infect Genet Evol. 2008;8:627–31.

8. Singh HB, Katoch VM, Natrajan M, Sharma VD, Chauhan DS, Lavania M, Sharma P, Sharma M, Katoch K, Benara S, Singh P. Improved protocol for PCR detection of *Mycobacterium leprae* in buffered formalin-fixed skin biopsies. Int J Lepr Other Mycobact Dis. 2004;72:175–8.
9. Martinez AN, Talhari C, Moraes MO, Talhari S. PCR-based techniques for leprosy diagnosis: from the laboratory to the clinic. PLoS Negl Trop Dis. 2014; 8:e2655.
10. Caleffi KR, Hirata RDC, Hirata MH, Calleffi ER, Siqueira VLDand Cardoso RD. Use of polymerase chain reactionto detect *Mycobacterium leprae* in urine. Braz, J Med Biol Res. 2012;45:153–7. PMCID: PMC3854251/PMID: 22286535.
11. Naaz F, Katoch K, Mohanty PS, Chauhan DS, Yadav VS, Kumar Amit, Shakya, Katara D, Babbanjee, Wasim M, Singh S. Use of RLEP-PCR as a Molecular Tool and Definitive Laboratory Test from Skin Smear Scrapings for Early Diagnosis of Leprosy in Field Situations. Indian J Lepr 2016, 88: 199–207.
12. Yoon KH, Cho SN, Lee MK, Abalos RM, Cellona RV, Fajardo TT Jr, Guido LS, Dela Cruz EC, Walsh GP, Kim JD. Evaluation of polymerase chain reaction amplification of *Mycobacterium leprae*-specific repetitive sequence in biopsy specimens from leprosy patients. J Clin Microbiol. 1993;31:895–9.
13. Williams DL, Gillis TP, Fiallo P, Job CK, Gelber RH, Hill C, Izumi S. Detection of *Mycobacterium leprae* and the potential for monitoring antileprosy drug therapy directly from skin biopsies by PCR. Mol Cell Probes. 1992;6:401–10.
14. Pathak VK, Singh I, Turankar RP, Lavania M, Ahuja M, Singh V, Sengupta U. Utility of multiplex PCR for early diagnosis and household contact surveillance for leprosy. Diagn Microbiol Infect Dis. 2019; 95:114855.
15. Banerjee S, Sarkar K, Gupta S, Mahapatra PS, Gupta S, Guha S, Bandhopadhayay D, Ghosal C, Paine SK, Dutta RN, Biswas N, Bhattacharya B. Multiplex PCR technique could be an alternative approach for early detection of leprosy among close contacts--a pilot study from India. BMC Infect Dis. 2010;252.
16. Kramme S, Bretzel G, Panning M, Kawuma J, Drosten C. Detection and quantification of *Mycobacterium leprae* in tissue samples by real-time PCR. Med Microbiol Immunol. 2004;193:189–93.
17. Santos AR, De Miranda AB, Sarno EN, Suffys PN, Degrave WM. Use of PCR-mediated amplification of *Mycobacterium leprae* DNA in different types of clinical samples for the diagnosis of leprosy. J Med Microbiol. 1993;39:298–304.
18. Rudeeaneksin J, Srisungngam S, Sawanpanyalert P, Sittiwakin T, Likanonsakul S, Pasadorn S, Palittapongarnpim P, Brennan PJ, Phetsuksiri B. Light Cycler real-time PCR for rapid detection and quantitation of *Mycobacterium leprae* in skin specimens. FEMS Immunol Med Microbiol. 2008;54:263–70.
19. Jiang H, Tsang L, Wang H, Liu C. Loop-mediated isothermal amplifcation (LAMP) assay targeting RLEP for detection of *Mycobacterium leprae* in leprosy patients. Int J Infect Dis. 2021;107:145–52.
20. Garg N, Sahu U, Kar S, Ahmad FJ. Development of a Loop-mediated isothermal amplifcation (LAMP) technique for specifc and early detection of *Mycobacterium leprae* in clinical samples. Sci Rep. 2021.
21. Joshi S, Sharma V, Ramesh V, Singh R, Salotra P. Development of a novel loop-mediated isothermal amplifcation assay for rapid detection of *Mycobacterium leprae* in clinical samples. Indian J Dermatol Venereol Leprol. 2021; 87:491–7.
22. Bezerra Da Cunha FM, Werneck MC, Scola RH, Werneck LC. Pure neural leprosy: diagnostic value of the polymerase chain reaction. Muscle Nerve. 2006;33:409–14.
23. Rodriguez G, Pinto R, Gomez Y, Rengifo ML, Estrada OL, Sarmiento M, Lopez F, Beltran-Alzate JC, Cardona-Castro N. Pure neuritic leprosy in patients from a high endemic region of Colombia. Lepr Rev. 2013;84:41–50.
24. Sandhika W, Adriaty D, Agusni I. Detection of *Mycobacterium leprae* in formalin-fixed paraffin-embedded sample by fite-faraco staining and polymerase chain reaction. Procedia Chemistry. 2016;18:231–6.

Section 3

Drug Therapy and Management of Leprosy

Multidrug Therapy for Leprosy

Chapter 13

Recommendation of World Health Organization (WHO) and National Leprosy Eradication Programme (NLEP), Govt of India

• Usha Khemani • Mohammad Adil

INTRODUCTION

Introduction of multidrug therapy (MDT) has been a huge success, with leprosy prevalence dropping from 5 million cases in 1980s to 177, 175 cases in 2019.[1] In the last 4 decades of MDT, 18 million people have been treated and registered prevalence has dropped by 95%.

This chapter deals with the recommendations and practical issues relating to the use of MDT recommended by WHO and NLEP. It shall outline when to start MDT, required investigative work-up before initiating MDT and follow-up of a leprosy affected person on MDT.

DEFINITION

Multidrug therapy (MDT): Multidrug therapy or combination therapy is the use of more than one drug for the treatment of a disease to avoid the selection and propagation of resistant mutants from the use of a single drug (monotherapy).[2] MDT has been in use effectively for other mycobacterial infections like tuberculosis. The evolution of MDT over the years has been summarized in Table 13.1.

Fixed duration therapy (FDT): The use of MDT leprosy is for a fixed time duration and not for the duration till bacteriological clearance is achieved or clinical lesions have resolved. The WHO Expert Committee in 1994 recommended for the first time a 'fixed duration therapy' for multibacillary leprosy with rifampicin, dapsone and clofazimine, for a period of 24 months only, irrespective of skin smear status. It was later reduced to 12 months in 1998.

RATIONALE OF MDT

Important reasons for WHO promoting MDT for leprosy are:

- **To minimize drug resistance:** It was observed that dapsone monotherapy leads to development of drug resistance. During the times of dapsone monotherapy, there were reports of up to 50% primary resistance and 19% secondary resistance to dapsone. When rifampicin was found to be highly bactericidal, its indiscriminate monotherapy led to fears that rifampicin-resistant strains would emerge and spread, rendering the best armament for leprosy to be ineffective. The chance of finding drug resistant mutants is 1 in 7 logs for rifampicin and 1 in 6 logs for dapsone and clofazimine. The risk of mutants with resistance to any two drugs decreases to 1 in 13 logs.[3]
- **To improve compliance:** The longer duration of treatment with monotherapies over many years, was associated with lower chances of compliance which led to defaults. Shorter treatment is cost efficient and less resource-consuming.

Table 13.1: Major milestones in the chemotherapy of leprosy

Year	*Milestone*
Till 1940s	Chaulmoogra oil for the treatment of leprosy in Indian subcontinent
1946	Cochrane used dapsone for the first time in India
1962	Clofazimine used for treatment by Browne and Hogerzeil in Nigeria
1963	Rifamycin reported effective in leprosy
1970	Rifampicin was reported to the most potent chemotherapeutic bactericidal agent against *Mycobacterium leprae*
1977	Primary dapsone resistance reported
1981	WHO study group on chemotherapy of leprosy recommended MDT for 24 months or smear negativity for MB leprosy and 6 months for PB disease
1983	National Leprosy Eradication Programme (NLEP) launched and adopts MDT
1994	WHO changes recommendation for MDT in MB disease for 24 months irrespective of smear positivity
1998	WHO shortens MDT for MB disease to 12 months and introduces ROM therapy for single skin-lesion leprosy.
2018	WHO recommends 3 drug therapy for all PB and MB patients

PB: Paucibacillary; MB: Multibacillary; WHO: World Health Organization, MDT: Multidrug therapy

- **Persisters:** Persisters are viable, drug-sensitive bacilli recovered in lepromatous leprosy patients despite treatment. One of the premise of introduction of MDT was that these combinations of anti-leprosy drugs may be able to eliminate such persisting organisms and thus significantly reduce the required duration of treatment.[4]

  Knowledge gap: There is uncertainty over the duration of treatment for leprosy patients with some experts arguing that patients with high bacillary load may need treatment longer than the standard 12 months. Similar may be the case where the patient has resistance to one or more drugs in the standard drug regimen. At the same time, there is paucity of robust controlled trials evaluating drug combinations incorporating the newer anti-leprosy drugs which are highly bactericidal and which could be the key for eradication of leprosy.

Treatment Modalities

Conventional MDT drugs:[4] The three principal drugs currently used for MDT recommended by WHO and NLEP are: dapsone, rifampicin and clofazimine. Dapsone is weakly bactericidal for *M. leprae* at a dose of 100 mg per day. Rifampicin is a very strong bactericidal drug, and the patient becomes non-infectious within a few days of treatment. As the drug is strongly bactericidal and the bacteria multiplies slowly, rifampicin may be administered monthly. Clofazimine is weakly bactericidal like dapsone but offers an excellent safety profile (Figs 13.1 and 13.2).

Dapsone: It is inexpensive and relatively nontoxic drug in the doses used for leprosy as a part of MDT. In that dosage dapsone is weakly bactericidal against *M. leprae*. Nonetheless, 100 mg/day results in peak serum levels that exceed the minimum inhibitory concentration (MIC) of dapsone against *M. leprae* by a factor of about 500. Such high levels over MIC will also inhibit the multiplication of mutants of *M. leprae* with low and moderate degrees of

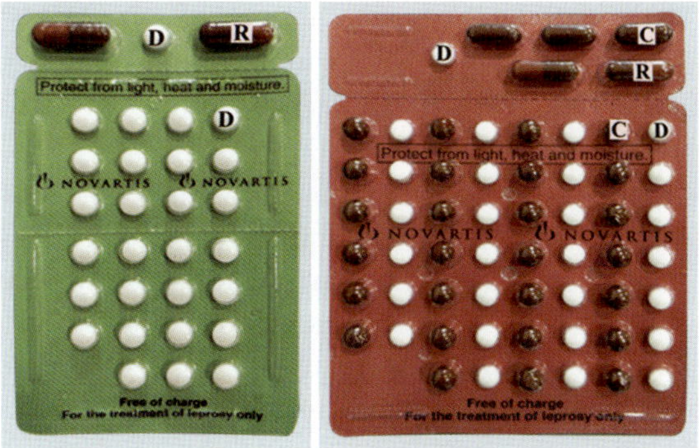

Fig. 13.1: WHO-MDT blister packs for adults

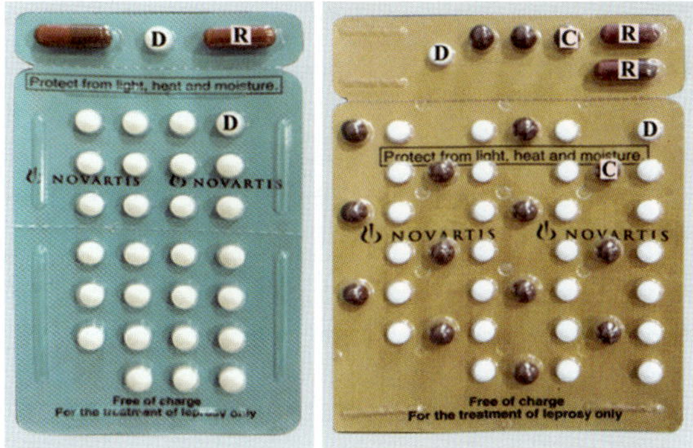

Fig. 13.2: WHO-MDT blister packs for children 10–14 years of age

dapsone resistance. The same dosage of dapsone should be used for leprosy, including during phases of reactions. Mild hemolytic anemia is common following treatment with the drug, but severe hemolytic anemia is rare except in patients with G-6-PD deficiency. Occasional cases of dapsone hypersensitivity and very rarely agranulocytosis have been reported.

Rifampicin: It is by far the most effective bactericidal drug against *M. leprae*. Its activity is greater than that of any other single anti-leprosy drug and plays a key role in MDT of leprosy. Rifampicin given as a monthly dose of 600 mg is highly bactericidal against *M. leprae*. The toxicity of the drug is relatively low, although occasional cases of renal failure, thrombocytopenia, influenza like syndrome and hepatitis have been reported. Its effect on the metabolism of other drugs, such as corticosteroids and oral contraceptives, is not an issue as it is administered monthly. A number of rifampicin derivatives with longer half-lives with high bactericidal effect have been prepared, such as rifabutin; however, at present, they are not recommended as a part of MDT.

Clofazimine: This drug dosage employed in the MDT (50 mg/day) for MB leprosy is virtually nontoxic. Pigmentation of the skin, particularly within skin lesions, is common, but it clears completely after treatment is discontinued. The higher doses (200–300 mg daily) of clofazimine sometimes used for the control of leprosy reactions may occasionally produce severe gastrointestinal side-effects. In the standard MB MDT regimen, clofazimine is given in doses of 300 mg once monthly, plus 50 mg daily which is well tolerated.

Newer drugs: Fluoroquinolones such as ofloxacin and moxifloxacin are effective against leprosy. Moxifloxacin has bactericidal activity equivalent to rifampicin. However, these are not recommended for children due to the risk to growth by its effect on cartilage. Minocycline is a tetracycline antibiotic with a potent bactericidal effect against leprosy bacilli. Clarithromycin is a macrolide and is a weaker bactericidal agent than minocycline. Animal studies have shown bedaquiline to be as effective as rifampicin. Other drugs that can be used are rifapentine, rifabutin, dihydrofolate reductase inhibitors (brodimoprim), fusidic acid and beta lactams. Some of these drugs are recommended by WHO to be used in combination for rifampicin resistant leprosy. However, at present none of these drugs are recommended by WHO or NLEP as a part of first line MDT for PB or MB leprosy.

Current Guidelines

WHO recommendation of regimen containing 3 drugs for all types of leprosy-2018: A modified case definition for leprosy was proposed by WHO in 2018, and classified it into paucibacillary (PB) and multibacillary (MB) groups (Table 13.2). Further, the WHO Guidelines Development Group recommended the use of the same 3 drug regimen (dapsone, rifampicin and clofazimine) for a period of 6 months in PB leprosy and 12 months in MB leprosy[5] (Table 13.3).

It was seen that the 3-drug regimen (rifampicin, dapsone and clofazimine) for 6 months offered a 10–14% benefit in clinical outcome at 12 months and 26% benefit at 24 months.[5] The risk of relapse was lower with the 3-drug regimen. The same 3-drug treatment for all cases of leprosy prevents misclassification of certain MB cases as PB and consequent undertreatment. Further, such a regimen offers operational ease. It must be noted that at present this uniform drug regimen is not currently being practiced by NLEP, India in its programme.

Pretreatment work-up: The WHO Guidelines Development Group (GDG) in December 2018 published the guidelines for the diagnosis, prevention and treatment of leprosy. The group

Table 13.2: Classification of leprosy according to WHO and NLEP

Catagory	*Definition of WHO*	*Definition of NLEP*
Paucibacillary (PB) case	A case of leprosy with 1–5 skin lesions and with negative slit skin smear	A case of leprosy with 1–5 skin lesions and/or with no nerve involvement or a single nerve involvement and/or with negative slit skin smear.
Multibacillary (MB) case	A case of leprosy with >5 skin lesions; or with involvement of nerves or with any neuritis irrespective of number of skin lesions; or with positive slit skin smear irrespective of number of skin lesions	A case of leprosy with >5 skin lesions and/or or with involvement of more than one nerve and/or with positive slit skin smear from any site irrespective of the number of skin lesions or number of nerves involved.

Table 13.3: MDT for leprosy: WHO recommendations (2018)

Age	*Drug*	*Dose and frequency*	*Duration*	
			PB	*MB*
Adult (>14 years)	Rifampicin	600 mg once a month	6 months	12 months
	Clofazimine	300 mg once a month, 50 mg daily		
	Dapsone	100 mg daily		
Children (10–14 years)	Rifampicin	450 mg once a month	6 months	12 months
	Clofazimine	150 mg once a month, 50 mg on alternate days		
	Dapsone	50 mg daily		
Children (<10 years or <40 kg)	Rifampicin	10 mg/kg once a month	6 months	12 months
	Clofazimine	100 mg once a month, 50 mg twice weekly		
	Dapsone	2 mg/kg daily		

concluded that the current methods of clinical examination with/without slit skin smear or histopathological examination of skin biopsies must be used for diagnosis. It also mentions that newer diagnostic methods such as ELISA or lateral flow assays offer no added benefit while PCR based assays lack standardization, and are difficult to perform at primary health care facilities, and are not widely available.

Follow-up: The drugs given once a month are recommended to be supervised by the health care worker. Thus, the patient attends the clinic every 28 days. This is referred to as 'a month'.[6] This visit is also used to check for compliance and early identification of complications. The standard PB MDT must be taken within 9 months and MB MDT within 18 months. WHO currently does not recommend follow-up of leprosy patients beyond the period of treatment. Patients are encouraged to visit health facilities if new signs or symptoms appear.

WHO MDT for Children

MDT blister packs are available for adults and children 10–14 years of age, while blister packs for younger children <10 years are not available. Also, MDT drugs in syrup formulations are not available. Fortunately, leprosy in children below 10 years is rare. At the same time, children of all age groups may find it difficult to swallow capsules or tablets, which is the most important cause of high treatment dropout rates of 10–20% in children.[7] (This is covered in detail in Section 4, Chapter 27).

Recommended MDT by NLEP

The NLEP-MDT regimen, while broadly following WHO recommendations, often had differences. Initially, between 1983–1994 rifampicin was given daily for initial 14 days as intensive treatment and MB MDT continued till smear negativity. The 24-month FDT was introduced in NLEP in 1994. The current 12-month regimen is in effect from 1998 (Table 13.4).

Current NLEP classification of leprosy follows the WHO classification except that involvement of a single nerve is classified as paucibacillary disease (Table 13.2). Nerve involvement was included in the classification criteria because around 5% of all leprosy cases in the country are of 'pure neuritic leprosy' and more than 60% of such cases present with involvement of more than one nerve.[8]

Table 13.4: NLEP: Recommended MDT for leprosy

Category	*Rifampicin*	*Dapsone*	*Clofazimine*	*Duration*
Adult-PB	600 mg once a month (supervised)	100 mg daily (unsupervised)	-	06 months
Adult MB	600 mg once a month (supervised)	100 mg daily (unsupervised)	300 mg once a month (supervised) 50mg daily (unsupervised)	12 months
Paediatric-PB (Children 10–14 years of age)	450 mg once a month (supervised)	50 mg daily (unsupervised)	-	06 months
Paediatric MB (Children 10–14 years of age)	450 mg once a month (supervised)	50 mg daily (unsupervised)	150 mg once a month (supervised) 50 mg alternate day (unsupervised)	12 months

VARIATIONS

Accompanied MDT (A-MDT)

WHO recommends that a full course of MDT may be provided to the patients on their first visit. The responsibility of helping to complete the treatment is delegated to someone close to the patient, hence, the term 'accompanied'. A-MDT ensures better access of MDT to leprosy patients such as mobile populations, migrant urban labourers, and people living in areas of civil strife or hard to reach areas or who may be unable to access the health facility easily again.[5] Such A-MDT was recommended and provided to leprosy patients across many parts of India during COVID-19 pandemic and the resulted lockdowns.[9,10] However, A-MDT has been criticised as the administration of monthly supervised dose of MDT is not possible, compliance may be affected due to lack of contact between health care provider and the patient.

Other variations of MDT: Apart from the MDT combinations currently recommended by WHO and NLEP, single dose ROM (rifampicin, ofloxacin and minocycline) for single skin-lesion leprosy was recommended by WHO in 1998. However, it was discontinued after 2005 and not recommended any more.

WHO-MDT in cases of drug resistance: The WHO also gave recommendations for patients with drug resistance (Table 13.5). Patients on WHO-MDT, if found resistant to rifampicin alone or in association with dapsone, should restart second-line treatment, irrespective of the clinical outcome with MDT. These guidelines are based on expert opinions, resistance patterns and known activity of the antibiotics, however, evidence on the effectiveness of such drug combinations based on studies in the field is still lacking.

Because fluoroquinolones are also effective against tuberculosis, a patient receiving second line therapy must be investigated for tuberculosis, and an appropriate regimen effective against both the diseases started, to avoid emergence of drug resistant strains. Patients receiving second line agents must also be monitored by electrocardiogram for QT interval prolongation and cardiac arrhythmias.[5]

MDT in Special Clinical Scenarios

Pregnancy and lactation: The standard WHO-MDT regimen is considered safe for the mother and child and any potential harm is outweighed by its benefit. Since leprosy tends to exacerbate during pregnancy, WHO recommends that MDT be continued unchanged during

Table 13.5: Recommended regimens for drug-resistant leprosy

Drug Resistance	*Treatment*	
	First 6 months (daily)	*Next 18 months (daily)*
Rifampicin	Ofloxacin 400 mg + Minocycline 100 mg + Clofazimine 50 mg	Ofloxacin 400 mg OR Minocycline 100 mg + Clofazimine 50 mg
	Ofloxacin 400 mg + Clarithromycin 500 mg + Clofazimine 50 mg	Ofloxacin 400 mg + Clofazimine 50 mg
Rifampicin + Ofloxacin	Clarithromycin 500 mg + Minocycline 100 mg + Clofazimine 50 mg	Clarithromycin 500 mg OR minocycline 100 mg + Clofazimine 50 mg

Ofloxacin 400 mg can be replaced by moxifloxacin 400 mg or levofloxacin 500 mg pregnancy. Though drugs may be excreted in breastmilk, no major adverse effects have been reported in babies except for skin discoloration due to clofazimine, which subsides after a few weeks of stopping treatment. Hence, MDT must be continued in breastfeeding women and alternative methods of feeding of newborn discouraged due to the risk of malnutrition in endemic countries. A-MDT may be provided to women who may find it difficult to reach the clinic for MDT during later stages of pregnancy and postpartum period.[11]

Concomitant tuberculosis (TB): The patient should be given anti-tubercular therapy along with MDT in cases of active TB-leprosy coinfection. As rifampicin is used in higher doses in TB, it must be used in the dose needed for tuberculosis and monthly dose of rifampicin in MDT can be omitted.

HIV Coinfection: Leprosy patients with HIV respond similarly to MDT as non-HIV patients. Thus, MDT may be continued with antiretroviral therapy in such patients.

Dapsone intolerance: If dapsone is not tolerated by the patient due to severe adverse effects, then it must be stopped immediately. No modification of regimen is needed except for addition of clofazimine if it is not already given.

Intolerance or refusal to use clofazimine: If MB patient refuses clofazimine on grounds of skin discoloration, then WHO model prescribing information for drugs used in leprosy, 1998 suggests the use of ofloxacin 400 mg/day or minocycline 100 mg/day for 12 months in place of clofazimine.[12]

Persistence of skin lesions: Persistence of skin lesions, appearance of new lesions or reappearance of lesions may be seen after release from treatment. This has been attributed to residual skin changes, lepra reactions or persistent antigenic stimulation due to bacterial antigens. Present guidelines recommend that no active intervention is needed, unless there are signs of new activity. Nonetheless, such lesions weaken the faith of the patient in the treatment and decrease the quality of life.[13] Cosmetic camouflage of visible skin lesions could help to overcome stigma and improve life quality index in these patients.[14] This issue has been dealth with in detail in Section 4, Chapter 21.

Patients with high bacillary load: At present both WHO and NLEP do not recommend any different regimen to MB patients with higher bacterial load, including those presenting as histoid leprosy. The same standard MDT MB of 12 months duration is recommended for all smear positive cases. This specific scenario is discussed in detail in Section 4, Chapter 17.

Adverse drug reactions to MDT: Although adverse drug reactions are not a major concern with MDT, early detection of such events is essential for patient safety and program implementation. The most common adverse effect is clofazimine induced pigmentation. Dapsone hypersensitivity syndrome (DHS) is a serious adverse effect seen in approximately 1–2% patients. The presence of HLA B*13:01 confers a significant risk for DHS.[15] At present, a test to identify this locus is not recommended by WHO or NLEP for leprosy patients in the program. If a patient develops a severe reaction to dapsone, the drug must be stopped and no further change in treatment is needed for MB patients. For PB patients, clofazimine may be added in place of dapsone.

Effect on nerve function impairment: Nerve function impairment is not affected and neuropathy is neither prevented nor halted by MDT.[16] It should be managed separately as required, while continuing MDT as necessary. Nerve thickening also takes many years to resolve in leprosy patients after completion of MDT.

SCOPE FOR FURTHER RESEARCH

The WHO MDT is still the most effective and safe treatment regimen for leprosy.[16] However, newer MDT regimens with bactericidal agents need to be evaluated for rapid and effective elimination of the bacteria. Mechanisms to identify and monitor drug resistance must be devised. The challenges faced by each country are unique and leprosy control programmes must be tailored to such needs. Integrated, country-owned leprosy roadmaps for each endemic country have been recognised as one of the strategic pillars of WHO Global Leprosy Strategy 2021–30.[17]

SUMMARY

- The National Leprosy Eradication Programme (NLEP), Govt of India, continues from 1998 to recommends 2 drug therapy (rifampicin 600 mg monthly and dapsone 100 mg daily) of 6 months for paucibacillary leprosy and 3 drug therapy (the above two drugs with clofazimine 300 mg monthly and 50 mg daily) of 12 months for multibacillary leprosy.
- World Health Organization (2018) recommends the same 3-drug therapy (consisting of rifampicin 600 mg monthly, dapsone 100 mg daily and clofazimine 300 mg monthly and 50 mg daily) for paucibacillary leprosy (for 6 months) and multibacillary leprosy (for 12 months).[18] These recommendations have not yet been taken up by many countries, including India.
- The WHO has provided guidelines for the management of patients of leprosy who are found to be resistant to rifampicin alone or in conjunction to dapsone. This regimen consists of 3-drug regimens for 6 months followed by 2-drug regimens for 18 months. These regimens use clofazimine with fluoroquinolones (ofloxacin/moxifloxacin), minocycline or clarithromycin.

REFERENCES

1. World Health Organization. Weekly epidemiological record no. 36. (Internet) 2020; 95: 417-40. (cited 2022 Mar 20) Available from: https://apps.who.int/iris/bitstream/handle/10665/334140/WER9536-eng-fre.pdf.
2. Naaz F, Mohanty PS, Bansal AK, Kumar D, Gupta UD. Challenges beyond elimination in leprosy. Int J Mycobacteriol 2017;6:222–8.
3. Chauhan D, Kamal R, Saxena A. Therapy of leprosy-present strategies and recent trends with immunotherapy. J Dermatol Res Ther 2020;6:093.
4. Chemotherapy of Leprosy for Control Programmes. A report of WHO study group. Technical report series 675. WHO 1982.
5. World Health Organization. Guidelines for the diagnosis, treatment and prevention of leprosy. New Delhi: WHO Regional Office for South-East Asia; 2017.
6. World Health Organization. Global Leprosy Programme. Global Leprosy Strategy 2016–2020: accelerating towards a leprosy-free world–Monitoring and evaluation guide. New Delhi: WHO Regional Office for South-East Asia; 2017.
7. Narang T, Kumar B. Leprosy in children. Indian J Paediatr Dermatol 2019;20:12–24.
8. Misra RS, Kataria JK. Classification. In: Kumar B, Kar HK, editors. IAL textbook of leprosy, 2nd ed. New Delhi: Jaypee publishers; 2017; p.254–62.
9. Bhardwaj A, Gupta SK, Narang T, Suneetha S, Pradhan S, Agarwal P, et al. Updates on management of leprosy in the context of COVID-19 pandemic: Recommendations by IADVL SIG Leprosy. Indian Dermatol Online J 2021;12:S24–30.
10. Rathod S, Suneetha S, Narang T, Bhardwaj A, Gupta SK, Kamoji SG, et al. Management of leprosy in the context of COVID-19 pandemic: Recommendations by SIG leprosy (IADVL academy). Indian Dermatol Online J 2020;11:345–8.

11. Butlin CR, Withington S. Chapter 3.2: Mothers and children with leprosy. In: Scollard DM, Gillis TP, editors. International textbook of leprosy (Internet). American Leprosy Missions; 2018. (cited 2022 Apr 04). p.1–34. Available from: https://m3u9w4p9.stackpathcdn.com/sites/default/files/ITL_3_2% 20FINAL.pdf.
12. World Health Organization. WHO Model Prescribing Information: Drugs used in leprosy. Geneva: WHO Library. 1998.
13. Narang T, Bishnoi A, Thakur V, Chatterjee D, Razmi TM, Kamat K, et al. Persistent plaques after release from treatment in slit-skin smear negative leprosy patients: Wait and watch or adopt a proactive approach. Dermatol Ther 2020;33:e14226.
14. Rao P, Vellala M, Potharaju AR, et al. Cosmetic camouflage of visible skin lesions enhances life quality indices in leprosy as in vitiligo patients: an effective stigma reduction strategy. Leprosy Review. 2020; 91 (4): 343–52.
15. Zhang FR, Liu H, Irwanto A, Fu XA, Li Y, Yu GQ, et al. HLA-B*13:01 and the dapsone hypersensitivity syndrome. N Engl J Med. 2013;369(17):1620–8. 10.1056/NEJMoa1213096.
16. Giesel LM, Pitta IJR, de Silveira RC, Andrade LR, Vital RT, da Costa Nery JA, et al. Clinical and neurophysiological features of leprosy patients with neuropathic pain. Am J Trop Med Hyg 2018;98:1609–13.
17. World Health Organization. Towards Zero Leprosy. Global Leprosy (Hansen's disease) Strategy 2021–2030. New Delhi: WHO Regional Office for South-East Asia; 2017.

Chapter 14

Practical Guidelines on Implementation of Chemoprophylaxis in Leprosy

• *Hemanta Kumar Kar* • *Reetu Agarwal*

INTRODUCTION

India though has achieved elimination of leprosy in 2005 with implementation of multidrug therapy, but we are far from eradicating this disease, as the annual new case detection rate (ANCR) shows very slow decline over last 17 years. This indicates that transmission of *M. leprae* is ongoing in the community, more so among contacts of newly diagnosed leprosy patients. Therefore, all contacts of newly diagnosed leprosy patients should be the main target in future control program strategy for the final eradication of this disease.

Awareness and steps on how to provide chemoprophylaxis to the contacts of newly diagnosed leprosy patient is the need of the hour. This chapter shall outline chemoprophylaxis in leprosy and steps of how to administer chemoprophylaxis to the eligible contacts.

DEFINITIONS

Chemoprophylaxis is 'administration of chemicals, including antibiotics, to prevent the development of an infection or the progression of an infection to active manifest disease'.[1] In case of a chronic infectious disease with long incubation period, like leprosy, such intervention among contacts may abort the progression of the disease in individuals who are already harbouring the organism asymptomatically.[1] Hence chemoprophylaxis in leprosy is aptly termed as post-exposure prophylaxis (PEP) as it is a preventative medical treatment and to be started immediately after exposure to pathogen *M. leprae,* but before development of the clinical disease among high risk people residing close to the index leprosy case.

At present single dose rifampicin (SDR) as a drug of PEP is recommended by WHO as it has shown efficacy in preventing leprosy in 60% of contacts in field trials in the landmark COLEP study conducted in Bangladesh.[3] As per the recommendation of expert group of ICMR in India, NLEP, Govt of India introduced this strategy in year 2016, especially in districts conducting LCDC (leprosy case detection campaigns), among contacts of all newly detected cases.[2]

CONTACTS OF INDEX CASE

Human beings are the largest known reservoir of leprosy, and the risk of transmission of leprosy is higher to people living in close vicinity of a known case of leprosy, referred to as 'contacts'.[4] However, development of clinical leprosy depends on several factors including specific cell-mediated immune (CMI) response of the individual against *M. leprae*, vaccination with BCG/MIP vaccines, specific genetic factors, closeness of contacts, endemicity of leprosy in the region and finally environmental and socioeconomic factors.[4]

Definition of Contacts[2]

An individual who has prolonged or interrupted contact with a newly detected leprosy case in the last one year is considered to be a 'contact'. There can be various types of contacts[2,5] of a leprosy index case. For the program point of view, at present the leprosy contacts are categorised into four types:

(i) Family contacts—comprise of all family members, except one/s who stays away for more than one year for study or work during last one year.
(ii) Household contacts—people who reside in the same house with the index case.
(iii) Neighborhood contacts—individuals residing in three houses on either side and three houses across the street from an index case house.
(iv) Social contacts—comprise of all people with whom the index case is in contact for more than 20 hours per week for a cumulative period of three months or more, e.g. peers at educational institutions, colleagues at work, religious associates, etc.

Eligibility Criteria for PEP[2]

Inclusion criteria:

(i) A person who has been living/working/having social activities for more than three months and 20 hours/week with a newly detected leprosy case in last one year.
(ii) Age more than two years.

Exclusion criteria:

(i) Pregnant women (PEP can be given after delivery)
(ii) People receiving rifampicin therapy for any other reason in last two years (for TB or leprosy treatment or as a contact of an index case)
(iii) People with history of liver disorder (jaundice, pain abdomen, pale conjunctiva, etc.)
(iv) People with possible signs and symptoms of leprosy and tuberculosis
(v) People with acute febrile illness.

Contact Tracing and Screening

Contact tracing by active and passive surveillance is tedious, requires motivation, financial aid, skilled man power and is an integral part of implementing chemoprophylaxis. Moreover, these methods are difficult to implement in remote geographical areas, especially hilly terrains, deserts and other non-approachable areas. There are various factors making the contact vulnerable to acquire leprosy infection like old age, non-compliance to BCG vaccination, genetically related individual, bacillary load of index case, etc. However, all these factors may not be equally applicable for all new cases developing from an 'index case' of leprosy.

Contact tracing is already known to leprosy programs over decades, much before the introduction of PEP with SDR. Case detection is mainly passive, with few periodic active outreach and routine household contact tracing. Suspect identification and their adherence is checked by volunteers like Accredited social health activist (ASHA), paramedical staff (village midwife) at field level. Contact screening is done by paramedical staff like auxiliary nurse midwife (ANM) at subcenter. The role of doctors is limited to the confirmation of unclear cases and management of complicated cases at higher levels.

Preparatory Activities for PEP

NLEP is now actively conducting PEP. Before starting in the target population sensitization and orientation meeting is being conducted for ASHA (accredited social health activist), MPW/PMW (paramedical worker), NMS (nonmedical supervisor), PHN (public health nurse) and medical officers(MO). IEC activities are being carried out one week before to create acceptability of chemoprophylaxis in community. Willingness to accept prophylactic dose with consent is essential for PEP. District leprosy officers (DLO) supervise the preparatory activities with support from medical officers posted in PHC of that area (Flowchart 14.1).

Dose of SDR[2]

All eligible contacts are given SDR. Depending on age/weight, the dose of **rifampicin** is as follows:

1. 600 mg for age 15 years and above
2. 450 mg for age 10–14 years
3. 300 mg for age 6 to 9 years and weight 20 kg or above
4. 10–15 mg/kg body weight for children under 20 kg/2 years and above

Oral administration of rifampicin should be supervised by health staff. In case child index case his/her contacts/classmates are to be examined in their houses (not in school) after collecting their home address from the school. PEP has to be given for children after taking informed consent from parent.

Flowchart 14.1: PEP with single dose rifampicin (SDR). Based on NLEP-LPEP operational guidelines (2019)

After confirmation of index case of leprosy PHC MO directs concerned MPW for action

↓

Household contacts and close contacts will be identified and screened for leprosy after taking informed consent.

↓

Any suspected case among contacts to be referred to MO for confirmation. All contacts except suspected one to be screened for exclusion criteria

↓

Contacts not meeting any exclusion criteria will be administered SDR after taking informed consent

↓

Suspected case if confirmed will be administered MDT and further of his/her contacts will be identified for PEP

↓

In case any contact is not available at home, exclusion criteria will be assessed by MPW in family members

SDR will be handed over to ASHA for administration with informed consent. All SDR administration is directly observed. If the index case is a child (2–14 years), home visit of classmates of the child living in same locality must be done to screen them for leprosy and checking eligibility for PEP. Informed consent has to be taken from parent of index child case as well as child contacts.

Safety/adverse Reaction and Management

Mild adverse reaction related to rifampicin like stomach upset, heartburn, nausea, headache, drowsiness or dizziness are managed by standard treatment protocol. Any severe adverse reaction must be intimated to MO and District Leprosy Officer (DLO) for referral and admission in nearest district hospital or tertiary care hospital.

Monitoring and Supervision

Medical Officer of PHC is responsible for ensuring screening of all contacts of every index case, strictly to follow guidelines of exclusion and inclusion criteria. Procurement of drug rifampicin is done by state/district as per requirement based on number of new index cases of that district.

Reporting

Health workers collect data from field/subcenters of the corresponding PHC. MO has to verify the completeness of the forms through random selection. District leprosy officers send data from all PHCs to state leprosy officer and finally to central leprosy division of Government of India.

Household and neighborhood contacts are at four times higher risk of acquiring the disease in comparison to general population.[4] If index case is multibacillary (MB) then household contacts are at 5–10 times higher risk of acquiring leprosy than neighbours.[6,7] The risk is 3–5 times higher for neighbors and social contacts; however, the risk decreases significantly to only 2–4 times higher than the outsiders if the index case is a paucibacillary (PB).[6,7]

There is no ideal screening laboratory test at present to detect individuals with subclinical infection. The currently available serodiagnostic tests have low specificity. Demonstration of antiphenolic glycolipid-1 (PGL-1) antibodies (IgM and IgG) among healthy contacts of leprosy patients has shown a consistent association with future development of the disease.[8] Evidence from a systematic review and meta-analysis of studies on the 'role of anti-PGL-1 antibodies in detecting future risk of developing the disease among healthy contacts of leprosy patients has demonstrated that seropositive individuals have three times greater risk of developing the disease than individuals who are seronegative.[8] However, in the available studies, the maximum sensitivity of this test was less than 40% , which carries a chance of missing more than half of the probable future cases if only this method is adopted to decide the targets for chemoprophylaxis. Moreover, because of probability of prolonged persistence of IgM anti-PGL-1 antibodies against these obligate intracellular bacteria, it may be difficult to differentiate between recent and old infections.[8] Hence, at present all the family and social contacts are provided blanket courage under the PEP program.

VARIATIONS OF PEP

Chemoprophylaxis by definition is protection conferred by use of antibiotics and as observed in the findings of the COLEP study it confers protection up to 57% for the first two years after given the dose and efficacy wanes off after 2 years.[3] The probable cause of medium effectiveness of SDR was short half-life of rifampicin (3 hours) hence, a single dose may not ensure cure of contacts with preclinical infection and that the protective effect of SDR wanes off after two years. This led to continuing search for a better chemoprophylactic regimen which would be efficacious as well as leave long lasting protective effect. For this reasons some researchers felt that rifapentine has a longer half-life in the body, so theoretically more suited than rifampicin.[9,10] Others supported the idea of using drug combinations in leprosy chemoprophylaxis. However, it should be mentioned here at present WHO and NLEP only recommend SDR-PEP for leprosy.

Possible Multidrug PEP Regimens

There was placebo controlled trials using ROM therapy (rifampicin 600 mg, ofloxacin 400 mg, minocycline100 mg in combination as a single dose) as chemoprophylaxis in leprosy.[11,12] The protective effect of ROM therapy observed in the studies was not superior to SDR as well as higher cost involved in implementation on wide scale, has put it out of favor as a chemoprophylactic regimen. Resistance has been documented with both rifampicin and ofloxacin[13] and minocycline cannot be administered in pregnant women and children were few other drawbacks. [13]

The experts from The Netherlands Leprosy Relief (NLR) (including the lead author, of this chapter) proposed a project labelled PEP ++,[14] with the goal of interrupting the transmission of leprosy. This project is a conglomeration of interrelated objectives; early detection of new cases by active measures and treatment, detection by an appropriate screening test and administration of PEP to preclinical cases, and also for high-risk contacts of a known case. With implementation of these measures, the transmission of *M. leprae* is expected to disrupt in a given community by next 5 years. The committee came to the conclusion and proposed rifampicin and moxifloxacin as tentative drugs for PEP++, given as 3 doses at 4 weekly intervals, in case moxifloxacin is contraindicated then clarithromycin can be used, especially in children.[14] The expected efficacy of the tentative PEP++ regimen would be 80–90%. The trial is on-going at present and results are awaited.

The protective effect of an optimal chemoprophylactic regimen can further be enhanced by combined immune-prophylaxis. The PEP++ project would be strengthened if combined chemoprophylaxis and immune-prophylaxis (with use of MiP vaccine) can be implemented in endemic areas for leprosy. Inclusion of screening of the subclinical household contacts who are the carriers of *M. leprae* would also be a firm step towards efficacy of PEP++. However, not a single diagnostic test is available presently with high sensitivity and specificity for detection of subclinical infection.

SUMMARY

- The fight against transmission of leprosy started in India with dapsone chemoprophylaxis from 1960s. Since then search for an ideal chemoprophylaxis regimen continues. Almost stagnant Annual new case detection rate (ANCDR) for leprosy is a cause of concern globally as well as in India. NLEP, India has included SDR-PEP as a prioritized strategy, as it is also a recommendation of WHO. At present, an enhanced chemoprophylaxis(PEP++) with a robust regimen consisting of two bactericidal drugs (rifampicin + clarithromycin) monthly once for three months among under global research trial in three countries (India, Brazil, and Indonesia). However, the repeat administration of chemoprophylactic agents may not be agreeable to many contacts, even if it is at the monthly intervals. Hence, some authors suggest preferable to continue the search for a single-dose chemoprophylactic regimen with high efficacy.[13]
- In summary, to achieve the goal of zero leprosy, prevention of transmission through implementation of PEP is an important initiative. There is a need to take it forward with the involvement of all stake-holders, including the leprosy affected and their family members.

REFERENCES

1. Smith CM, Smith WCS. MILEP2 Study Group. Chemoprophylaxis is effective in the prevention of leprosy in endemic countries: a systematic review and meta-analysis. Mucosal immunology of leprosy. J Infect Dis. 2000;41:137–42.
2. National Leprosy Eradication Programme, Post Exposure Chemoprophylaxis, Operational guidelines 2019, Central Leprosy Division, Directorate of Health and Family Welfare, Government of India.
3. Moet FJ, Oskam L, Faber R, et al. A study on transmission and a trial of chemoprophylaxis in contacts of leprosy patients: design, methodology and recruitment findings of COLEP. Lepr Rev. 2004;75:376–88.
4. Transmission of leprosy. Available at: http://www.who.int/lep/transmission/en/index4.html#.V8A_aA9Emps
5. Palit A, Kar HK. Prevention of transmission of leprosy: The current scenario. Indian J Dermatol Venereol Leprol. 2020;86:115-23.
6. Chaptini C, Marshman G. Leprosy: a review on elimination, reducing the disease burden, and future research. Lepr Rev. 2015;86:307–15.
7. Deps PD, Guedes BVS, Filho JB et al. Characteristics of known leprosy contact in a high endemic area in Brazil. Lepr Rev. 2006;77:34–40.
8. Penna MLF, Penna GO, Rodrigues LC. Anti-PGL-1 positivity as a risk marker for the development of leprosy among contacts of leprosy patients: Systematic review and meta-analysis. PLoS Negl Trop Dis. 2016;10:e0004703.
9. Saunderson PR. Chemotherapy of leprosy. In: Kumar B, Kar HK, editors. IAL textbook of leprosy. 2nd edn. New Delhi: Jaypee Publishers; 2016.p.-441–7.
10. Barth-Jaeggi T, Steinmann P, Mieras L et al. Leprosy Post-Exposure Prophylaxis (LPEP) programme: study protocol for evaluating the feasibility and impact on case detection rates of contact tracing and single dose rifampicin. BMJ Open. 2016;6:e013633.
11. Ji B, Sow S, Perani E *et al*. Bactericidal activity of single-dose combination of ofloxacin plus minocycline, with or without rifampicin, against *M. leprae* in mice and in lepromatous patients. Antimicrobial Agents Chemother. 1998;42:1115–20.
12. Diletto C, Blank L. Leprosy chemoprophylaxis in Micronesia. Lepr Rev. 2000; 71: S21–5.
13. Oskam L, Bakker MI. Report of the workshop on the use of chemoprophylaxis in the control of leprosy held in Amsterdam, the Netherlands on 14 December, 2006. Lepr Rev. 2007;78:173–85.
14. Mieras LF, Taal AT, van Brakel WH, et al. An enhanced regimen as post-exposure chemoprophylaxis for leprosy: PEP++. BMC Infect Dis 2018;18:506.

Chapter 15

MDT Regimens of Leprosy: Modifications, Extension and Additional Dosing

• Ashwini PK • Sejal Thakkar • Priti P Shah • P Narasimha Rao

INTRODUCTION

Leprosy scenario has significantly changed after a historical step of introduction of multi-drug therapy (MDT) by WHO in 1982.[1] Implementation of MDT has reduced the prevalence rate thereby achieving reduction of leprosy in most countries including India.[2] In spite of achieving elimination target in 2005, India still contributes more than half of the total new cases (where 60% being multibacillary type) every year and has few high endemic pockets, which shows that leprosy transmission has continued in spite of intense and dedicated efforts.[3] Amongst 2,990 relapsed cases reported in 2020 after completion of MDT, 498 cases were from India.[2] Occurrence of new leprosy cases, especially with high bacillary load, as well as relapsed cases and emergence of antimicrobial resistance (AMR) points the need to re-evaluate the efficacy of MDT and its duration, especially when we are looking forward to achieve the goal of 'zero leprosy' by 2030.

MDT REGIMENS RECOMMENDED BY WHO/NLEP

After MDT was introduced in 1982, it was revised periodically by WHO.[1] Journey of leprosy management moved through various milestones over years, like changes in criteria for paucibacillary (PB) and multibacillary (MB) (from smear status to number of lesions), changes in duration of regimens for MB leprosy; from treatment till smear negativity to fixed duration multidrug therapy (FDT) (Table 15.1).

As mentioned in Table 15.1, WHO/NLEP introduced 24 months fixed duration FDT for multi bacillary (MB) patients in 1994. In 1998, FDT was further reduced to 12 months on WHO recommendation.[4] WHO came out with new 'Guidelines for the diagnosis, and prevention of leprosy' in 2018, proposing a common drug regimen for both 6-month (PB) and 12-month (MB) FDT (Table 15.2). Discussed in detail in Chapter 13.

Advantages and limitations of FDT: The introduction of MDT has a substantial role in reducing number of leprosy cases globally. MDT in general proved to be effective in reducing bacterial load in newly diagnosed MB patients and the 12-months FDT was found to be effective in reducing relapse rates.[5,6] Even though MDT has considerably changed the global leprosy scenario, some of the patients continue to show positive BI at the end of 12 or 24-month FDT and may show either clinical or bacteriological activity or both.[3] This is because MB patients, especially polar lepromatous and histoid leprosy, have an overtly impaired immune system which results in slower bacterial clearance. In spite of such varied disease activity, all leprosy patients are 'released from treatment' once they complete FDT,

<table>
<tr><th colspan="3">Table 15.1: Periodical updates for leprosy management since introduction of MDT</th></tr>
<tr><th>Period</th><th>WHO Classification</th><th>WHO MDT regimens</th></tr>
<tr><td>1982</td><td>PB: BI<2+
MB: BI≥2+</td><td rowspan="2">PB: Rifampicin 600 mg once a month (supervised) + dapsone 100 mg daily (unsupervised) for 6 months
MB: Rifampicin 600 mg once a month, clofazimine 300 mg once a month (supervised) + clofazimine 50 mg daily + dapsone 100 mg daily (unsupervised) for at least two years or till smear negativity, whichever is later</td></tr>
<tr><td>1988</td><td>PB: BI=0
MB: BI≥1+</td></tr>
<tr><td>1994</td><td>PB: BI=0
MB: BI≥1+</td><td>PB: Same (RMP + Dapsone)-6 packs
MB: Same (RMP + Dapsone + Clofazimine) for a fixed duration of 24 months</td></tr>
<tr><td>1998</td><td>SLPB: 1 skin lesion
PB: 2–5 skin lesions
MB: >5 skin lesions</td><td>SLPB: Single supervised dose of rifampicin 600 mg + ofloxacin 400 mg + minocycline 100 mg
PB: Same (RMP + Dapsone)-6 packs
MB: Same (RMP + Dapsone + Clofazimine) for a fixed duration of 12 months</td></tr>
<tr><td>2000 proposal</td><td rowspan="3">PB: 1–5 skin lesions
MB:>5 skin lesions</td><td>A-MDT: Assisted MDT-complete supply of MDT drugs given to the patient at the time of diagnoses</td></tr>
<tr><td>2002 proposal</td><td>U-MDT: Uniform MDT of 6 months of MB MDT for both PB and MB cases</td></tr>
<tr><td>2018</td><td>Same regimen for PB and MB patients: Rifampicin 600 mg once a month, clofazimine 300 mg once a month (supervised) + clofazimine 50 mg daily + dapsone 100 mg daily (unsupervised)
PB: for 6 months
MB: for 12 months</td></tr>
</table>

WHO: World Health Organization, MDT: Multidrug therapy, MB: Multibacillary, PB: Paucibacillary, BI: Bacillary index, A-MDT: Accompanied MDT, U-MDT: Uniform MDT, RMP: Rifampicin, ROM: Rifampicin, ofloxacin, minocycline, SLPB: Single lesion paucibacillary leprosy

<table>
<tr><th colspan="4">Table 15.2: WHO recommended anti-leprosy treatment regimen–2018</th></tr>
<tr><th>Age</th><th>Drugs</th><th>Dosage and frequency</th><th>Duration MB/PB</th></tr>
<tr><td rowspan="3">Adult</td><td>Rifampicin</td><td>600 mg once a month</td><td>12 months/6 months</td></tr>
<tr><td>Clofazimine</td><td>300 mg once a month and 50 mg daily</td><td></td></tr>
<tr><td>Dapsone</td><td>100 mg daily</td><td></td></tr>
<tr><td rowspan="3">Children (10–14 years)</td><td>Rifampicin</td><td>450 mg once a month</td><td>12 months/6 months</td></tr>
<tr><td>Clofazimine</td><td>150 mg once a month and 50 mg alternate days</td><td></td></tr>
<tr><td>Dapsone</td><td>50 mg daily</td><td>12 months/6 months</td></tr>
<tr><td rowspan="3">Children (< 10 years or <40 kg wt)</td><td>Rifampicin</td><td>10 mg/kg once a month</td><td></td></tr>
<tr><td>Clofazimine</td><td>100 mg once a month, 50 mg twice a week</td><td></td></tr>
<tr><td>Dapsone</td><td>50 mg daily</td><td></td></tr>
</table>

WHO: World Health Organization, MB: Multibacillary, PB: Paucibacillary as completion of duration as per the present criteria is the end point of therapy, without any consideration for clinical signs and symptoms or skin smear status.

Situations Where Additional MDT is Recommended by WHO

Leprosy patients are believed to be cured and released from treatment at the end of completion of FDT at the field level, where clinical or bacteriological activity are not taken into account. Situation would be different, especially in MB leprosy, if they were to be taken in consideration for treatment end point, as done for other diseases, e.g. tuberculosis. A study has observed that many MB patients may still be clinically active and continue to be smear positive even after completion of FDT, even after 12 months of follow up.[7] Such patients can harbour viable bacilli, which when multiply can precipitate relapse of leprosy. Moreover, these patients could continue to act as agents for transmitting infection in community.[8] In addition, many MB patients may have active granuloma on histopathology even after completion of FDT, indicating delayed resolution.[7,9]

For these reasons, WHO in its publication mentions 'if a programme can identify patients with high bacterial index and those at the risk of developing reactions/neuritis by clinical and/or bacteriological examination, than such selected patients may be kept on surveillance for 1–2 years to diagnose deterioration and reactions as early as possible' In addition it also mentions that 'patients not showing improvement,with evidence of deterioration, will need an additional 12 months of MDT for multibacillary leprosy.[10]

Extended MDT in such needy leprosy patients will help in reducing the rate of relapse as well as development of additional disability. The benefit, may weigh higher than the cost of extended MDT.[11] Few studies from Brazil have found the significant response with extended MDT in patients who did not respond to standard FDT for MB Patients.[12,13]

Guidelines on MDT from Some Developed Countries

Looking at the diverse severity and clinical presentations associated with leprosy, there is a need to look beyond the WHO recommended duration of FDT, at least in some special situations. Moreover, it is important to note that the practice of extending MDT beyond the WHO recommended duration or modifications by certain country health associations/agencies in its implementation is not new or unknown. Here are some of the recommendations and modifications in MDT regimen for leprosy in practice at present, in few developed countries.

Japan: The Japanese guidelines for leprosy recommend a longer treatment based on the baseline BI. The recommendation for MB patients with BI >3 at baseline is 2 years of treatment with MB-MDT regimen. In case BI is still positive after 2 years, one year of MB-MDT is added (3 years in total), followed by maintenance therapy with dapsone and clofazimine until BI negativity and resolution of active lesions. In case of patients with BI <3, WHO MB-MDT is recommended but however, if BI continues to be positive or active lesions persist after completion of 1 year, additional therapy with MB-MDT for one more year is recommended.[14]

USA: The US National Hansen's disease programme (NHDP) recommendations are for daily rifampicin, and for longer duration of treatment than the WHO's recommendations. NHDP justifies it by stating that 'treatment that is more intensive and of longer duration is medically preferable' and adds that 'WHO's recommendations are due to cost considerations for developing countries'.[15] As a result, in the United States, the recommended regimen by the NHDP involves a longer duration of treatment because of fewer cost restrictions.[16] NHDP recommends for PB patients dapsone and rifampicin (2 drugs) for 12 months; and for MB patients dapsone, rifampicin and clofazimine (3 drugs) for 24 months. However, importantly in both these regimens rifampicin is given daily. The relapse rate for this regimen is extremely low.[17]

UK: In the UK the type of regimen that a patient receives is determined by combining their Ridley-Jopling classification, skin smear result and biopsy findings. Paucibacillary treatment is given for 6 months to TT and BT patients with negative slit skin smears. Multibacillary treatment is given to smear positive BT, BL and LL patients for 12 months. Patients with an initial bacterial index above 4 need 24 months of treatment.[18]

By the above practices followed in developed countries we can note that a) modification and extension of regimen for leprosy is not uncommon in many countries for better outcomes b) Cost considerations of treatment plays an important part deciding the drug regimen and its duration (FDT), as MDT strips are being supplied by WHO free of charge to all developing countries. With leprosy numbers decreasing globally including India, combined with improved economic conditions, it is time to consider modifications in MDT regimen and duration, especially for subsets of patients with severe forms of disease. Below are some of the conditions where a trained and qualified leprosy specialist or leprologist could consider extension of MDT.

Situations where scrutiny on adequacy of FDT regimen is needed are (Flowchart 15.1)

a. **Patients with persistent disease activity:** Persistent disease activity or nonresponders can be identified by persistent active skin lesions and/or persistent high/increasing bacillary

Flowchart 15.1: Algorithmic approach for a patient of leprosy treated with FDT-MDT

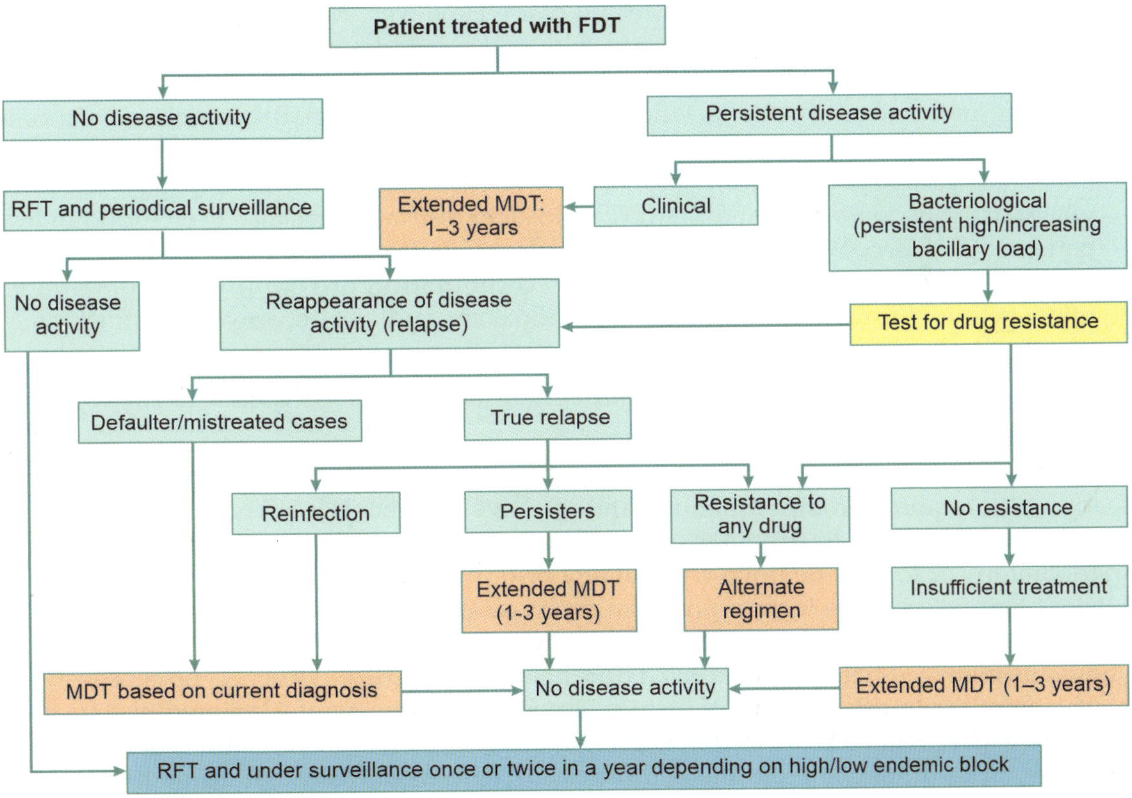

(FDT: Fixed duration therapy, MDT: Multidrug therapy)

load even after completion of FDT.[19] As already mentioned in such patients who have persistent clinical/bacteriological activity after 12 months of MDT, should be provided additional MDT for 12 months.

b. **Relapse** (refer to Chapter 19: Diagnosis and Management of a Case of Relapse)
Any activity (clinical, bacteriological or histopathological) in a patient who has completed MDT, will prompt a clinician to rule out relapse. World Health Organization (WHO) has defined relapse as 'the re-currence of the disease at any time after the completion of a full course of treatment with WHO recommended MDT'. It is diagnosed by the appearance of definite new skin lesions and/or an increase in BI by two or more units at any single site compared to BI taken from the same site at a previous examination.[20]

Patients diagnosed as a relapse case can be treated either with MDT or other newer agents, with or without MDT, depending on the clinical status of the patient as well as underlying cause for the relapse. As per present WHO guidelines, all the relapsed patients must be screened for the drug resistance. Sample of slit skin smear and skin biopsy can be sent for exploring mutations for particular drugs.[21] Patient with relapse must be started with MDT without waiting for the reports. The present WHO guidelines recommend that relapsed cases *with no AMR* should be retreated with standard WHO PB-MDT or MB-MDT, depending on the type of the disease (PB/MB). The recommended drug therapy for relapsed patients with confirmed AMR should be by 'alternative regimen' recommended by WHO, based on the drug resistance patterns (Refer to Chapter 16).

c. **Patients with antimicrobial resistance (AMR)**
Inadequate or irregular treatment can be a culprit in producing resistant strains, which leads to treatment failure, in MDT treated cases. However, WHO in 2017 has suggested, although may not be feasible at present, to test all newly diagnosed MB patients who are smear positive with BI ≥2+ for AMR.[21] India is one of the countries which contributes to a significant number of patients who relapsed due to resistance. Rifampicin resistance is found to be prevalent in significant number of relapsed (secondary resistance) as well as new cases (primary resistance). It may be found in combination with dapsone resistance where patients do not respond to MDT. Ofloxacin resistance has also been found in few patients.[22] For all confirmed cases of rifampicin resistance WHO recommends alternative therapy regimen which includes various combination of rifampicin, clofazimine, minocycline, ofloxacin/moxifloxacin/levofloxacin and clarithromycin, lasting for 24 months.[23]

In addition, the subset of MB leprosy patients in whom there is a need to check for the adequacy of WHO MDT (FDT) are:

Histoid leprosy: Histoid leprosy, an uncommon variant of leprosy having very high bacillary load, which requires prompt diagnosis and effective treatment. It is known that it usually occurs in patients due to irregular or inadequate therapy, dapsone resistance or dapsone monotherapy or to arise de novo without any prior history of any anti leprosy treatment.[24] Histoid leprosy patients form a potential reservoir of infection in the community due to their high bacillary load. It is pertinent to point out that while WHO recommends that it should be managed with standard fixed duration of MB MDT only, there is no consensus on extension of treatment duration of histoid leprosy.[25] The review of 62 treated histoid cases reported excellent clinical outcomes with regimens which included variations of rifampicin, dapsone, clofazimine, minocycline and ofloxacin, with most treatment duration lasting 12 or 24 months.[24–26]

Recurrent/Chronic ENL

Patients with chronic/recurrent ENLs with/without persistent neuritis, who are not responding to steroids or have become corticosteroid dependent, can respond well to extended course of MDT after completion of recommended regimen.[27,28] Addition of ofloxacin to WHO-MB MDT has demonstrated a high cure rate and tolerability in a small case series of leprosy patients over an 8-year period.[29]

MB Patients with Comorbidities

MB patients with immunocompromised conditions (renal transplant,[30] liver transplant,[31] cancer, human immunodeficiency virus infection, etc.) having MB leprosy may require modified/extended MDT.

SUMMARY

For the leprosy elimination strategy, it was assumed that MDT would reduce transmission of *M. leprae*, but there is no convincing evidence for this as data showing the impact of MDT on transmission are not readily available because leprosy has a long incubation period. With leprosy being in the 'post-elimination phase' the expressions, concepts and priorities have also changed. Leprosy at present may no longer be affecting large groups of people (populations) but is seen as a disease that affects small groups or clusters. This change in perspective provides an opportunity to ensure that each person with leprosy can be given the best opportunity to be a healthy' member of their community, with total cure from the disease. Such care of leprosy patients in India is possible at present as the leprosy prevalence has fallen to less than seventy thousand in India in 2022; which was close to 5 million in 1982. To achieve this goal, leprosy patients must be diagnosed early and prescribed appropriate MDT to achieve cure and freedom from disease in each and every case, thus prevent disability and reduce chances of spread of infection in the community. Patients with persistent disease activity at the end of FDT, especially those with the high initial BI and polar leprosy forms must be evaluated for bacterial resistance, kept under surveillance and ideally be treated till the cessation of all clinical activity/smear negativity.

REFERENCES

1. Daumerie D. Implementation of MDT-Successive steps. In: Sansarricq H, editor. Multidrug therapy against leprosy: Development and implementation over the past 25 years. Geneva: WHO Library Cataloguing-in-Publication Data; 2004. pp. 45–57.
2. WER 2021: WHO. Weekly epidemiological record. 2021;96:421–44.
3. Malathi M, Thappa DM. Fixed-duration therapy in leprosy: limitations and opportunities. Indian J Dermatol. 2013;58:93.
4. WHO expert committee on leprosy. WHO Tech Rep Ser; 1998. p. 874.
5. Kumar A, Girdhar A, Girdhar BK. Twelve months fixed duration WHO multidrug therapy for multibacillary leprosy: incidence of relapses in Agra field-based cohort study. Indian J Med Res. 2013;138:536–40.
6. Ji B. Why multidrug therapy for multibacillary leprosy can be shortened to 12 months. Lep Rev. 1998;69;106–9.
7. Job CK, Jayakumar J, Aschhoff M. Delayed resolution versus treatment failure in paucibacillary leprosy patients under six months fixed duration multidrug therapy. Indian J Lepr. 1997;2:131–42.
8. Singh I, Sengupta U. Drug resistance in *Mycobacterium leprae* in the context of zero leprosy. Indian Dermatol Online J. 2021;12:791–5.
9. Mathew D, Kishore BN, Shwethadri GK, Sukumar, Shetty NJ. An evaluation of clinical and histopathological status in paucibacillary leprosy patients after completion of fixed duration therapy. Indian J Lepr. 2004;76:11–8.
10. MDT—questions and answers. Revised 1997. Action programme for the elimination of leprosy World Health Organisation. WHO/LEP/97.8.

11. Lemaster JW, Shwe T, Butlin CR, Roche PW. Prediction of 'highly skin smear positive' cases among MB leprosy patients using clinical parameters. Leprosy review. 2001;72:23–8.
12. Lastória JC, Putinatti MSMA, Diório SM, Trino LM, Padovani CR. Índices baciloscópicos e morfológico na hanseníase após doze doses do esquema poliquimioterápico (PQT/OMS) Hansen Int. 2006;31:15–21.
13. Nascimento ACMD, Dos Santos DF, Antunes DE, Gonçalves MA, Santana MAO, Dornelas BC, Goulart LR, Goulart IMB. Leprosy Relapse: A Retrospective Study on Epidemiologic, Clinical, and Therapeutic Aspects at a Brazilian Referral Center. Int J Infect Dis. 2022 May;118:44–51. doi: 10.1016/j.ijid.2022.01.009. Epub 2022 Jan 10. PMID: 35017109.
14. Goto M, Nogam R, Okano Y, Gidoh M, Yotsu R, Ishida Y, et al. Ad Hoc Committee on Treatment Guideline and Judgment of Cure; Japanese Leprosy Association. [Guidelines for the treatment of Hansen's disease in Japan (third edition)]. Nihon Hansenbyo Gakkai Zasi. 2013;82:143–84.
15. Available at: https://www.hrsa.gov/hansens-disease/diagnosis/recommended-treatment [Last accessed on 2 Aug 2023].
16. Maymone MBC, Venkatesh S, Laughter M, Abdat R, Hugh J, Dacso MM, et al. Leprosy: Treatment and management of complications. J Am Acad Dermatol. 2020;83:17–30.
17. Dacso MM, Jacobson RR, Scollard DM, Stryjewska BM, Prestigiacomo JF. Evaluation of multi-drug therapy for leprosy in the United States using daily rifampin. South Med J. 2011;104:689–94.
18. Public Health-England (PHE) Memorandum on leprosy 2012, on behalf of the Panel of Leprosy Opinion May 2013 Wellington House, London SE1 8UG. Available at: www.gov.uk/phe [Last accessed on 2 Aug 2023].
19. Gupta UD, Katoch K, Singh HB, Natrajan M, Katoch VM. Persister studies in leprosy patients after multi-drug treatment. Int J Lepr Other Mycobact Dis. 2005;73:100–4.
20. Girdhar BK, A Girdhar, A Kumar. Relapses in multibacillary leprosy patients: effect of length of therapy. Lepr Rev. 2000;71:144–53.
21. Guidelines for Global Surveillance of Drug Resistance in Leprosy. New Delhi: World Health Organization, Regional Office for South-East Asia; 2017. Licence: CC BY-NC-SA 3.0 IGO.
22. Cambau E, Saunderson P, Matsuoka M, Cole ST, Kai M, Suffys P, et al. WHO surveillance network of antimicrobial resistance in leprosy. Antimicrobial resistance in leprosy: results of the first prospective open survey conducted by a WHO surveillance network for the period 2009–15. Clin Microbiol Infect. 2018;24:1305–10.
23. WHO Guidelines for the diagnosis, treatment and prevention of leprosy 2018.
24. Gupta N, Mathur R, Sharma A, et al. The Burden of Histoid Leprosy in Post Elimination Era. Indian J Lepr. 2022;94:219–226.
25. Bartos G, Sheuring R, Combs A, Rivlin D. Treatment of histoid leprosy: a lack of consensus. Int J Dermatol. 2020;59:1264–9.
26. Kaur I, Dogra S, De D, Saikia UN. Histoid leprosy: a retrospective study of 40 cases from India. Br J Dermatol. 2009;160:305–10.
27. Narang T, Bishnoi A, Dogra S, Saikia UN, Kavita. Alternate anti-leprosy regimen for multidrug therapy refractory leprosy: A retrospective study from a tertiary care center in North India. Am J Trop Med Hyg. 2019;100:24–30.
28. Lastória JC, Almeida TSC, Putinatti MSMA, Padovani CR. Effectiveness of the retreatment of patients with multibacillary leprosy and episodes of erythema nodosum leprosum and/or persistent neuritis: a single-center experience. An Bras Dermatol. 2018;93:181–4.
29. Faust L, Klowak M, MacRae, Kopalakrishnan CS, Showler AJ, Boggild AK. Ofloxacin-Containing Multidrug Therapy in Ambulatory Leprosy Patients: A Case Series. J Cutan Med Surg. 2020;25:45–52.
30. Guditi S, Ram R, Ismal KM, Sahay M, Dakshinamurthy KV, Girish N, *et al*. Leprosy in a renal transplant recipient: review of the literature. Transpl Infect Dis. 2009 Dec;11(6):557–62.
31. Trindade MA, Palermo ML, Pagliari C, Valente N, Naafs B, Massarollo PC, et al. Leprosy in transplant recipients: report of a case after liver transplantation and review of the literature. Transpl Infect Dis. 2011;13(1):63–9.

Chapter 16

Management of Antimicrobial Resistance in Leprosy

• Ajeet Singh • Neel Prabha

INTRODUCTION

Drug resistance in leprosy is a rising public health problem. Dapsone resistance has been reported in leprosy since the early 1960s. According to the data between 2009 and 2015 from 19 countries, rifampicin resistance was found in 5.1% of relapse cases and 2% of new cases.[1] Clofazimine and quinolone resistance have also been reported.

In India, data between 2011 and 2015 showed rifampicin resistance in 3.5%, dapsone resistance in 2.3%, and ofloxacin resistance in 2.3% of new cases.[2] In relapse cases, rifampicin resistance was found in 8.2%, dapsone resistance in 4.8%, and ofloxacin resistance in 2.3% of cases. Drug resistance has been speculated to be responsible for chronic erythema nodosum leprosum (ENL) and steroid nonresponsive type 1 lepra reaction.[3]

All these factors highlight the need for continuous surveillance and early drug resistance detection in patients treated with multidrug therapy. This chapter will entail the steps on when to suspect and what are the tools available for confirmation of antimicrobial resistance (AMR), followed by available treatment options for the management of AMR.

TYPES OF DRUG RESISTANCE[4]

***Primary resistance*:** An untreated leprosy case who is infected with a drug-resistant *Mycobacterium leprae* strain. The patient is a new leprosy case, unresponsive to the standard WHO-MDT regimen.

***Secondary resistance*:** Secondary drug resistance occurs when *M. leprae* was initially susceptible to a particular drug, develop resistance to it after exposure to that drug. This can happen due to various reasons like inadequate and incomplete treatment with MDT.

CURRENT KNOWLEDGE AND KNOWLEDGE GAP ON THE SUBJECT

Screening of new MB cases with high bacillary load and relapse cases from endemic countries has revealed a rise in primary and secondary resistance to rifampicin and ofloxacin. In addition to this, there are reports of rifampicin-resistant in leprosy cases with lepra reactions. The importance of AMR leprosy in the patients is that the resistant strains released from these cases might be responsible for spread of the resistant strains of *M. leprae* in the endemic area.[5]

When to Suspect AMR?

Drug resistance should be suspected in the following cases:

1. Newly diagnosed cases of leprosy not responding to treatment and MI positive even after 5–6 months of MB-MDT.

2. Relapse case: Relapse is defined as re-currence of leprosy that is not because of reactions at any time after completion of recommended WHO-MDT regimen.[1] Diagnostic features are: new skin lesions and/or an increase in BI by 2 or more units from the same site at the previous examination.
3. Recurrent erythema nodosum leprosum: is defined as 2nd or subsequent episodes of type 2 reaction developing 28 days or more after stopping ENL treatment.
4. Chronic erythema nodosum leprosum is defined as ENL for ≥ 24 weeks; during this period, either the patient required treatment continuously or any treatment-free period had been 27 days or less.[3]

Testing Methods

Available diagnostic tools for the detection of antimicrobial resistance: Detection of drug resistance can be done by various drug susceptibility testing methods

In vivo* method to detect resistant strains of *M. leprae

- ***Mouse foot pad assay*:** Detects drug resistant *M. leprae* strains by determining *M. leprae* growth pattern in mouse footpad (MFP). Shepard and Chang developed it in 1962.[6] It is the gold standard tool for drug susceptibility testing in leprosy. By this method, in 1964, Pettit and Rees reported the first bacteriological proof of dapsone resistance in leprosy.[7] First, rifampicin and ofloxacin resistance were reported by this technique in 1976 and 1994, respectively.[8] MFP method requires 5×10^3 viable bacilli from patient for inoculation in each footpad for drug susceptibility testing. For this reason, it often fails to grow bacilli in footpad due to the requirement of significant number of viable bacilli in patient's biopsy. Overall, MFP assay is laborious, expensive and time consuming and for this reason facilities for MFP assay are available in very few research institutes in India. Nonetheless, MFP is the only method to prove the link between novel mutation with drug resistance.

In vitro* methods to detect resistant strains of *M. leprae

- ***PCR-DNA sequencing:*** Mutation detection by PCR-DNA sequencing is fast and provides comprehensive data to monitor the global resistance level. This method is being used by researchers internationally.[4] Mutations is identified based on PCR amplification of drug resistance determining regions (DRDR) of *rpoB*, *folP* and *gyrA* genes which are associated with rifampicin, dapsone and ofloxacin followed by Sanger sequencing of PCR product. Identified mutations has already been proven to be associated with resistance by MFP. Mutations identified in *rpoB* gene is responsible for rifampicin resistance. Missense mutations observed at the amino acid positions 438, 441, 451 and 456 and insertion of nucleotide between 439 and 440 confers rifampicin resistance. Mutations observed in *folP* gene at the amino acid positions 53 and 55 are responsible for conferring resistance for dapsone. Mutations observed in *gyrA* gene at amino acid positions 89 and 91 confers ofloxacin resistance.
- ***DNA microarray*:** It is a simple and rapid method. In this method, a series of oligonucleotides probes are used. These probes correspond to each mutation detected in *folP*, *rpoB* and *gyr A* genes. This method is executed using multiplex PCR amplifying the DRDR region of target genes from clinical samples followed by amplicons labels with biotin. These amplicons are hybridized with probes on slide known as leprosy drug susceptibility testing (LDS-DA), and are detected by an avidin-biotin horseradish peroxidase reaction then the result is analyzed in dots or signals form on the slides.[3]
- ***Real-time PCR-based high-resolution melting analysis:*** This method is a novel and simple post-PCR step. In this method, for the detection of sequence variants, the thermal

properties of amplicons are used. The amplified DNA is denatured in precise temperature increments becomes single stranded and producing melt curves. These melt curves have features that are dependent upon nucleotide sequence.[4] Drug susceptible and resistant DNA fragment generates different melt curves, based on these melt curve analysis reporting can be done.

- ***Genotype ® Leprae DR Kit*:** It is a commercially available kit from Hain Lifesciences, Nehren, Germany. This test uses same technology as described in DNA microarray section, except that probes are pre-hybridized on the nitrocellulose membrane (Fig. 16.1).

Existing SOPs Regarding AMR Surveillance

WHO Guidelines for Surveillance

The main aim of surveillance is to detect secondary as well as primary dapsone, rifampicin, and ofloxacin resistance in leprosy patients, who relapsed after completion of WHO recommended MB-MDT regime, all suspected retreatment cases and MB cases with high bacillary load (BI>2+).[9]

The components of the surveillance system are:

1. The first component is regarding the systematic collection of samples in the field. It includes identifying relapse cases, retreatment cases and new MB cases with high BI (>2+) collecting samples from them, and transporting samples to the respective reference laboratory.

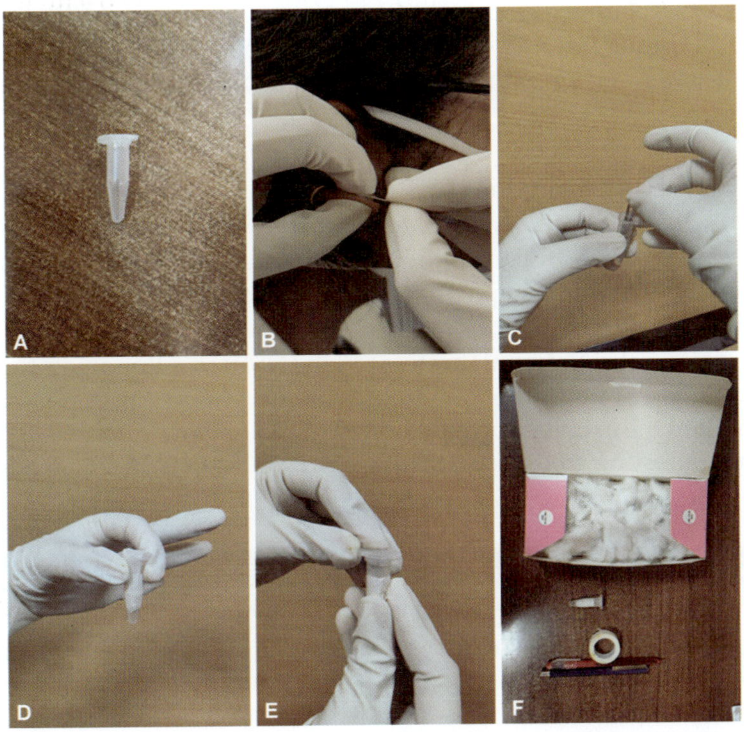

Fig. 16.1: Method of sample collection by slit skin smear. Steps of slit skin smear tissue fluid collection for AMR (A) Microcentrifuge tube with 70% ethanol; (B) Slit skin tissue fluid is taken with the help of 15 number blade (C) Tissue fluid transferred into the tube by rinsing thoroughly (D) Capping and labeling; (E) Reassuring the cap is secured (F) Proceed with packaging

2. The second component is testing the collected samples for dapsone, rifampicin, and ofloxacin resistance.

WHO recommendation for resistance testing in leprosy is mentioned in Table 16.1. Method of sample collection by slit skin smear is shown in Fig. 16.1.

NLEP Guidelines for Surveillance

Govt of India and NLEP have published 'National guidelines for surveillance of AMR in leprosy' in 2013.[2] The objectives of the AMR surveillance system are: (a) To establish a nationwide robust surveillance system for AMR (b) To estimate burden and monitor trends of AMR in leprosy among new and relapse cases. (c) To provide evidence-based inputs for program intervention.

There are 3 phases of AMR surveillance. These are preparatory, appraisal, and implementation phases. The health facilities are divided into 3 levels. Level 1: Health facility where leprosy patients are diagnosed and treated. Level 2: Health facility where facility of sample collection for AMR by slit skin smear method is available. Level 3: Health facility where facility for skin biopsy is available

NLEP–Criteria for selection of patients for AMR surveillance:

1. AMR testing should be done for relpase cases in any part of the country.

2. 20% of new MB cases should be tested for presence of *M. leprae* by skin smears. Of these tested samples of new MB cases, those found to have BI equal to or more than 2+, at least one site, should be sent for AMR. Apex laboratory for AMR testing.

3. PB patients are to be included in AMR testing. Process of AMR testing is mentioned in Flowchart 16.1. Under the AMR surveillance system, six apex laboratories have been identified and all states and union territories are linked to these labs (Table 16.2).

MANAGEMENT

Treatment of AMR cases is mentioned in Table 16.3:

Plans of NLEP, India for dealing with the AMR in leprosy: At present there are only few designated apex laboratories for anti-microbial resistance testing for leprosy in India. In addition, there is a need to build capacity of staff to suspect resistance, collect and transport samples to AMR labs.

Keeping this in view, the National Strategic Plan (NSP) and Roadmap for leprosy 2023–27 recognizes that AMR as one of the key areas of intervention for these years. It is looking forward to strengthen the existing system and also develop new system in all states and union territories to ensure testing to detect AMR in leprosy. It envisages to make surveillance of

Table 16.1: WHO recommendations for antimicrobial resistance testing in leprosy

New cases	New cases who are smear positive (BI more than 2 +) are to be tested
Retreatment cases	All retreatment cases have to be tested for secondary resistance except transferred in cases unless they are considered at risk for resistance due to irregular treatment
Testing for drugs	PCR plus sequencing for folP1, rpoB, and gyrA gene mutations
Sample for testing	Two SSS samples from the site having BI 2+ or more should be taken. Earlobe being the preferred site, together with the most prominent skin lesion Or One skin biopsy from a prominent lesion having BI 2+ or more

Flowchart 16.1: Process of AMR testing

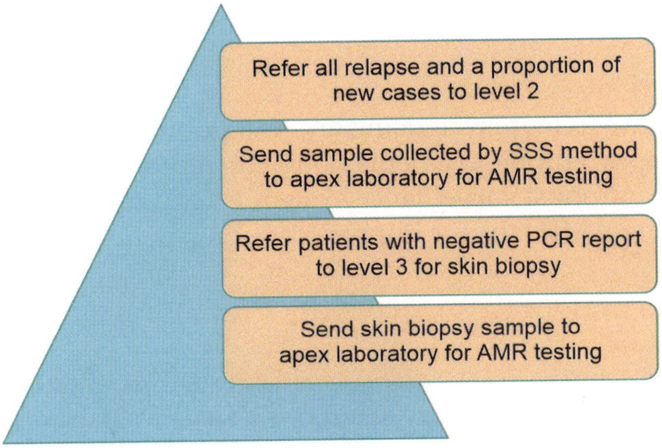

Table 16.2: Apex laboratories for AMR testing and allotted states and UTs

	Laboratory	*Allotted states and UTs*
1.	Central Leprosy Training Research Institute, Chengalpattu, Tamil Nadu	Kerala, Andaman and Nicobar, Lakshadweep, Puducherry
2.	National JALMA institute for Leprosy and other Mycobacterial diseases, Agra, UP	Uttar Pradesh, West Bengal, Assam, Tripura, Nagaland, Meghalaya, Gujarat, Rajasthan, Bihar
3.	Schieffelin Institute for Health Research and Leprosy Centre, Karigiri, Tamil Nadu	Tamil Nadu, Goa, Karnataka
4.	LEPRA-Blue Peter Public Health Research Centre, Telangana	Andhra Pradesh, Telangana, Maharashtra, Odisha, Madhya Pradesh
5.	Regional Leprosy Training and Research Institute, Raipur, Chhattisgarh	Chhattisgarh, Manipur, Mizoram, Sikkim, Arunachal Pradesh, Jharkhand, Dadra and Nagar Haveli, Daman and Diu
6.	Stanley Browne Lab, Leprosy Hospital, New Delhi	Delhi, Uttarakhand, Chandigarh, Haryana, Punjab, Jammu and Kashmir, Leh Ladakh, Himachal Pradesh

Table 16.3: Recommended regimes for drug–resistant cases in leprosy[10]

Name of resistant drug	*Treatment*	
	First 6 months	*Following 18 months*
Rifampicin or rifampicin plus dapsone	Clofazimine 50 mg/day plus minocycline 100 mg/day plus ofloxacin 400 mg/day	Clofazimine 50 mg/day plus minocycline 100 mg/day or ofloxacin 400 mg/day
	Clofazimine 50 mg/day plus ofloxacin 400 mg/day plus clarithromycin 500 mg/day	Clofazimine 50 mg/day plus ofloxacin 400 mg/day
Rifampicin and ofloxacin	Clofazimine 50 mg/day plus minocycline 100 mg/day plus clarithromycin 500 mg/day	Clofazimine 50 mg/day plus minocycline 100 mg/day or clarithromycin 500 mg/day
Dapsone	Standard WHO-MB-MDT, with follow-up at the end of treatment and should be examined regularly for possible relapse	

AMR a routine activity and data thus collected to be analyzed and used for administrative and technical planning of related activities.

CONCLUSION

Antimicrobial resistance in leprosy is rising and is a public health concern. Drug resistance is responsible for relapse, chronic erythema nodosum leprosum, and steroid nonresponsive type 1 lepra reaction. A robust surveillance system is required to deal with this problem in India by strengthening AMR labs for improved testing, confirming and reporting of drug resistance.

REFERENCES

1. Cambau et al. Antimicrobial resistance in leprosy: results of the first prospective open survey conducted by a WHO surveillance network for the period 2009–15. Clin Microbiol Infect. 2018;24:1305–10.
2. National guidelines for surveillance of antimicrobial resistance in leprosy. Available from https://dghs.gov.in/WriteReadData/userfiles/file/Leprosy%20New/AMR%20Guidelines%20in%20Leprosy.pdf
3. Narang T, Kamat D, Thakur V, et al. Equal rates of drug resistance in leprosy cases with relapse and recurrent/chronic Type 2 reaction: time to revise the guidelines for drug-resistance testing in leprosy? *ClinExpDermatol.* 2022;47:297–302.
4. Lavania M, Sengupta U. Drug resistance in leprosy. In: Sardana K and Khurana A eds. Jopling's handbook of leprosy 6th edn. New Delhi: CBS Publishers; 2020. p.228–35.
5. Singh I, Sengupta U. Drug Resistance in *Mycobacterium leprae* in the Context of Zero Leprosy. Indian Dermatol Online J. 2021;12:791–5.
6. Shepard CC, Chang YT. Effect of several anti-leprosy drugs on multiplication of human leprosy bacilli in footpads of mice. Proc SocExpBiol Med. 1962;109:636–8.
7. Pettit JHS, Rees RJW. Sulphone resistance in leprosy. An experimental and clinical study. *Lancet.*1964;2:673–4.
8. Jacobson RR, Hastings RC. Rifampicin resistant leprosy. Lancet 1976;2:1304–5.
9. WHO. A Guide for Surveillance of Antimicrobial Resistancein Leprosy. 2017 update. Delhi: World Health Organization, 2017.
10. Guidelines for the Diagnosis, Treatment and Prevention of Leprosy. Available from: https://apps.who.int/iris/bitstream/handle/10665/274127/9789290226383-eng.pdf.

Section 4

Management of Special Scenarios in Leprosy

Chapter 17

Management of High Bacteriological Index Leprosy Patients

• Tarun Narang • Vinod Kumar Hanumanthu

INTRODUCTION

Over the past decade there is a concern about the increase in the number of new cases presenting with smear positivity globally, including India. According to the WHO Weekly Epidemiology Record published annually, there is an observed increase globally in multibacillary (MB) forms of leprosy over the last few years. The proportion of MB cases in India which stands at 58.1% in 2021 has risen to 61% in the year 2023,[1] which indirectly points to the magnitude of the pool of infection in the community, as MB leprosy patients carry a higher risk of transmitting the disease than PB leprosy patients.[2]

Epidemiological significance of MB leprosy cases with high bacteriological index

Patients with initial high bacteriological index (BI) can be considered as an important subgroup of MB leprosy. Many patients with an initial high BI continue to have persistent or clinically active skin lesions and high BI even at the end of a year of fixed-duration treatment (FDT). These patients are at higher risk of recurrence that may be caused by an endogenous relapse or exogenous reinfection, or even both simultaneously.[3,4] Studies from Cebu, Bamako, Mali, and Agra have observed relapse frequencies ranging from 17 to 39% in patients with high initial BI.[5,6] Although the current WHO MDT regimes are effective in the majority of leprosy patients, the fixed duration treatment of 12 months may not be adequate in this subgroup of patients as observed in a study where viable bacilli in the mice footpads were demonstrated in 16% of BL/LL patients who had completed 12 months of MDT.[7]

The high BI group also includes patients with polar lepromatous leprosy (LLp), who are anergic to *M. leprae* and incapable of either killing or clearing the bacilli after treatment. A single untreated LL patient is known to shed as many as ten million viable bacilli per day in nasal discharges.[8,9] If inadequately treated, they may continue to shed bacilli even after being released from treatment (FDT). This makes them epidemiologically an important source of infection maintaining disease transmission in the community.[10] Transmission of leprosy cannot be effectively interrupted by confining attention to the management of contacts without adequate treatment of the sources of infection.

DEFINITION

According to WHO operational classification, leprosy is categorized into the pauci-bacillary (PB) and multi-bacillary (MB) groups. MB group includes a subset of patients with **initial high BI**, i.e. BI ≥3, and these are the cases that are the cases of concern as recent evidence indicates that the risk of transmission is highest among the contacts of high BI patients.[11]

POSSIBLE RISKS AND COMPLICATIONS

Leprosy reactions are significantly more frequent in MB patients with a high BI.[12] Reactional episodes can lead to nerve function impairment and disabilities, LL spectrum and high BI are established risk factors for ENL (erythema nodosum leprosum) episodes, also known as type 2 reactions.[12] In a recent study from India, about 74.2% of MDT-refractory leprosy patients, had ENL and half of these had chronic or recurrent ENL.[13] A change from the standard MDT regimen to an alternative regimen of minocycline, ofloxacin, and clofazimine led to a faster steroid tapering with no reactional episodes after completion of treatment.[13] These observations indicate that effective antimicrobial therapy can reduce and control ENL episodes. Similar observations were also seen in studies that used immunotherapy with MIP or BCG with MDT in patients with high BI.[14,15]

Patients with high bacillary load continue to suffer from reactions even after RFT; hence, there is an urgent need to follow up with these patients, and a possibility of relapse or drug resistance triggering reaction phenomena should be evaluated and managed.[16] Thus, it is essential that we identify this subset of patients with high BI. The reintroduction and quality control of slit skin smear (SSS) services are crucial for identifying and diagnosing patients with initial high BI, in addition to long-term monitoring and follow-up.

Need for Separate Guidelines for the Management of MB Leprosy with High BI

With significant reduction in leprosy prevalence, it is time for individualized treatment based on specific parameters of the diseases is offered to the leprosy affected. Unfortunately, despite advances in immunogenetics and immunopathogenesis of leprosy, the same has not translated into improved anti-leprosy drug therapy beyond the WHO-MDT guidelines which is in force for over four decades. Nevertheless, guidelines of few countries, such as Japan and US deal explicitly with managing high BI patients. The Japanese guidelines acknowledge that for MB leprosy with high BI, 12 months of treatment is insufficient and recommend 2 years of treatment with MB-MDT for patients with BI >3 at baseline.[17] The guidelines further state that when the BI becomes negative and there are no active lesions after 2 years, no maintenance therapy is required. However, if the BI is still positive, an additional year of MB-MDT is advocated (3 years in total), followed by maintenance therapy with dapsone and clofazimine until BI negativity and resolution of active lesions. In the case of MB patients with a BI <3, WHO MB-MDT is recommended and if the BI is still positive or active lesions persist after completion of MB-MDT for one-year, additional therapy with MB-MDT for one more year is recommended.[17]

The National Hansen's Disease Program (NHDP), USA recommends a 2 years regimen of daily rifampicin, dapsone, and clofazimine for all MB leprosy cases and in this area of low endemicity, they have observed very low relapse rates and minimum adverse effects with the daily rifampicin regimen.[18]

Based on the current situation in high leprosy load countries such as India, Brazil and Indonesia, there is a need to review treatment strategies adopted, especially with regard to initial high BI cases. Based on the review of literature and observations in various published studies, following options can be considered for the management of this subset of patients.

MANAGEMENT OPTIONS

Longer Duration for Treatment or Treatment till Smear Negativity

The number of new multibacillary (MB) cases globally has shown little or no decline since 2005 despite the use of MDT given to MB patients for 12 months.[19] This contrasts with examples of dramatic success following prolonged antimicrobial treatment. A demonstrable 16–20% annual decline in the new case detection rate of LL and MB cases was seen following antimicrobial chemotherapy given till smear negativity, and such declines were also observed in countries where dapsone or MDT was given to LL patients until smear negativity as observed in studies at Uele (in DR Congo), Karigiri (in India) and Weifang/Shandong (in China).[20,21] The most rapid decline in the incidence rate of leprosy was demonstrated in the Federated States of Micronesia (FSM), where integrated and expert skin camps for all conditions were combined with MDT given till skin smear negativity, plus annual mass multidrug administration in hyperendemic areas using ROM (rifampicin + ofloxacin + minocycline). An 84% decline of new leprosy cases within only two years was demonstrated there.[22] All these successes in low-income areas share one common characteristic. They all used prolonged antimicrobial protection of patients with high BI, first with dapsone during the period from the 1950s until the 1980s and then with MDT from the 1980s until 1998. Only in 1998 did a fixed duration of MDT (12 months) replaced more prolonged MDT. Thereafter, following an incubation period of some years, the decline in the number of new cases detected each year showed stagnation. In contrast, transmission of leprosy is observed in areas across the globe where patients were not treated until smear negativity, with only a slow decline in new case detection rates.

In a study from Agra, India, some patients were treated with 2-year MDT and others until smear-negativity (generally 5 years). At follow-up after 4 years of completion of treatment, no difference in the relapse rate was observed in the two cohorts, but when follow-up was extended beyond 4 years, relapse rates were significantly higher ($P<0.01$) in high BI (>4+) patients receiving two-year MDT than those treated to smear negativity.[6] A longer duration of treatment for 24 months (according to the WHO recommendation prior to 1998), or preferably till smear negativity (according to the WHO recommendation prior to 1988) will help in interrupting transmission, reducing the number of relapses or recurrences, and decreasing the episodes of reactions and neuritis in this subset of patients.

Better Treatment Regimens with More Bactericidal Drugs

Daily Rifampicin

Rifampicin is the backbone of the current WHO-MDT regimens and is the major bactericidal antimicrobial in MDT responsible for killing *M. leprae* in leprosy patients. It is estimated that a newly diagnosed LL patient could harbor as many as 10^{12} *M. leprae* per gram of tissue.[23] It is known that bacterial mutation to drug resistance occurs spontaneously and the frequency of drug-resistant mutants increases with the increase in bacterial load. Resistant mutants therefore can occur in frequencies typically ranging from 1 in 100 to 1 in a million viable bacilli. Mouse footpad measurements show that monthly rifampicin is less effective than daily rifampicin, and even daily clofazimine.[24] Based on the observed high frequency of recurrence in patients with high BI, once a month rifampicin dosing seems inadequate for this subset of patients. When MDT was first introduced in 1982 the number of leprosy patients on antimicrobial treatment globally was over 12 million, at which time the high cost of daily use of rifampicin influenced the decision to adopt monthly doses of rifampicin in MDT.[25] Now the number of leprosy patients on antimicrobial treatment globally has decreased to a <2 lakh, and it seems reasonable to implement an effective regimen with daily rifampicin that is more bactericidal. For building a fairer and healthier world, it would be good to allow endemic countries such as India, Brazil and Indonesia, home to more than 75% of the world's patients on antimicrobial treatment have an option of using regimen with daily rifampicin, which is being used in the United States, especially for high BI cases. It would be worthwhile to study the effects of a daily rifampicin containing MDT regimen versus conventional monthly rifampicin MB MDT on bacillary clearance, reactions, drug resistance, and recurrence rate.

Newer Drug Regimens

The WHO-MDT has been quite successful in bringing down the incidence rate of new cases of leprosy significantly wherever it was continued until smear negativity, as discussed above. Nevertheless, a reliably 'curative' regimen remains desirable. Various alternative drugs have been studied including fluoroquinolones like ofloxacin and moxifloxacin, minocycline, clarithromycin, ansamycins, etc.[26]

A study done at Mumbai observed that moxifloxacin-based regimens were found to be effective with a rapid decline in BI along with clinical improvement, although, a few reactional episodes were observed.[27] In a case series of MDT nonresponsive patients from India, a change from the standard MDT regimen to an alternative treatment (ALT) regimen of daily minocycline, ofloxacin, and clofazimine given for 24 months led to a faster drop in BI, quicker steroid tapering with no reactional episodes after completion of treatment.[13] The faster or more effective clearance was also seen in another case series from India, where more patients achieved a BI of zero after 2 years of ALT as compared to fixed MDT (12 months).[28] Newer drugs and regimens with strong bactericidal activity hold great promise but multicentric studies would help confirm their efficacy and safety in the short-term as well as their long-term effect in preventing reactions and recurrence. Their role in reducing transmission could also be studied by comparing a population using a newer regimen with a similar population using MDT.

Immunotherapeutic Vaccines (BCG, MIP) as Adjuncts to MDT

Mycobacterium indicus pranii (MIP) or BCG vaccines as immunotherapy are useful in MB patients with high bacterial load as they enhance bacterial clearance by upregulating the specific immune response or by nonspecific "trained immunity".[29,30] It was seen that the MIP/BCG vaccines led to a faster reduction in bacillary load, histopathological resolution of granuloma along with the decrease in the frequency and severity of type 2 reactions without exacerbating type 1 reactions and neuritis.[29,31] Studies from India have shown the efficacy and safety of MIP and BCG in the management of leprosy and the prevention of type 2 leprosy reactions and associated neuritis.[14,15] Hence, immunotherapy with MIP and BCG which are readily available in India can be used consistently as an adjunct to MDT in management of patients with high bacterial load. However, the dose and frequency of administration need to be standardised, as different field studies have used these vaccines in varying intervals of 3–6 months. The broad availability and cost of the MIP vaccine remain as issues to be resolved.

Post MDT–ROM

Ensuring adherence with prolonged MDT can be challenging. Hence, monthly dosing schedules with more powerful bactericidal drug combinations can be one option for high BI patients after completion of WHO MDT schedules as supervised monthly doses. Rifampicin + ofloxacin + minocycline (ROM), which is a WHO recommended drug combination, has seen the longest and most widespread use. Other combinations of potently bactericidal drugs can also be used for monthly post-MDT chemoprophylaxis. Rifapentine (P) + moxifloxacin (Mo) + minocycline (Mi) (PMM), sometimes with the addition of clarithromycin (Cl), are known to be used in centres of excellence in endemic countries.[32] Prolonged anti-microbial protection in Karigiri, Uele and Shandong resulted in a 16–20% annual decline in incidence rate of leprosy.[33,34] Post-MDT chemoprophylaxis with such once-a-month regime for patients can be managed easily and may not affect the drug compliance. It would take care of the prolonged bacillary shedding in patients with high BI and helps to check transmission from these important reservoirs of leprosy.

SUMMARY

High BI patients should be considered as the "Cases of Consequence" as far as leprosy transmission is concerned. Adequate management of these cases will help in ending transmission and achieving our goal of a leprosy-free world. The current WHO-MDT regimen for MB leprosy still follows the 12-month treatment adopted in 1998 for all MB patients, irrespective of their BI. Patients with a high BI continue to suffer from reactions and recurrences, often leading to disability and disfiguration. There is a need to look beyond 'fixed duration therapy' with monthly rifampicin in this group of patients, and to consider longer or more bactericidal regimens. Improved policies and guidelines are needed for the identification, diagnosis and management of initial high BI patients, to treat them effectively as well as to prevent community transmission of leprosy.

REFERENCES

1. World Health Organization (WHO) Weekly Epidemiological Record. No 37, 15th September 2023.
2. Quilter EEV, Butlin CR, Singh S, Alam K, Lockwood DNJ. Patients with skin smear positive leprosy in Bangladesh are the main risk factor for leprosy development: 21-year follow-up in the household contact study (COCOA). PLoS Negl Trop Dis. 2020;14(10):e0008687.
3. Malathi M, Thappa DM. Fixed-duration therapy in leprosy: limitations and opportunities. Indian J Dermatol. 2013;58(2):93–100.
4. Almeida JG, Jesudasan K, Christian M, Chacko CJ. Relapse rates in lepromatous leprosy according to treatment regularity. Int J Lepr Other Mycobact Dis. 1986;54(1):16–20.
5. Jamet P, Ji B. Relapse after long-term follow up of multibacillary patients treated by WHO multidrug regimen. Marchoux Chemotherapy Study Group. Int J Lepr Other Mycobact Dis. 1995;63(2):195–201.
6. Girdhar BK, Girdhar A, Kumar A. Relapses in multibacillary leprosy patients: effect of length of therapy. Lepr Rev. 2000;71(2):144–53.
7. Shetty VP, Wakade A, Antia NH. A high incidence of viable *Mycobacterium leprae* in post-MDT recurrent lesions in tuberculoid leprosy patients. Lepr Rev. 2001;72(3):337–44.
8. Dharmendra N, Sen N. Frequency of the presence of the leprosy bacillus in nasal smears of leprosy patients. Int J Lepr. 1948;16(2):286.
9. Hambridge T, Nanjan Chandran SL, Geluk A, Saunderson P, Richardus JH. *Mycobacterium leprae* transmission characteristics during the declining stages of leprosy incidence: A systematic review. PLoS Negl Trop Dis. 2021;15(5):e0009436.
10. Ploemacher T, Faber WR, Menke H, Rutten V, Pieters T. Reservoirs and transmission routes of leprosy; A systematic review. PLoS Negl Trop Dis. 2020;14(4):e0008276.
11. Leprosy: Global consultation of National Leprosy Programme managers, partners and affected persons on Global Leprosy Strategy 2021–2030: Report of the virtual meeting 26–30 October 2020. New Delhi: World Health Organization, Regional Office for South-East Asia; 2017.
12. Pandhi D, Chhabra N. New insights in the pathogenesis of type 1 and type 2 lepra reaction. Indian J Dermatol Venereol Leprol. 2013;79(6):739–49.
13. Narang T, Bishnoi A, Dogra S, Saikia UN, Kavita. Alternate Anti-Leprosy Regimen for Multidrug Therapy Refractory Leprosy: A Retrospective Study from a Tertiary Care Center in North India. Am J Trop Med Hyg. 2019;100(1):24–30.
14. Narang T, Kaur I, Kumar B, Radotra BD, Dogra S. Comparative evaluation of immunotherapeutic efficacy

of BCG and mw vaccines in patients of borderline lepromatous and lepromatous leprosy. Int J Lepr Other Mycobact Dis. 2005;73(2):105–14.

15. Zaheer SA, Misra RS, Sharma AK, Beena KR, Kar HK, Mukherjee A, et al. Immunotherapy with Mycobacterium w vaccine decreases the incidence and severity of type 2 (ENL) reactions. Lepr Rev. 1993;64(1):7–14.
16. Save MP, Dighe AR, Natrajan M, Shetty VP. Association of viable *Mycobacterium leprae* with Type 1 reaction in leprosy. Lepr Rev. 2016;87(1):78–92.
17. Goto M, Nogam R, Okano Y, Gidoh M, Yotsu R, Ishida Y, et al. [Guidelines for the treatment of Hansen's disease in Japan (third edition)]. Nihon Hansenbyo Gakkai Zasshi. 2013;82(3):143–84.
18. Dacso MM, Jacobson RR, Scollard DM, Stryjewska BM, Prestigiacomo JF. Evaluation of multi-drug therapy for leprosy in the United States using daily rifampin. South Med J. 2011;104(10):689–94.
19. Towards zero leprosy Global Leprosy (Hansen's disease) Strategy 2021–2030.
20. Li HY, Weng XM, Li T, Zheng DY, Mao ZM, Ran SP, et al. Long-term effect of leprosy control in two Prefectures of China, 1955–1993. Int J Lepr Other Mycobact Dis. 1995;63(2):213–21.
21. Norman G, Raja Samuel Bhushanam JD, Samuel P. Trends in leprosy over fifty years in Gudiyatham Taluk, Vellore, Tamil Nadu. Indian J Lepr. 2006;78(2):167–85.
22. Diletto C, Blanc L, Levy L. Leprosy chemoprophylaxis in Micronesia. Lepr Rev. 2000;71 Suppl:S21–3; discussion S4–5.
23. Pinheiro RO, de Souza Salles J, Sarno EN, Sampaio EP. *Mycobacterium leprae*-host-cell interactions and genetic determinants in leprosy: an overview. Future Microbiol. 2011 Feb;6(2):217–30. doi: 10.2217/fmb.10.173. PMID: 21366421; PMCID: PMC3123826.
24. Almeida JG. How effective is monthly rifampin? Int J Lepr Other Mycobact Dis. 1992;60(1):81–2.
25. Gelber RH, Grosset J. The chemotherapy of leprosy: an interpretive history. Lepr Rev. 2012;83(3):221–40.
26. Lavania M, Darlong J, Singh I, Ahuja M, Turankar RP, Pathak VK, et al. Analysis of bacteriological Index between fixed multidrug therapy and new WHO recommended alternative regimen with ofloxacin, minocycline and clofazimine of rifampicin resistant cases from the hospitals of The Leprosy Mission, India. J Glob Antimicrob Resist. 2020;23:275–7.
27. Ganapati R, Pai VV, Khanolkar S, Shinde M. Clinical trials with Moxifloxacin based regimens in leprosy. A Preliminary Communication. Revista de LEPROLOGIA. Enero-Abril 2009;XXVII:1.49–55.
28. Villahermosa LG, Fajardo TT, Jr., Abalos RM, Cellona RV, Balagon MV, Dela Cruz EC, *et al*. Parallel assessment of 24 monthly doses of rifampin, ofloxacin, and minocycline versus two years of World Health Organization multi-drug therapy for multi-bacillary leprosy. Am J Trop Med Hyg. 2004;70(2):197–200.
29. Natarajan M, Katoch K, Bagga AK, Katoch VM. Histological changes with combined chemotherapy and immunotherapy in highly bacillated lepromatous leprosy. Acta Leprol. 1992;8(2):79–86.
30. Convit J, Aranzazu N, Ulrich M, Pinardi ME, Reyes O, Alvarado J. Immunotherapy with a mixture of *Mycobacterium leprae* and BCG in different forms of leprosy and in Mitsuda-negative contacts. Int J Lepr Other Mycobact Dis. 1982;50(4):415–24.
31. Talwar GP. An immunotherapeutic vaccine for multibacillary leprosy. Int Rev Immunol. 1999;18(3):229–49.
32. Ji B, Grosset J. Combination of rifapentine-moxifloxacin-minocycline (PMM) for the treatment of leprosy. Lepr Rev. 2000;71 Suppl:S81–7.
33. Li HY, Pan YL, Wang Y. Leprosy control in Shandong Province, China, 1955–1983; some epidemiological features. Int J Lepr Other Mycobact Dis. 1985;53(1):79–85.
34. Balagon MF, Cellona RV, Cruz E, Burgos JA, Abalos RM, Walsh GP, et al. Long-term relapse risk of multibacillary leprosy after completion of 2 years of multiple drug therapy (WHO-MDT) in Cebu, Philippines. Am J Trop Med Hyg. 2009;81(5):895–9.

Chapter 18

Management of Defaulters in Leprosy

• Shagufta Rather • Faizan Younus Shah

INTRODUCTION

The multidrug therapy (MDT) is very efficient in curing leprosy, subject to patient compliance and treatment completion. Unfortunately, a significant proportion of patients default in treatment due to a number of personal, psychological, social, logistic, adverse drug events and health service factors. The proportion of defaulters worldwide has been seen to be as high as 10% in case of paucibacillary leprosy and even higher (up to 30%) for multibacillary leprosy.[1] In the year 2016–17, about 5.5% of leprosy patients defaulted in India.[2] Given the vast population of the country, even a small percentage of defaulters can have a significant negative impact on leprosy program. Noncompliance with treatment contributes to drug resistance, treatment failure and increased incidence of disabilities and deformities. A motivated and well-informed patient is more likely to comply with treatment course; thus, the importance of patient counseling cannot be over-emphasized. A defaulter is a patient who fails to complete treatment within a prescribed time frame, either by failing to take the drugs regularly or by not attending the treatment centers. Treatment default in leprosy leads to progression of the disease and to disabilities. The aim of this chapter is to provide most relevant practical points in the management of defaulters in leprosy.

DEFINITIONS

Defaulter: World Health Organization (WHO) defines a defaulter in leprosy as a person who has not collected treatment for 12 consecutive months for any reason, despite all the attempts to trace the patient.

A more practical and relevant operational definition, used by national leprosy eradication program (NLEP) India, classifies a patient as defaulter if the scheduled 6-month treatment for paucibacillary (PB) leprosy and 12 months treatment for multibacillary (MB) leprosy is not completed within 9 months and 18 months, respectively.[1] In other words, if a patient has missed treatment for 3 months in case of PB leprosy or 6 months in case of MB leprosy at any time, it is not possible for them to complete treatment in allotted time and they should be declared as defaulter.

Defaulters are a significant hurdle to leprosy eradication programs not just because they can act as a constant source of infection in the community but also because they are more likely to end up with disabilities and deformities; thus, adding to the morbidity resulting from leprosy.

Interruption from treatment: Interruption of treatment is defined as duration of treatment exceeding 7 months for paucibacillary (PB) leprosy and more than 13 months for multibacillary (MB) leprosy.[3] Patients who interrupt treatment and are habitual of missing clinic appointments are more likely to default in the long run. A special attention and check should be kept on these patients who have interrupted treatment at any stage so that they can be counseled to continue treatment before they turn into defaulters. As already mentioned above, counseling should be done so that PB-MDT (Rifampicin 600 mg once a month and dapsone 100 mg daily) of 6 months should be completed within 9 months; and MB-MDT (rifampicin 600 mg and clofazimine 300 mg once a month; dapsone 100 mg and clofazimine 50 mg daily) of 12 months should be completed within 18 months.

Risk factors for defaulting from leprosy treatment/ influencing MDT adherence: The treatment adherence and completion vary widely globally and several factors contribute to adherence to treatment schedule and to default. Factors contributing to defaulting, irregularity and non-compliance have been grouped as: personal factors (patients-related elements, condition-related elements, financial factors, social determinants), treatment factors, and health system factors.[4–6] (Fig. 18.1) There are multiple variables related to the condition of the patient, health system and drug related factors which can influence the treatment adherence. Other factors that need to be considered are summarized in Box 18.1.

Defaulting from treatment has several consequences as outlined in the (Fig. 18.2).

METHODS OF EVALUATING ADHERENCE TO MDT TREATMENT

As per WHO, the proportion of MDT default rates should be a commonly used measure of MDT adherence in leprosy and this can be utilized as an aberrant measure to distinguish

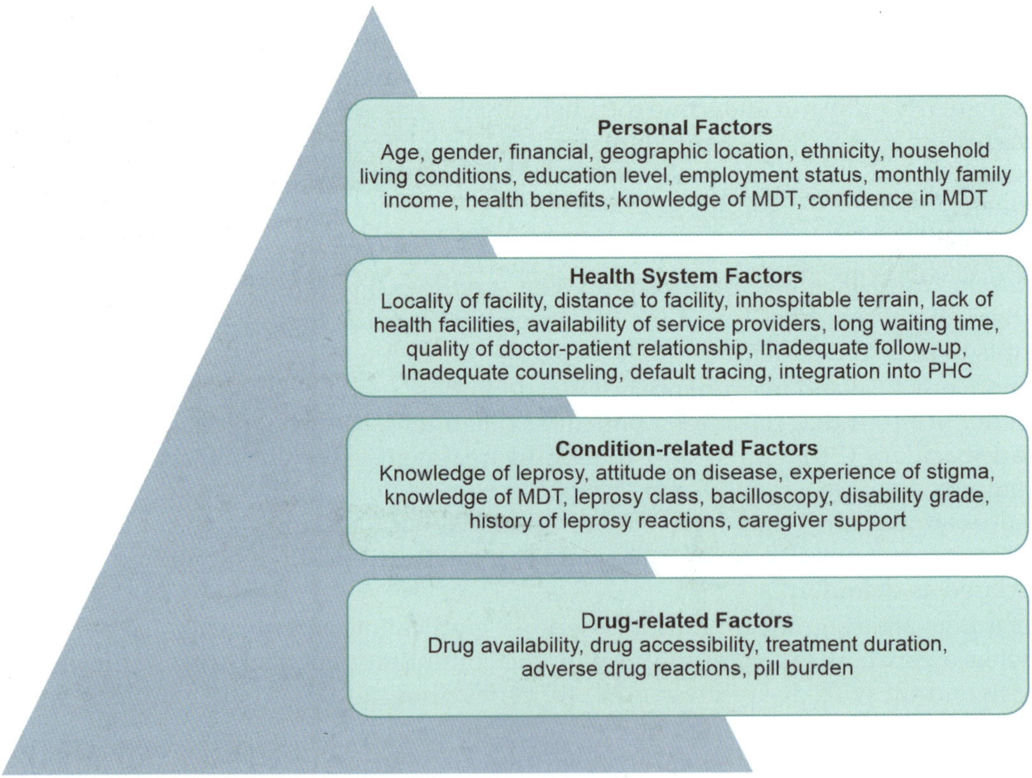

Fig. 18.1: Factors contributing to defaulting, irregularity and noncompliance

Box 18.1: Questions to be asked to understand the effect of individual factors[14,15]

- Seasonal variables: month of registration
- Clinical condition at registration: presence of a visible patch on the face and presence of visible impairment, as measured by WHO disability grade.
- Treatment history: previous treatment with dapsone monotherapy.
- Leprosy and treatment type: Lower default rate has been observed in ROM treatment of leprosy than that of standard MDT for both PB and MB leprosy.
- Time of default: About half of defaulters do so in the first months.
- The severity of disease may also play a role as seen through the observation that patients who completed treatment had more nerve involvement and others have less nerve involvement. The possible risk of disability due to nerve involvement might have driven them to understand the need to complete treatment.
- Nerve involvement
- Number of skin lesions

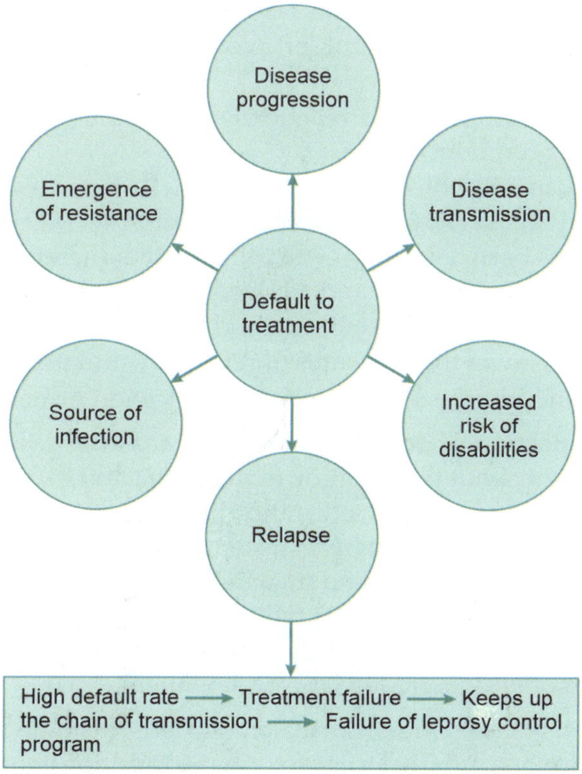

Fig. 18.2: Consequences of Default to Treatment

patients who are yet to finish their treatment as planned and as a measure of the quality of leprosy services. There is no standard method for estimation of treatment adherence and the strategies could be arranged into (a) direct and (b) indirect techniques.

Direct measures: These are costly, difficult to the service provider and include:

- Laboratory analysis of blood, urine or other body fluids for measurement of concentrations of a drug or drug metabolite.
- Detection or measurement in blood of a biologic marker added to the drug formulation.

The most famous techniques are:

- Urine spot test: A habitually utilized direct measure of MDT adherence in leprosy treatment is testing urine samples for dapsone, which is taken every day in the course of MDT. This test is said to be more specific and considered the method of choice when rapidity and reproducibility are the major objectives.[7] It is easily performed in field conditions[8] and that results correspond with those of the D:C proportion test.[7,9,10] Test is negative after roughly three missed doses of dapsone.[11] Some researchers have utilized the urine spot test in field conditions and greater part report significant degrees of non-adherence among patients with leprosy.
- Dapsone: Creatinine (D : C) proportion test: Found to have greater sensitivity than the urine spot test in distinguishing non-adherence.
- Measuring biological markers

Indirect measures: These include pill counts, questionnaires and analysis of pharmacy records.

- Number of pills: Tallying the pill count left with patient is the most widely recognized technique used to quantify adherence.
- Assessment of clinical response and reactions: are simple to utilize but susceptible to deception and an exaggeration.
- Analysis of pharmacy records: Blister packs have likewise been utilized to gauge adherence and are prescribed by the WHO as an approach to improve MDT adherence. Pharmacy-related information has been helpful in evaluating MDT adherence in a health system that utilizes electronic medicinal records and a closed pharmacy system.
- Medication refill rates: This is an exact method of determining adherence in a closed pharmacy framework, given that the rates of refill are estimated frequently.
- Utilizing questionnaires like the 8-Item Morisky Medication Adherence Scale (MMAS-8).[12]

Steps for reducing proportion of defaulters: Some of measures which can be practiced are: (a) education of the patient about the duration of treatment and (b) the need for continuation of treatment despite relief in symptoms, education about continuation of treatment in event of lepra reaction or minor adverse effects. (c) The leprosy clinic should ensure regular supply of MDT and meticulous record keeping and tracking in case of loss of patient. (d) In addition, the patient should be advised to bring empty blister pack used during previous month at every clinic visit. (e) Random tablet count by healthcare workers is recommended at least once in 2 months and more frequently in case of defaulters.

Accompanied MDT (A-MDT): Under normal conditions, a single blister pack is given to patient which suffices for one month. Drugs for greater duration should be given to patients who cannot visit the healthcare facility on a monthly basis. This will ensure better compliance in patients who live at long distances from healthcare facility, nomadic and patients from far flung areas which face road blocks due to bad weather. In exceptional cases, there is a provision for providing full treatment supply at the time of diagnosis. This is known as accompanied MDT, as in this a close relative or friend of the patient takes the responsibility of helping the patient complete treatment course. This method has been widely recommended and found to be very practical and beneficial during the COVID-19 pandemic across the world.[13] Nonetheless, it undermines the importance of regular contact between healthcare workers and patient which is crucial not just for treatment but for early recognition of complications, deformities and leprosy reactions.[7]

Tracing the patient: A patient who does not visit the healthcare facility on two successive visits is at risk for defaulting treatment. It is the duty of the healthcare work to trace every such patient and on successful tracing, the patient should be counselled and convinced to continue treatment. Involving the family of the patient can reinforce the patient's desire and motivation to continue treatment. NLEP provides a guidance regarding actions that can be taken in case of patients who are not reporting for appointments (Table 18.1).

Apart from above clinician driven steps, following programmatic steps need to be taken in order to reduce the default (Table 18.2).

Table 18.1: Tracing the defaulting patient: Situations and suggested actions

S.No	Situation	Action
1.	Patient's family is residing at registered address but patient has temporarily moved out	Advise the patient's family to inform patient to collect medicines immediately on returning.
2.	Patient available at registered address but not collecting medicines	Patient should be counseled intensely and patient retrieval should be tried. Accompanied MDT (A-MDT) can be given if the patient is motivated but regular follow up should be ensured.
3.	Patient obstinate and does not agree to take treatment	Continue counseling but give medicines only if the patient agrees to take the medicine and follow up regularly

Table 18.2: Programmatic Strategies to tackle default to treatment (abridged)

Core issues	Activities	Monitoring and performance indicators
Increased number of defaulters	Strengthen the mechanism for defaulter tracing	• Provide training and strengthen the use of district register to trace patients missing an MDT dose • Develop SMS reminder system for patients who are missing doses • Follow up mechanism to be introduced utilizing health officers/ ASHA workers with adequate emphasis on privacy and confidentiality
	Develop mechanisms to promote privacy and confidentiality of patient information	• Develop a mechanism to inform the relevant medical officer regarding the defaulters in his/her area • Developing a defaulter notification form and develop a quarterly return on defaulter tracing • Initiate incentive schemes for defaulters returning to treatment • Develop a guide emphasizing causes for defaulting and possible remedies • Strengthening the mechanism to keep track of patients and send them back for treatment before they default treatment • Improve the counseling methods and increase knowledge of patients and collect proper contact numbers • Improve lab facilities. • Maintain a separate relapse register at clinic level • Ensure availability of thalidomide/ROM/Azathioprine therapy through leprosy clinics.

(Contd.)

Table 18.2: Programmatic Strategies to tackle default to treatment (abridged) *(Contd.)*

Core issues	*Activities*	*Monitoring and performance indicators*
Quality of Leprosy services at some dermatology clinics Problems in MDT supply (shortages, record keeping, distribution and extended treatment)	Ensuring prompt start and adherence to treatment, including working towards improved treatment regimens	• Development of standards for record keeping at individual level, clinic level, regional level and central level. • Establish a computerized record keeping system at all dermatology units • Ensure availability of free-of-charge WHO distributed MDT for all leprosy patients, including those cared for by the private sector and implement A-MDT, when required • Update the operational guidelines/manual for leprosy with the help of dermatology faculty. • Issue a circular making chief pharmacist responsible for MDT stock management • Disseminate information on treatment guidelines to all dermatologists/ pharmacists • Implementation of a reaction guidelines. • Consider the introduction of direct observation of treatment by the healthcare workers (DOT) for all leprosy cases or at the very least for all paediatric cases • Strengthen the use of disability assessment forms, contact tracing forms, clinic registers, district registers and referral forms,
Non-availability of counseling services	Strengthen counseling services and health education for patients and their families	• Entrust a designated staff member to engage in counseling of leprosy patients and families in the clinic and MO. • Provide hands-on training in counseling to relevant staff • Develop a counseling guide and flash cards • Prepare training materials for counseling
Non-availability of a proper Health information management system (HIMS) and a geographical information system (GIS) for mapping of leprosy cases	Strengthening surveillance and health information systems for program monitoring and evaluation (including geographical information systems)	• Develop an online web-based human information management system (HIMS) for leprosy • Establish a web-based patient management system for dermatology clinics and integrate it with the HIMS • Train MO's in dermatology clinics, Regional epidemiologists (RE's) and health officer leprosy control for data entry at clinic level and district level • Develop a GPS app based mapping system for leprosy patients (with a complete geographical information system for leprosy) • Train RE's and PHI LC's/ Range PHI's in GIS-based mapping of cases. • Development and maintenance of a comprehensive database (include follow-up of patients/defaulters details/ GPS location

TREATMENT FOR DEFAULTERS

When a defaulter returns for treatment, the patient should be examined once again and receive a fresh classification, as paucibacillary or multibacillary and treated accordingly. New nerve involvement not recorded in any previous examination and appearance of any lepromatous nodules should be noted. However, prior to starting treatment, the patient should be counseled regarding the importance of treatment completion and every effort should be made to ensure that the patient completes treatment.

Clinical outcome post default: Following things need to be monitored while planning treatment of defaulter. (A) Skin lesions healed in spite of defaulting. (B) Disease parameters that could not be cured and remained status quo, without deformity. (C) Developed either grade 1 or grade 2 disabilities. (D) Developed type 1 or type 2 reactions.

CONCLUSION

To prevent leprosy control program from failing due to the increase in number of defaulters, irregular/inadequate monitoring of MDT administration, and treatment of leprosy patients by doctors in private setup with no facilities for follow-up, there should be a good liaison between field level workers, public health personnel and clinicians. Special focus should be on underserved populations, those who live in difficult to reach geographical areas and migrant population.

REFERENCES

1. Kumar A, Girdhar A, Chakma JK, Girdhar BK. WHO multidrug therapy for leprosy: epidemiology of default in treatment in Agra district, Uttar Pradesh, India. Biomed Res Int. 2015;2015:705804.
2. NLEP–Progress Report for the Year 2016–17, Central Leprosy Division. New Delhi: Directorate General of Health Services, Nirman Bhawan; New Delhi; 2017. [Last accessed on 2019 Apr 05]. Available from: http://nlep.nic.in/pdf/Annual%20report_%202016-17_rev.pdf.
3. Heukelbach J, André Chichava O, Oliveira ARd, Häfner K, Walther F, Alencar CHMd, *et al.* Interruption and Defaulting of Multidrug Therapy against Leprosy: Population-Based Study in Brazil's Savannah Region. PLoS Negl Trop Dis 2011:5:e1031.
4. KarS, PalR, BharatiDR. Understanding non-compliance with WHO Multidrug therapy among leprosy patients in Assam, India. J Neuro Sci Rural Practice. 2010;1:9–13.
5. Ferreira SM, Ignotti E, Gamba MA. Clinical and laboratory characteristics in the retreatment of leprosy relapse. Revista Brasileira de Epidemiologia. 2012;15:573–81.
6. Ferreira SM, Ignotti E, Gamba MA. Factors associated to relapse of leprosy in Mato Grosso, Central-Western Brazil. Revista de Saude Publica. 2011;45:756–64.
7. Bhatnagar PI, Kumar BH, Kaur S, Kaur I, Seghal S. Dapsone drug compliance study among leprosy patients: a comparison between qualitative and quantitative methods. Indian J Lepr. 1989;61:373–8.
8. Yoder LJ, Guitrau M, Jacobson R. Comparison of a urine spot test and blood tests as indicators of patient compliance. Indian J Lepr. 1991;63:195–202.
9. Kumar A, Balakrishnan S. Monitoring the regularity of self administration of dapsone by leprosy patients. Lepr India. 1982;54:664–70.
10. Naik SS. Comparative value of Dapsone" spot test" and Dapsone" tile test" in leprosy control programme. Indian J Lepr. 1984;56:847–51.
11. Huikeshoven H, Madarang MG. Spot test for detection of dapsone in urine: an assessment of its validity and interpretation in monitoring dapsone self administration. Int J Lep. 1986;54:21–4.
12. Morisky DE. Predictive validity of a medication adherence measure for hypertension control. J Clin Hypertens. 2008;10:348–54.

13. Bhardwaj A, Gupta SK, Narang T, Suneetha S, Pradhan S, Agarwal P, Suvirya S, Gupta A, Chhabra N, Rao AG, Ashwini PK, Jandhyala S, Rathod S, Rao PN, Dogra S. Updates on Management of Leprosy in the Context of COVID-19 Pandemic: Recommendations by IADVL SIG Leprosy. Indian Dermatol Online J. 2021;12:S24–S30.
14. Kumar A, Girdhar A, Chakma JK, Girdhar BK. WHO multidrug therapy for leprosy: epidemiology of default in treatment in Agra district, Uttar Pradesh, India. Biomed Res Int. 2015;2015:705804.
15. Mushtaq S, Dogra D, Faizi N, Dogra N. Profile of Defaulters and Pattern of Treatment Default among Leprosy Patients at a Tertiary Care Hospital: A 10-Year Analysis. Indian Dermatol Online J. 2020;11: 355–60.

Chapter 19

Diagnosis and Management of a Case of Relapse

• P Narasimha Rao • Sujai Suneetha • Akshay Ambasana

INTRODUCTION

The World Health Organization (WHO) has raised a concern regarding the rise in the number of relapsed cases of leprosy in the world, with Brazil, India and Indonesia leading in numbers.[1] As per recent data, there were 2990 cases of relapse from a total of 10,432 retreated cases worldwide. India with 498 recorded relapsed cases stood at 2nd place only after Brazil with 1,153 cases.[2] Due to the slow growing nature of the organism, incidents of relapse tend to occur 10–15 years after completion of treatment. Practically, long duration follow-up studies are less feasible. For this reason, most of the studies involving the use of WHO recommended or shorter duration of MDT usually lacks this longer duration follow up, making it difficult to comment on actual long-term rates of leprosy relapses. Relapse rate is often taken as an indicator of the success of an ongoing leprosy program and effectiveness of MDT. Relapse could also be a strong pointer to drug resistance. In this chapter, attention is given to the practical aspects of relapse—its prevention, identification and management.

CURRENT KNOWLEDGE

Definition

Over the years, a number of different definitions of relapse have been proposed by the WHO, by researchers and in National Leprosy Programme guidelines. However, a more recent WHO document (2017) defines relapse as: '*A patient who has completed a full course of treatment for leprosy in the past and who returns with signs and symptoms of the disease that are not deemed to be due to a reaction according to the clinician*'.[3]

A surveillance period of 2 years and 5 years respectively for PB and MB has been advocated by WHO as lepra reactions are more common during this period.[4] Relapses however are likely to occur in the post-surveillance period as well. It is important to note that at present, surveillance and follow-up of patients after completion of MDT is not a part of the guidelines of NLEP in India, and patients are expected to self-report in case of any post RFT problem.[5] A relapse could be the result of the reactivation of previous infection or can be due to reinfection, which is possible in endemic areas (Fig. 19.1). Various predisposing factors for relapse are depicted in Box 19.1.

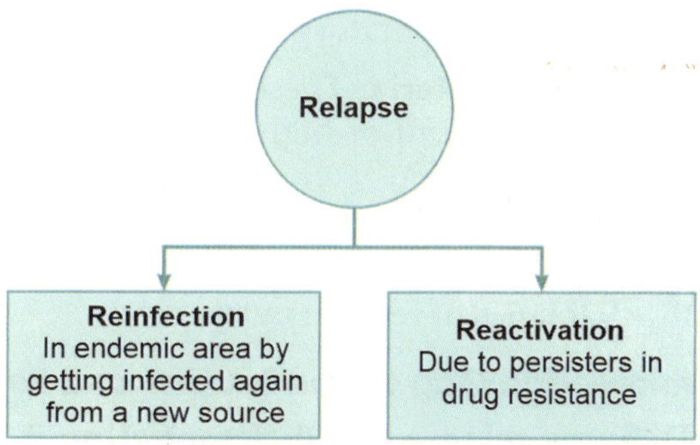

Fig. 19.1: Causes of relapse

Box 19.1: Predisposing factors for relapse

Dapsone monotherapy: From its discovery in 1945 and until the late 1970s, dapsone was used as monotherapy resulting in drug resistance. Its initial usage in low dosage coupled with irregular treatment played a role in inducing drug resistance and relapse.[11] On the other hand relapse was found to be rarer in those on MDT regimens.[12]

Reinfection: Molecular epidemiological studies suggest that most relapses are a result of reinfection rather than reactivation of previous disease. In endemic countries these relapsed cases can act as an important source of infection in the community, hence prevention and detection of these cases become a priority.

Drug resistance to drugs used in MDT: Besides dapsone resistance, resistance to rifampicin and ofloxacin are also rising in newly diagnosed MB cases in endemic countries. Quinolone resistance is also rising and reaching almost to the level of dapsone resistance. Given this, only a clear indication for use of quinolones can justify its use.[13] Studies in India reveal that MDT resistance ranges from 3.9 to 8.1 %. Rifampicin and ofloxacin resistance are on the rise in newly diagnosed case as well as in relapsed cases.[14] All these factors predispose to relapse.

Irregular treatment: WHO has recommended 9 months and 18 months as the stipulated time to complete the course of MDT in PB and MB leprosy respectively. Irregularly treated patients; patients who have had modified regimen; or have taken more than the stipulated 9 and 18 months to complete the treatment tends to show higher relapse rate.

Insufficient treatment: This may occur if a MB patient is wrongly diagnosed as PB and receives a weaker regimen of PB MDT. It can also occur when the patient fails to take the full course of prescribed MDT.

High initial BI: A few studies have stated that the risk of relapse is directly correlated with the initial bacillary load of the patient and a BI ≥3 is associated with a 10–20% relapse.[15] Prabu et al. observed higher proportion of relapse in patients with grade 2 disability (G2D).[16]

Recurrent/Chronic ENL: In one North Indian study, drug resistance was found to be 16.2% in relapsed cases and 16.6% in patients with chronic and recurrent ENL. This comparable numbers of drug resistance in relapsed cases and ENL requires further studies for more insight on the possible influence of recurrent ENL (and drug resistance) on relapse.[17,18]

Criteria for Relapse

Various clinical and laboratory criteria have been proposed in order to identify a relapse. The widely accepted criteria for the diagnosis of relapse proposed by Ramu et al. in 1995 included: appearance of new skin and nerve lesions; positive skin smears for AFB in previously negative cases; and an increase in BI by two logs at any site over the previous BI in two successive examinations in bacteriologically positive cases during surveillance.[6]

In comparison, a recent study from Brazil considered the following additional criteria for relapse.[7]

Clinical criteria: These include, reactivation of preexisting lesions; development of new lesions; new areas of sensory loss or altered sensation; new neural alteration; evolving lesions or symptomatic outbreaks which do not respond to treatment for lepra reactions including other anti-inflammatory treatment.

Laboratory criteria: These include, the presence of solid stained, non-granular bacilli in smears; persistent or higher bacillary DNA load in qPCR tests; and a raised or persistent anti-PGL-1 ELISA.

With advances in facilities for the above investigation, these new criteria may be considered. Overall, however, the clinical criteria and skin smear finding are of primary importance in the diagnosis of relapse in leprosy.

Knowledge Gap on the Subject and Recommendation

Defining relapse and differentiating it from reaction: As mentioned already, there is no consensus on the definition of relapse in leprosy. The WHO definition of relapse makes no reference to the post-RFT surveillance period and so any post-RFT events that occur either during the surveillance or thereafter that are proved not to be lepra reactions, are to be labeled as relapse.

Relapse needs to be differentiated from late lepra reactions in post RFT patients with which it has common features. Table 19.1 outlines a few ways to differentiate relapse from reaction.[8]

Lesions in leprosy continue to improve and resolve for years, even after stopping the treatment.[9] Being a chronic disease, during treatment as well as in the post-RFT period patients may develop reactions or present with recurrent or late lepra reaction. In general, studies report a lower percentage of relapse with longer duration of MDT.[7]

Understanding the link between relapse and drug resistance and addressing it: In some of the suspected cases of relapse, resistance to commonly used anti-leprosy drugs has been reported. For this reason, it is important to identify relapse of leprosy early to prevent transmission of such drug resistant strains in the community. The following strategies may be followed to check the transmission of resistant strains in endemic areas: [10]

1. Empowerment of the field level setup for the early diagnosis of relapse; differentiate it from reaction and for molecular screening of organism for any drug resistance.
2. Molecular screening of all the newly diagnosed MB cases for primary drug resistance to dapsone, rifampicin, ofloxacin and clarithromycin.
3. All the close contacts of the drug resistance leprosy patient should be screened for transmission of the resistant strain.
4. Complete and adequate treatment of a resistant case with an effective alternate regimen.
5. Taking the long incubation period in consideration, long-term follow-up of up to 10 years is required in leprosy for the early detection of relapse.

DIAGNOSIS OF RELAPSE

Clinical Features

New skin lesions, reactivation of preexisting lesions, new areas with sensory loss and symptoms similar to reactional outbreaks; which do not respond to anti-inflammatory

Table 19.1: Differentiation between relapse and reaction[8]

Criteria	*Relapse*	*Reaction*
Time since completion of treatment	Usually more than 3 years	Usually less than 3 years
Progression of signs and symptoms	Slow	Fast
Site of skin lesions	In new places	Over old patches
Pain, tenderness and swelling	No	Yes—skin and nerves
Damage	Occurs slowly	Sudden onset
General condition	Not affected	Affected in form of constitutional symptoms
Nerve to damage	New peripheral nerves may involved	Previously involved nerves may get affected
Improvement with immunosuppressive drugs	No improvement	Improves rapidly with corticosteroids
Precipitating factors	No associated history of any precipitating factors	Usually there is history of precipitating factors like pregnancy, acute infection, etc.

treatment in a patient who has completed MDT are the main clinical features to look for in relapse. As new skin lesions and reactivation of preexisting lesions may occur during reactions, it needs to be differentiated from relapse (Table 19.1).

Before labeling the case as a relapse, the possibility of inadequate or irregular therapy should be ruled out, and such cases retreated. The WHO uses the term *'Retreatment after loss to follow up'* for a patient diagnosed with leprosy who has abandoned treatment before its completion and returns to the healthcare facility to complete treatment.[19] When a patient continues to develop new signs and symptoms while on MDT, drug resistance should be suspected and such cases should be differentiated from relapse.

Histopathology of Relapsed Lesions

In MB leprosy: Skin biopsy of the suspected lesion may reveal small clumps of previously formed foamy macrophages along with newly formed spindle shaped young macrophages with pink granular cytoplasm as small and large foci. Solidly stained bacilli reappear in previously AFB-negative lesions or lesions with granular bacilli. In well-established relapse lesions collections of spindle shaped, young/immature macrophages overgrow and obscure the foamy changes. Solid stained AFBs can be found packed within macrophages, Schwann cells and endothelial cells. Skin adnexa can become atrophic and scanty with neural changes in the form of perineural thickening, fibrosis and reduction in dermal nerves.[20]

In PB leprosy: Newly formed lymphohistiocytic and epithelioid granuloma can be seen at the site of previously resolved and healed lesions. It may start in fibrosed nerves or in the arrector pili muscle cells as a tiny focus of epithelioid cells and lymphocytes which gradually expand to involve the surrounding dermis. Rare solid stained bacilli can reappear in fibrosed nerves. Fully developed granuloma can involve a large portion of dermis making it difficult to distinguish from the original lesion.[20]

Serological Tests in Relapse

The following serological tests can be useful in diagnosing a case of relapse, but are not confirmatory. The level of serum IgM antibodies to phenolic glycolipid 1 (PGL-1) are raised significantly in LL patients during relapse. Tuberculoid (TT) and BT patients who relapse as BL or LL show a rise in serum PGL-1 and anti-35 kD antibodies.[4]

Serological tests have also been useful as a tool in identifying patients at higher risk of relapse and in predicting relapse. The dipstick assay for anti-PGL-1 antibodies has be used to identify the patients with higher risk of relapse.[21] Natural Disaccharide-O-Bovine serum antigen-based ELISA test (NDO-BSA-ELISA) is also a helpful method to identify early infection and prediction of relapse, particularly in cured leprosy patients.[22] Change in the proportion of Th1 and Th2 type of interleukin (IL) profile is helpful in prediction of type of relapsed leprosy. Rise in interferon (IFN)-gamma, IL-2 and IgG2 antibodies with lepromin positivity are changes of Th1 type immune response which is suggestive of upregulation of CMI, seen when BL/LL patient relapse as TT/BT. On other hand rise in IL-4, IL-5, IL-6, IL-10 and IgG1 along with lepromin negativity are changes of Th2 type of immune response expected when there is downregulation of CMI and consequent PB leprosy patients relapsing with MB disease.

Relapse can be confirmed by a combined approach of clinical examination, skin smears, histopathology and serological tests. The details of tools that may be required is as suggested in Table 19.2.

Table 19.2: Tools for diagnosing relapse

Aspect	*Equipment*	*Purpose*
Clinical	Camera	Periodic clinical photographic record
	Graded Mono-filaments	Fine and protective touch perception charting
Bacteriological	Stains and other essential chemicals	For Acid-fast stain,
	Microscope	To calculate BI and MI
Imaging	Ultrasonography machine	To note the integrity of nerves and measure nerve thickness/ CSA
	With doppler	To check for any abnormal neural blood flow
Histopathology	A well-functioning pathology lab	To diagnose and compare histopathology. (H & E and modified Fite stains)

How to Investigate Relapse?

- **History and clinical examination:** Obtain a detailed history including treatment history to evaluate if the patient has completed the course of MDT in the specified period regularly. Carry out a detailed clinical examination which includes morphology of the skin lesions, nerve palpation, sensory testing (ST) and voluntary muscle tests (VMT).
- **Skin smears:** Perform slit skin smears from routine sites like the earlobe and selective site smears from the edge of the suspected skin lesions. Skin smear examination, when positive, should be compared with the recent smears done and the smears at baseline. Solid staining bacilli in the smear are more reliable indicators and specific for relapse; however, it has low sensitivity. Since bacilli are rarely detected in paucibacillary (PB) forms, a negative smear does not mean the absence of relapse.[23]
- **Histopathology:** Perform a 4–6 mm punch biopsy from the active edge of the suspected relapse lesion. Study the morphological changes on the Hematoxylin and Eosin (H & E) stained sections and the presence of AFB on the Fite-Faraco stained section. The details of the findings in a case of relapse are mentioned in the section on diagnosis of relapse. Histopathology gives a more precise diagnosis according to Ridley-Jopling classification. Additionally, ZN stain, modified Fite stain and even DNA-PCR studies can also be performed simultaneously which are useful in diagnosing relapse.
- The use of serological tests to predict or diagnose relapse is still limited to testing in research laboratories.

The approach to the patient suspected with relapse is outlined in Fig. 19.2.

MANAGEMENT OF A CASE OF RELAPSE

i. **In drug susceptible individuals**

In case of relapse in a patient who was once successfully treated with conventional MDT, the patient should be treated with another standard course of MDT according to the WHO classification unless secondary drug resistance is proven. When a PB or MB patient relapses with MB disease a 12-month course of MB MDT can be administered. However, when a PB patient relapses with PB disease it may be better to give a 12-month course of MB MDT. Patients with a high initial BI >3+ have a higher (10–20 %) chance of relapse and these patients may benefit from a longer duration treatment (for 24 months or until smear negativity), though long-term follow-up studies are required for more clarity on such patients.[24,25]

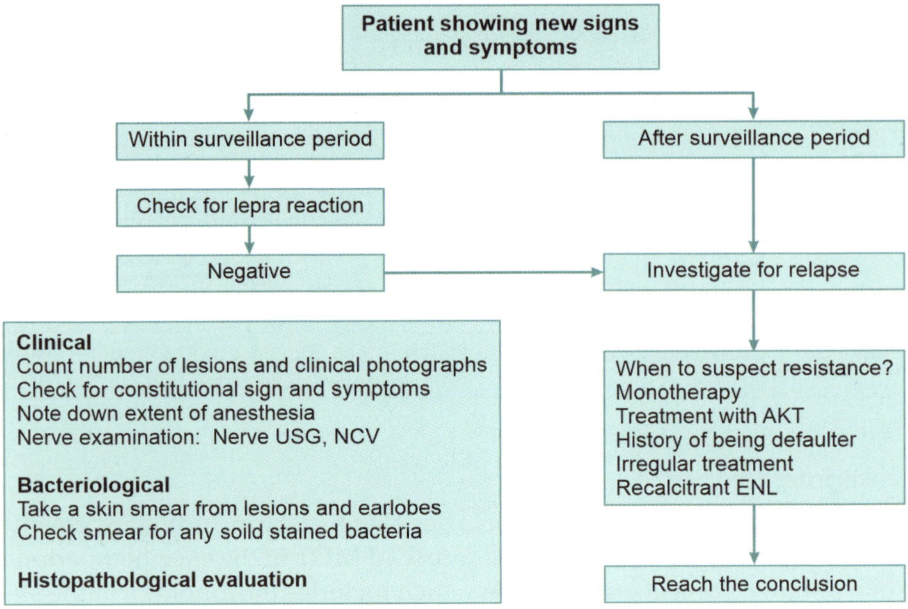

Fig. 19.2: Approach to the patient suspected with relapse

ii. **In individuals with antimicrobial resistance**[13,26] **(Table 19.3).**
Antimicrobial resistance (AMR) is one of the key areas of concern of the global leprosy strategy. At present surveillance for drug resistance among retreatment cases in leprosy is being carried out by National and international laboratories and Sentinel centers identified for performing the testing. However, there are only few such centers to check for drug resistance in India at present.

Table 19.3: Treatment of leprosy in drug resistance

Suspected drug resistance	*Treatment*		*Total duration of treatment*
Dapsone	Monthly supervised dose Rifampicin Clofazimine	Daily unsupervised dose Clofazimine	12 months
Rifampicin	Intensive phase × daily × 6 months Either 2 of Following for 6 months Clarithromycin Minocycline Quinolone + Clofazimine	Maintenance phase × daily × 18 months Continuation of either one drug from intensive phase. + Clofazimine daily	24 months
Rifampicin plus ofloxacin	Either 2 of following for 6 months Clarithromycin Minocycline + Clofazimine	Maintenance phase × 18 months Continuation of either one drug from intensive phase. + Clofazimine daily	24 months

- Dapsone resistance–in case of dapsone resistance in a PB relapse, only dapsone has to be withdrawn from the WHO-MB-MDT, patient should be treated with single monthly dose of rifampicin (600 mg) and clofazimine (300 mg), along with daily 50 mg clofazimine.
- Rifampicin resistance–In a case of MB relapse the patient should receive the following alternate regimen for 24 months-Initial 6 months phase of using at least two of the following second-line drugs [1. Clarithromycin, 2. Minocycline or 3. Quinolone (ofloxacin/levofloxacin/moxifloxacin)] with daily 50 mg clofazimine followed by another 18 months phase with continuation of one of the second-line drug along with 50 mg clofazimine.
- Rifampicin plus ofloxacin resistance: Here also the patients are treated for 24 months. Clofazimine, clarithromycin and minocycline are used for initial 6 months followed by either of clarithromycin or minocycline with additional clofazimine for another 18 months.

iii. Prevention of relapse

Based on the available knowledge on the risk factors for relapse the following measures may be taken to prevent the occurrence of relapse:

- Patients who received dapsone monotherapy in the past may be given a 12-month course of MB MDT.
- Ensure that all new patients are properly classified into PB and MB leprosy; that they are administered the appropriate regimen; and that it is taken regularly for the specified period. Ensure that MB leprosy patients are not misclassified as PB leprosy and given a less effective regimen.
- In patients with a baseline high BI of 3+ or more, some workers/researchers suggest that they may be treated with 24 months of MB MDT or until smear negativity (which was the 1982 MDT recommendation of WHO).
- Wherever possible in MB patients carry out drug resistance studies, especially in those with high initial BI.
- When patients develop recurrent ENL after the completion of the FDT of 12 months it may be beneficial to continue MB MDT for a further 6 months to 1 year. Moreover, use of daily clofazimine in antireaction dosage would help manage both the ENL as well as prevent relapse.

Practical challenges in diagnosing and management: For an accurate diagnosis of relapse, it is important that proper case charts and investigations are recorded and stored for each patient. Charting of skin lesions, serial skin smear examination and skin biopsy records; at baseline, at the time of RFT and at follow-up would help in arriving at a definitive diagnosis of relapse. In the field much will depend on the eliciting a proper treatment history. With skin smears being done away in the national program, it is important that skin smears are continued to be done in medical colleges and tertiary centres considering how important it is in diagnosing relapse.

As the availability of serological tests to predict or diagnose relapse is still limited at present, there is a need to further develop and bring such tests to point-of-care in due course. Developing a screening tool for relapse with high specificity and sensitivity is vital.

The current WHO policy is to release patients from treatment (RFT) after completion of fixed duration MDT (FDT) even when there are clinical and bacteriological signs of activity. Sometimes, this continued activity can be a practical problem as it can be mistaken as a relapse.

SUMMARY

- Relapse is a key indicator of the efficacy of a treatment regimen.
- Risk factors for relapse include insufficient or irregular treatment and drug resistance which need to be recognized and addressed. Proper classification, effective treatment regimen and good patient adherence/treatment compliance can play a key role in preventing relapse.
- Early post-RFT events include lepra reactions and it is important to differentiate it from relapse.
- Good clinical history taking that includes a detailed treatment history is vital before labelling a case of relapse. This combined with dependable skin smear services can help in the accurate diagnosis of relapse.

REFERENCES

1. Nery JAC, Sales AM, Hacker MAVB, Moraes MO, Maia RC, Sarno EN, et al. Low rate of relapse after twelve-dose multidrug therapy for Hansen's disease: A 20-year cohort study in a Brazilian reference center. PLoS Negl Trop Dis 2021;15(5): e0009382.
2. World Health Organization. Organisation mondiale de la Santé. (2021). Weekly Epidemiological Record, 2021, vol. 96, 36 [full issue]. Weekly Epidemiological Record = Relevé épidémiologique hebdomadaire, 96 (36), 421–44. World Health Organization = Organisation mondiale de la Santé. https://apps.who.int/iris/handle/10665/345048.
3. WHO. A guide for surveillance of antimicrobial resistance in leprosy. 2017 update. Delhi: World Health Organization; 2017.
4. Kaimal S, Thappa DM. Relapse in leprosy. Indian J Dermatol Venereol Leprol 2009; 75:126–35.
5. NLEP, Disability prevention and medical rehabilitation, Guidelines for primary, secondary and tertiary level care, CLD, DGHS, MHandFW, Govt of India. 2012.
6. Ramu G. Clinical features and diagnosis of relapses in leprosy. Indian J Lepr. 1995;67(1):45–59.
7. Nascimento AC, Dos Santos DF, Antunes DE, Gonçalves MA, Santana MA, Dornelas BD, Goulart LR, Goulart IM. Leprosy Relapse: A Retrospective Study on Epidemiologic, Clinical, and Therapeutic Aspects at a Brazilian Referral Center. Int J Infect Dis. 2022:44–51.
8. Pannikar VK, Jesudasan K, Vijaykumaran P, Christian M. Relapse or late reversal reaction? Int. J Lepr. 1989;57(2):526–8.
9. Lockwood DNJ, Butlin CR, Penna GO. Current leprosy multi-drug treatment duration for MB patients (12 months) produces good clinical outcomes over many years; Lepr Rev; 2021;92;2;97–101.
10. Singh I, Sengupta U. Drug resistance in *Mycobacterium leprae* in the context of zero leprosy. Indian Dermatol Online J 2021;12:791–5.
11. Singh S, Kumar A, Nath G, Singh T, Mishra M. Resistance to anti leprosy drugs in multibacillary leprosy: A cross sectional study from a tertiary care centre in eastern Uttar Pradesh, India. Indian J Dermatol Venereol Leprol. 2018; 84:275–9.
12. Hambridge T, Nanjan Chandran SL, Geluk A, Saunderson P, Richardus JH. *Mycobacterium leprae* transmission characteristics during the declining stages of leprosy incidence: a systematic review. PLoS Neglected Tropical Diseases. 2021;15(5):e0009436.
13. World Health Organization. Guidelines for the diagnosis, treatment and prevention of leprosy. https://www.who.int/lep/resources/9789290226383/ en/. Published October 2018.
14. Lavania M, Jadhav RS, Chaitanya VS, Turankar R, Selvasekhar A, Das L, Darlong F, Hambroom UK, Kumar S, Sengupta U. Drug resistance patterns in Mycobacterium leprae isolates from relapsed leprosy patients attending The Leprosy Mission (TLM) Hospitals in India. Leprosy review. 2014;85(3):177–85.
15. Saar M, Hanus I, Huber K, Beissner M, Löscher T, Bretzel G. Report on an unusual case of leprosy from Germany: just an exception of the rule? Infection. 2019;47(6):1065–9.
16. Prabu R, Manickam P, Mahalingam VN, Jayasree P, Selvaraj V, Mehendale SM. Relapse and deformity among 2177 leprosy patients released from treatment with MDT between 2005 and 2010 in South India: A retrospective cohort study. Lepr Rev. 2015;86(4):345–55.

17. Arora P, Sardana K, Agarwal A, Lavania M. Resistance as a cause for chronic steroid dependent ENL-a novel paradigm with potential implications in management. Leprosy Review 2019;90(2):201–5.
18. Narang T, Kamat D, Thakur V, Lavania M, Singh I, Ahuja M, Dogra S. Equal rates of drug resistance in leprosy cases with relapse and recurrent/chronic Type 2 reaction: time to revise the guidelines for drug resistance testing in leprosy? Clinical and experimental dermatology 2022;47(2):297–302.
19. A guide for surveillance of antimicrobial resistance in leprosy: WHO 2017 update.
20. Job CK. Histopathological features of relapsed leprosy. Indian J Lepr. 1995;67(1):69–80. PMID:
21. Bührer-Sékula S, Cunha MG, Foss NT, Oskam L, Faber WR, Klatser PR. Dipstick assay to identify leprosy patients who have an increased risk of relapse. Trop Med Int Health. 2001;6(4):317–23.
22. Wu Q, Yin Y, Zhang L, *et al*. A study on a possibility of predicting early relapse in leprosy using a ND-O-BSA based ELISA. Int J Lepr Other Mycobact Dis. 2002;70(1):1–8.
23. Ule Belotti NC, Tonelli Nardi SM, Arco Paschoal VD, Martins Montanha JO, Paro Pedro Hd, Gazetta CE. Laboratory diagnosis of leprosy: Two staining methods from bacilloscopy and rapid ml flow test. Int J Mycobacteriol 2021;10:393–7.
24. Girdhar BK, Girdhar A, Kumar A. Relapses in multibacillary leprosy patients: effect of length of therapy. Lepr Rev. 2000;71(2):144–53.
25. Norman G, Joseph G, Richard J. Relapses in multibacillary patients treated with multi-drug therapy until smear negativity: findings after twenty years. Int J Lepr Other Mycobact Dis. 2004;72(1):1–7.
26. Neto FBA, Feitosa RDB, da Silva MS. Daily Moxifloxacin, Clarithromycin, Minocycline, and Clofazimine in Nonresponsiveness Leprosy Cases to Recommended Treatment Regimen. Int J Trop Dis 2020;3:035.

Chapter

20 Pure Neuritic Leprosy and Silent Neuritis

• Santoshdev P Rathod • P Narasimha Rao • Gauri Mahabal

INTRODUCTION

Pure neuritic leprosy (PNL) is a distinct type of leprosy in which there is nerve involvement in absence of skin lesions.[1,2] It is more frequently described from Indian subcontinent and has been recognized as a separate entity by the Indian Association of Leprologist's Classification of Leprosy of 1955 and 1981.[3,4] It is often difficult to diagnose this type of leprosy in the field due to the overlapping features with other peripheral neuropathies in absence of classic cutaneous lesions of leprosy. The lack of skin lesions often causes a delay in the diagnosis of PNL, which can lead to disability.

DEFINITIONS

Pure neuritic leprosy (PNL): it is defined as leprosy involving the peripheral nerve trunks in the absence of cutaneous signs.[3]

Criteria for Definition

- Essentially there should be thickened and/or tender peripheral (including cutaneous) nerves, with sensory impairment in the distribution area of the nerve, with or without motor impairment.
  And
- Typical skin lesions of leprosy should be absent
  And
- Slit skin smear should be negative for AFB

Current Available Knowledge on the Subject

Reported incidence varies from 4–17%.[1] It has been reported to be more common in men and in the 15–30 age group.[5] Published epidemiologic data by World Health Organization and National leprosy eradication program (NLEP) of India statistics don't include estimate of this subset of leprosy patients[2]. In the DermLep study conducted in India, pure neuritic leprosy (PNL) was the subset of leprosy in 5.06% of total patients.[6]

CLINICAL PRESENTATION

PNL presents with insidious development of sensory symptoms in form of paresthesia or numbness which are often most dominant and common along the area of distribution of the effected nerve. In addition, nerve thickening is palpably evident. However, there is large variation in the data as clinical evaluation of neural thickening requires skill and experience.[7]

With single nerve trunk involvement being the usual presentation, leprosy remains one of the most common causes of mononeuritis multiplex in the endemic countries of leprosy, wherein disease process affects one nerve at a time but eventually asymmetrical neuropathy involving multiple (≥2) nerves occurs. Due to the peripheral nerve involvement, sensory, autonomic and motor symptoms can occur (Box 20.1). While any peripheral nerve can be effected; ulnar, median, common peroneal, posterior tibial and sural nerves are the commonly affected nerves. Selective involvement of the facial nerve branches has also been reported.[8] In addition, there is a variable degree of 'neuritis' along with NFI in cases of PNL. Unfortunately, many patients of PNL also present with grade 2 disabilities at the time of initial diagnosis.

DIAGNOSIS

Generally, most of the PNL patients usually present to the general practitioners or neurologists, as there are no skin lesions. A proportion of them present with visible disability, e.g. a nonhealing ulcer or flexion deformity of a finger. One should keep high index of suspicion and always consider PNL as possible diagnosis if a person presents with clinical symptoms and/or signs suggestive of unilateral neuropathy in high endemic zones for leprosy.

Although nerve thickening is a pointer to PNL, there are other rare conditions in which a patient presents thickened nerves. Some of the conditions with peripheral nerve thickening are neurofibromatosis, pachydermo-periostosis, primary amyloidosis, familial hypertrophic interstitial neuropathy, recurrent or chronic progressive polyneuritis.

As already mentioned, while PNL can present as mononeuritis, other causes for mononeuritis multiplex need to be considered/ruled out in all suspected cases, which are vasculitis, lymphomas, polyarteritis nodosa, rheumatoid arthritis and diabetes mellites. In fact, mononeuritis in clinical practice is observed more commonly due to these causes than due to leprosy. However, in these conditions, unlike in PNL, the peripheral nerve thickening is absent.

Testing Methodology

Patient's whole body should be examined for typical leprosy skin lesions/patches. Classically there is absence of leprosy skin lesions/patches. A thorough peripheral nerve palpation and sensory testing should be done with SW monofilaments. Voluntary muscle testing should be done in all cases. Nerve conduction studies should be performed in all suspected cases of PNL wherever possible. (Table 20.1). In all suspected cases of PNL it is ideal to perform following routine investigations, Fasting and postprandial bloods sugar levels, Serum HBA1c levels, testing for HIV, HBsAg, and serology for syphilis. Always perform skin smear and skin biopsy from the hypoaesthetic skin of suspected PNL patients. Imaging of the effected nerve trunk and the spine would help rule out entrapment neuropathy, nerve sheath tumors and other causes. HRUS of peripheral nerve would help confirm the thickening of nerve and assess its integrity. Nerve biopsy can be performed for confirming the diagnosis of PNL.

Slit skin smear (SSS): By definition skin smear should be negative in pure neuritic leprosy. Hence to confirm it, it is advisable to perform SSS from standard sites in all suspected PNL

Box 20.1: Symptoms due to peripheral nerve involvement

***Sensory*:** Paresthesia or hypo/anesthesia, observed along the area of distribution of the effected nerve.

***Motor*:** Weakness/ paralysis of muscles supplied by the effected nerve, depending on the severity of nerve involvement.

***Autonomic*:** Variable degree of hypo/anhidrosis, xerosis, fissuring and ulcers along nerve distribution, depending on the severity of nerve involvement.

Table 20.1: Nerve conduction study	
Testing modality	***Salient features***
Electrophysiological studies	Reduction in the amplitude of motor and sensitive responses more than the decrease in velocity of nerve conduction is supportive diagnostic finding. Patterns seen on nerve conduction study: 1. Subclinical neuropathy (electroclinical dissociation). 2. Mononeuritis multiplex or mononeuritis (clinically and electrophysiologically). 3. Mosaic pattern of combined demyelinating and axonal changes (in electrophysiology).
Nerve conduction studies are dealt with in greater detail in Section 2, Chapter 9.	

cases. In case the skin smear is positive for AFB, the case should be considered as lepromatous form of leprosy.

Fine needle aspiration cytology (FNAC): In situations where nerve biopsy cannot be performed, FNAC of the nerve can be performed which is a less invasive and relatively safe diagnostic method. However, usage of mycobacterial antigen specific antibodies can further enhance diagnostic accuracy.[9]

Nerve biopsy: Nerve biopsy is the gold standard for diagnosis of PNL. To avoid the risk of motor nerve damage and residual effects preferably a pure sensory nerve supplying the area of involvement should be selected for biopsy. Nerve biopsy from PNL demonstrate the presence of epithelioid cell granuloma, perineural expansion, endoneural infiltrate, endoneural and perineural fibrosis and a reduction in the number of myelinated nerve fibers. However, low sensitivity and poor sampling are some of the risks of nerve biopsy. Use of immunolabeling of LAM or PGL-1 and DNA PCR (Refer to Chapter 12: 'Molecular Diagnosis of Leprosy' for further details) in the biopsy specimens is confirmatory. (Technique of nerve biopsy is described in detail in Section 2, Chapter 8).

Imaging studies: High resolution ultrasonography (HRUS) is useful tool to confirm and assess the enlargement of nerves. It has higher sensitivity than clinical examination and it also assists in identifying the location and extent of involvement. When combined with color doppler study, the presence of increased vascularity of nerves, suggests lepra reaction. (HRUS is described in detail in Section 2, Chapter 10).

Other investigations: Serological tests like detection of antibodies against PGL-1 are good for prediction of response to therapy but they are not specific for PNL. Some workers[10,11] have proposed diagnostic criteria using qPCR on skin biopsy sample, slit skin smear samples and ELISA anti-PGL 1. However, they are not practiced widely at present.

MANAGEMENT OF PURE NEURITIC LEPROSY

The management of PNL can be discussed under following:

a. Providing appropriate MDT.
b. Management of neuritis and disability.

MDT for PNL

The classification of PNL into PB and MB leprosy for therapeutic purposes, is not straightforward as there are no skin lesions to count. Hence, it should be based on the count of nerves involved. However, there are differences in the WHO and NLEP-India guidelines for grouping of patients based on the count of nerve lesions.

As per the NLEP Training Manual for Medical Officers (2019), all the patients with involvement of one peripheral nerve should be considered as PB leprosy, while those with >1 peripheral nerve involvement should be considered as MB leprosy. However, the WHO Guidelines for the Diagnosis, Treatment and Prevention of Leprosy (2018), considers a case of leprosy with nerve involvement, including pure neuritis or any number of skin lesions and neuritis as MB case; which infers that all PNL cases should be considered only as MB leprosy, irrespective of number of nerves involved.

In other words, as per NLEP-India recommendation, a case of PNL with a single nerve involvement should only receive PB MDT, while WHO recommends MB MDT to all cases of PNL, irrespective of number involved.

Many clinicians and workers tend to follow the WHO recommendation and consider all cases of PNL as MB for therapeutic purposes, as the assessment of nerve involvement by palpation is subjective and a greater number of nerves can be observed to be involved when methods like HRUS are used.

As per current WHO recommendation, a 3-drug regimen of rifampicin, dapsone and clofazimine may be used for all leprosy patients, with a duration of treatment of 6 months for PB leprosy and of 12 months for MB leprosy. It should be noted that MDT does not halt the progression of nerve damage and patient may also develop disability after successful completion of MDT.

Management of Neuritis

All PNL cases have an associated clinical or subclinical neuritis. When neuritis is manifest, and/ or associated with NFI, such cases should be managed with corticosteroids in doses as required for management of type 1 reaction. In cases of motor NFI of recent onset (<6 months duration), appropriate steroid therapy would help to regain lost function, when given along with physiotherapy. However, the role of prophylactic use of steroids in patients of PNL is debatable.[12] (Management of type 1 reaction is elaborated in Section 4; Chapter 23 and principles of physiotherapy in leprosy is discussed in Section 5, Chapter 28).

Management of Disability

In almost all patients of PNL there will be associated anesthesia or hypoesthesia (grade 1 disability) of the limb involved. In some patients it would have, unfortunately, progressed to grade 2 disability. All patients should be advised about self-care measures and care of anesthetic limb which are discussed elsewhere in this book. Those with G2D should be advised specific preventive and remedial measures, including physiotherapy and supports. (*see* Section 5, Chapters 29 and 30).

SUMMARY

It is important to arrive at a correct diagnosis of PNL for its effective management and prevention of disabilities. The management of PNL includes provision of MDT along with the control of neuritis with corticosteroids.[9] The primary goal of treatment of neuritis is to provide adequate dose and duration of analgesics and corticosteroids to relieve the patient's symptoms and prevent nerve damage. When nerve function impairment is less than 6 months old, rapid improvement of nerve function can occur with such therapy. However, physiotherapy has an important role in recovery. Nonetheless, regeneration and recovery of function following severe nerve damage takes several months and sometimes does not occur at all.[13]

Silent Neuritis

When patients with leprosy have abnormal nerve conduction studies without any clinical evidence of mechanosensory and/or motor impairment in an area of a limb innervated by one or more nerves is categorized as "subclinical neuropathy."[13] However, when a leprosy patient develops a new NFI or worsening of existing sensory or motor nerve function without overt signs or symptoms of inflammation of nerve/s involved it is called ***Silent neuritis or neuropathy***.[14] It may also occur in patients with other forms of leprosy apart from pure neuritic leprosy.

Terms like 'quiet nerve paralysis', 'silent nerve paralyses' are used interchangeably with silent neuritis, which point to neuropathy with motor impairment, but without complaints of nerve pain, paresthesia or nerve tenderness on palpation. It does not refer to the chronic insidious destructive neuropathy of lepromatous leprosy, but rather to the episodes of neuropathy that cause clinical nerve damage within a relatively short period of weeks to months.

Pathophysiology, while not very clear, lies in the way how *M. leprae* affect nerves. In the initial stages it affects nerves without activating the inflammatory process, and in the later stages when the bacillus promotes Schwann cell (SC) parasitism altering nerve function. Essentially it is a condition in which sensory or sensory-motor nerve dysfunction occurs without clinical symptoms of pain associated with acute neuritis and evolves indolently and passes usually unnoticed by the patient till he/she develops manifest NFI.

Studies have reported that when nerve function was assessed for sensations using a nylon filament and VMT performed to test to motor function, as many as 7% of newly presenting patients had silent nerve paralysis at their initial examination, and 75% of all silent nerve paralysis episodes occurred during the first year of MDT.[13]

Therefore, due to lack of obvious symptoms, it can be easily missed if thorough nerve function assessment is not done at every follow-up. Hence, it is vital to have a high index of suspicion and perform periodical detailed neurological evaluation at every visit for the identification and management of silent neuritis and resulting NFI. When observed, it should be managed with steroid therapy in doses as recommended for other types of leprous neuritis.

REFERENCES

1. Kumar B, Kaur I, Dogra S, Kumaran MS. Pure neuritic leprosy in India: an appraisal. Int J Lepr Other Mycobact Dis. 2004;72(3):284–90.
2. Narang T, Vinay K, Kumar S, Dogra S. A critical appraisal on pure neuritic leprosy from India after achieving WHO global target of leprosy elimination. Lepr Rev. 2016;87(4):456–63.
3. Cinical histopathological and immunological features of the five type classification approved by the Indian association of leprologists. Lepr India 1982;54:22–5.
4. Rao PN, Suneetha S. Pure neuritic leprosy: Current status and relevance. Indian J Dermatol Venereol Leprol. 2016;82(3):252–61.
5. Mendiratta, V Khan A, Jain A. Primary neuritic leprosy: A reappraisal at a tertiary care hospital. Indian J Lep 2006;78(3), 261–7.
6. Rao PN, Rathod S, Suneetha S, Dogra S, Gupta SK, Vora R, et al. The DermLep Study I: Results of Prospective Nation-Wide Survey of the Number and Profile of Leprosy Patients seen by Dermatologists in India. Indian Dermatol Online J. 2020;11(5):701–7.
7. Mafoyane NA, Jacyk WK, Lotz, BP. Primary neuritic leprosy in a black South African. Lepr Rev; 1992:63(3), 277–81.
8. Lima PO, Cunha FM, Gonçalves HS, Aires MA, De Almeida RL, Kerr LR. Correlation between clinical tests and electroneuromyography for the diagnosis of leprosy neuropathy. Lepr Rev. 2016;87(1):60–70.
9. Narang T, Vinay K, Kumar S, Dogra S. A critical appraisal on pure neuritic leprosy from India after achieving WHO global target of leprosy elimination. Lepr Rev 2016;87(4), 456–63.
10. Santos DFd, Mendonça MR, Antunes DE, Sabino EFP, Pereira RC, et al. Revisiting primary neural leprosy: Clinical, serological, molecular, and neurophysiological aspects. PLoS Negl Trop Dis 2017;11(11): e0006086.

11. Wilder-Smith E. Diagnosis of pure neuritic leprosy. Neurol J Southeast Asia 2002; 7: 61–3.
12. Kumar B. Pure or Primary neuritic Leprosy (PNL). Lepr Rev. 2016;87(4):450–5.
13. Ebenezer GJ, Scollard DM. Treatment and Evaluation Advances in Leprosy Neuropathy. Neurotherapeutics 2021;18(4), 2337–50.
14. Van Brakel W, Cross H, Declercq E, Deepak S, Lockwood D, Saunderson P, et al. ILEP Technical Commission. Review of leprosy research evidence (2002–2009) and implications for current policy and practice. Lepr Rev 2010;81(3):228–75.

Chapter

21 Visible Skin Lesions of Leprosy: Issues and Management

• P Narasimha Rao • Santoshdev P Rathod

INTRODUCTION

With most countries achieving the global elimination target and decline in the number of leprosy patients, healthcare providers (HCP) are now faced with the unique challenge to address the needs of patients released-from-treatment (RFT) one of which is the 'persisting skin lesions.' While this is a common occurrence, very few studies are available on this aspect, hence the magnitude of the problem is not fully known. However, a retrospective the study done in India observed that about 15% of RFT patients complain of persistent skin lesions.[1]

There are two aspects to these persistent skin patches. First, a patient who has visited the HCP for the presence of skin patch for its management would expect that all skin lesions to disappear with a successful treatment. While they are concerned about the presence of skin patches while on treatment, their incomplete regression and/or non-disappearance after completion of MDT, disappoint them greatly. Their persistence, especially on exposed areas of skin would be a cause of embarrassment for the patient, and as they look forward to a healthy blemish-less skin posttreatment. Hence, many a person affected seek advice on remedial measures and management options for them, both while on MDT and more often, after RFT. Second, these persistent lesions being visible contributes to 'enacted stigma' by the community on the individual. In addition, it also leads to 'anticipated stigma' which refers to expectations of stigma experiences happening in the future, which occurs in individuals with such visible skin conditions.[2] Therefore, management of active or residual skin lesions on face and exposed parts of the body assume great importance in the fight against stigma. This chapter outlines the management and required work-up for the patients with persistent skin lesions.

DEFINITIONS

- **Persistent skin lesions of leprosy**: These are skin lesions that do not improve and remain visible after completing their scheduled duration of MDT or even after patient has become smear negative.[1]
- **Anticipated stigma**: It is defined as belief that prejudice, discrimination and stereotyping will be directed at the self from others in the future.[2]
- **Enacted stigma**: Also known as external stigma and discrimination, refers to the experience of unfair treatment by others.[3,4]
- **Cosmetic camouflage:** The art of concealing a discoloration, blemish or scar with the application of specialist camouflage creams that are matched to the surrounding skin tone.[5]
- **Release from treatment (RFT) case:** A person who has completed a full course of treatment with WHO recommended MDT of required duration.

CURRENT AVAILABLE KNOWLEDGE ON THE SUBJECT

According to *the dermlep study*, active or persistent skin lesions were the most common reason to consult a dermatologist in 21.2% patients following release from treatment.[6] Persistent skin patches of leprosy can occur on any part of the body, but when persist for a long time on face cause greatest distress to the patient. While persistent hypopigmented patches are the common occurrence, they can occasionally be hyperpigmented or atrophic skin patches as well. Facial patches of leprosy can be of varying morphology ranging from hypopigmented to pale macules to red raised patches. The erythema is pronounced due to type 1 lepra reaction, which may present and persist very late, for many years following RFT. Moreover, some of these regressed facial skin patches become obvious as they become erythematous on exposure to sunlight. As these reactions and changes are known to occur more commonly on face, these may remain noticeable for months and years, with associated erythema on and off on residual hypopigmentation. Recent comparative DLQI studies have shown that leprosy patients experience similar level of stigma and deterioration of quality of life, as vitiligo patients.[7]

Approach to a patient with persistent hypopigmented/ erythematous patches: Patients complaining of persistent lesions following RFT, should be first ascertained if this is an active ongoing disease or 'residual effect' of leprosy. Check if baseline charting/topographic drawings and mapping the skin lesions of the patient are available. In clinical practice; unavailability of such baseline charting of skin lesions is a major drawback. Check if the lesions have increased from the baseline, decreased or are static in nature. Rule out on-going late type-1 lepra reaction and if present, institute appropriate treatment. This is because, when type 1 reaction is controlled, the skin patches become less obvious.

If in doubt, perform skin biopsy to rule out ongoing disease or lepra reaction, which requires continuation of anti-leprosy MDT and/or treatment of type 1 reaction (Box 21.1).

Cosmetic Camouflage

It works on the principles of 'protective concealment' that is to disguise an object in plain view, for the purpose of concealing it from something or someone.[5] Cosmetic camouflage is a great tool which can help improve the patient's appearance considerably, thereby improving self-esteem and quality of life. Most camouflage cosmetics should be inert, fragrance free, specially designed to be hypoallergenic and gentle on the skin.[5]

Cosmetic camouflage (Fig. 21.1) can be considered and offered for all patients of leprosy with visible skin patches on face and exposed area of body, to reduce stigma as mentioned below:

a. For hypopigmented or raised skin patches on face and exposed areas in *patients with active disease*
b. For *'residual skin patches'* of any kind on face and exposed areas of body *in RFT patients*
c. For *Hyper-pigmented skin patches*, including those due to clofazimine induced pigmentation.
d. For all patients with *persistent facial erythema*, on active or inactive skin patches.

Box 21.1: Features suggestive of 'type 1 reaction' in a skin patch

- Lesional erythema
- Lesional hyperalgesia upon stroking the lesion
- Associated neuritis

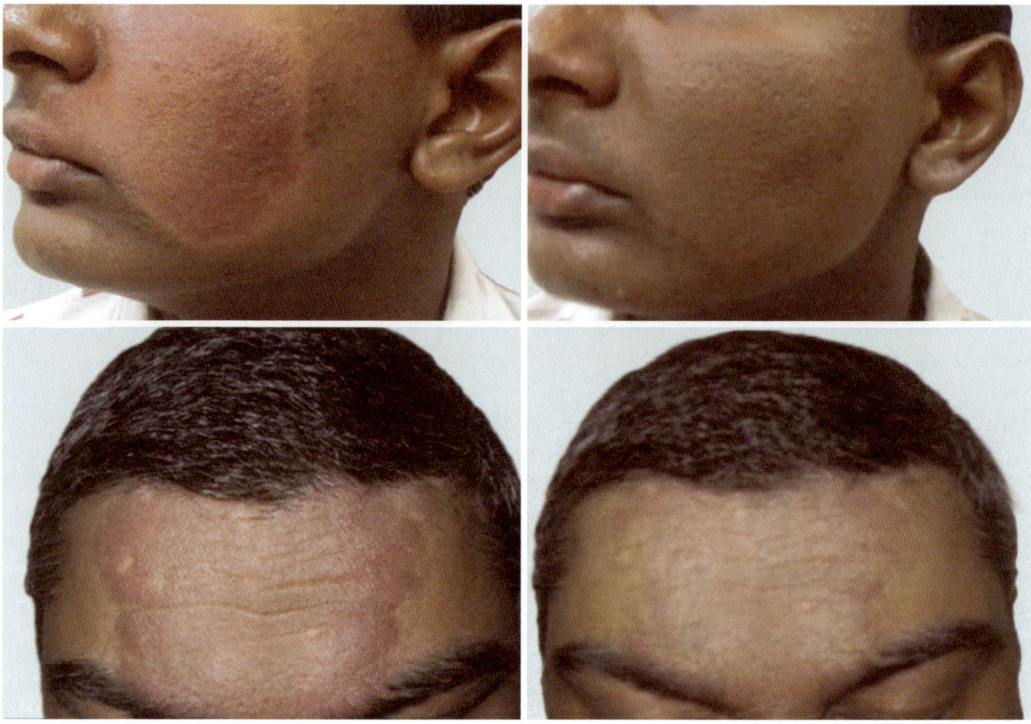

Fig. 21.1: Patients with facial lesions before and after application of camouflage.[7] (*Courtesy:* From the open access publication in leprosy review by Rao PN, Vellala M, Potharaju AR, Kiran KU. Cosmetic camouflage of visible skin lesions enhances life quality indices in leprosy as in vitiligo patients: an effective stigma reduction strategy; Lepr Rev; 2020;91:343–52.)

Available tools are camouflage kit and erythema regressing lotions

a. Dermacolor camouflage creme kit (Kryolan, USA): This kit is available in various shades and these shades can be mixed to achieve desired skin type matching the natural appearance and proper color match with the adjoining skin.[8] Basically, it is a temporary make up and removable after the use. Such a camouflage is more suitable for facial and neck lesions. It can be fixed using a powder to make it stay for long hours, and can be reapplied as and when required. Such a make-up takes about 5–10 minutes to cover a patch of size of a palm. Patients need to be educated about the use of camouflage and demonstrated how to apply the camouflage product on the skin lesion.

   In the Indian market, domestic cosmetic products, e.g. (a) Forever face-concealer palette (Fig. 21.2), (b) Lakme color corrector, are available for camouflage of skin lesions.

b. Topical agents for management of persistent erythema

   Topical brimonidine gel 0.33% lotion is used for control of persistent facial erythema, and it is widely used in patients of rosacea.[9] It can be of benefit if used in leprosy patient with facial patches with persistent erythema. After application the effect of brimonidine starts within 30 minutes and maximum effect is achieved after 3–6 hours and fades after 10–12 hours. However, there are few reports of rebound erythema after 12 hours. As such there is no published literature or studies of brimonidine gel use for control of erythematous lesions over face in leprosy but it has good a potential for use in patients of leprosy with stigmatising erythematous facial patches.

In addition, off-label and anecdotal use of topical tacrolimus and short duration topical corticosteroids also have been suggested for control of edema and erythema of facial patches of leprosy.[10]

Of all the above methods, cosmetic camouflage is a simple, safe, repeatable method and without any adverse effects, which hides the skin blemishes effectively. It should be promoted and offered to all patients with visible patches of leprosy, both while on anti-leprosy treatment and also for RFT patients with persistent skin lesions, as it significantly improves the quality of life and reduces stigma associated with them.

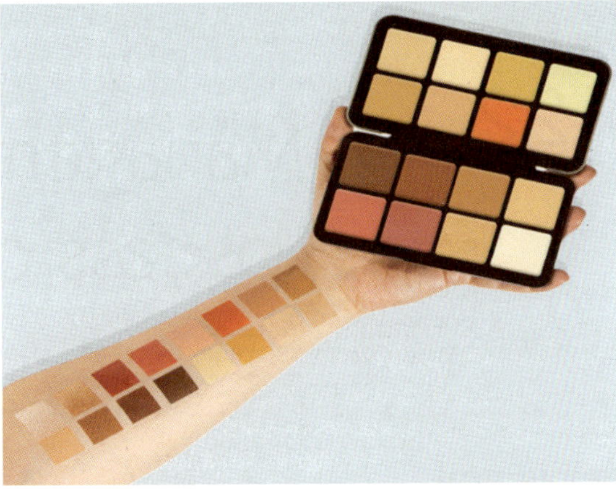

Fig. 21.2: Pallet containing various shades of camouflage

SUMMARY

Looking good and blemish free is a normal universal desire of human beings, it applies to leprosy affected as well. While a lot of attention was paid to treatment and management of leprosy the disease, little attention has gone into management of residual blemishes of leprosy affected. Self-image and appearance has a very powerful role in affecting social interactions with people, and patients with low self-image due to disfigurements experience stigma from society on a day-to-day basis. While this chapter emphasized on management of facial patches, same methods can be used for visible skin patches on other areas of body such as arms or hands. Covering skin defects of contour and color, which are visible signs of the disease with camouflage minimizes stigmatization. Moreover, cosmetic camouflage improves the quality of life of patients without interfering with the treatment.[7]

REFERENCES

1. Narang T, Bishnoi A, Thakur V, et al. Persistent plaques after release from treatment in slit-skin smear negative leprosy patients: Wait and watch or adopt a proactive approach? Dermatologic Therapy. 2020;e14226.
2. van Brakel WH. Measuring leprosy stigma—a preliminary review of the leprosy literature. Int J Lepr Other Mycobact Dis. 2003;71: 190–7.
3. Quinn DM, Chaudoir SR. Living with a concealable stigmatized identity: the impact of anticipated stigma, centrality, salience, and cultural stigma on psychological distress and health. J Pers Soc Psychol. 2009;97:634–51.
4. Gray AJ. Stigma in psychiatry. J R Soc Med. 2002;95:72–6.
5. Antoniou C, Stefanaki C. Cosmetic camouflage. J Cosmet Dermatol, 2006; 5: 297–301.
6. Rao PN, Suneetha S, Rathod SP, et al. Dermlep Study Part 3: Post-RFT events in leprosy patients presenting to dermatologists. Indian Dermatol Online J. 2022;13:340–5.
7. Rao PN, Vellala M, Potharaju AR, Kiran KU. Cosmetic camouflage of visible skin lesions enhances life quality indices in leprosy as in vitiligo patients: an effective stigma reduction strategy; Lepr Rev; 2020;91:343–52.
8. Kryolan professional makeup-dermacolor; https://in.kryolan.com/product-lines/dermacolor/palettes. [accessed 2020 June 18].
9. Jackson JM, Knuckles M, Minni JP, Johnson SM, Belasco KT. The role of brimonidine tartrate gel in the treatment of rosacea. Clin Cosmet Investig Dermatol. 2015;8:529–38.
10. Safa G, Darrieux L, Coic A, Tisseau L. Type 1 leprosy reversal reaction treated with topical tacrolimus along with systemic corticosteroids. Indian J Med Sci. 2009;63:359–62.

Chapter 22

Management of Nerve Abscess due to Leprosy

• Vivek M Pai • Preethi B Nayak

INTRODUCTION

Leprosy is a disease of the skin and nerves. The reservoir of *Mycobacterium leprae* in nerve tissue is Schwann cell. Neuropathy due to leprosy is still diagnosed and treated late, leading to permanent disability in about 25% of patients.[1] Nerve abscess is an uncommon presentation of leprosy. The presence of a fluctuant swelling on or within a fusiform swollen peripheral nerve suggests a nerve abscess. Usually, patients with nerve abscess tend to belong to tuberculoid end of the spectrum, and often some nerve function impairment will be present. Moreover, tuberculoid (paucibacillary) patients with type 1 reaction have a higher tendency to develop nerve abscess.[2–4] When it occurs in association with type 1 reaction, the nerve abscess is usually solitary, but can rarely be multiple along the course of a nerve or involving multiple nerves, especially in pure-neural leprosy patients. It may also be rarely seen in a patient with type 2 (ENL) reaction in lepromatous leprosy.

CURRENT KNOWLEDGE

Ulnar nerve is the most common nerve involved, followed by lateral popliteal, median and posterior tibial nerves. Nonetheless, nerve abscess can be observed in any involved cutaneous nerve, e.g. great auricular nerve, supratrochlear, radial cutaneous nerve. Nerve abscesses could be single or multiple. There are reports of multiple abscesses in a single nerve as well as multiple abscesses involving various nerve trunks. Nerve abscesses in leprosy are usually "cold abscesses", similar to those in tuberculosis. The size of the abscess ranges from very small (minute microabscesses) to very large 'giant' abscesses, many centimeters long and wide. However, the presence of the abscess or it growing in size does not indicate disease activity. Left alone, smaller abscesses tend to subside on their own while larger abscesses often do not do so. They are relatively painless, or in few patients may have only mild nerve pain. Intraneural abscess can be associated with significant nerve function impairment depending on its location in the nerve due to pressure effects. Extent of nerve function impairment is irrespective of nerve abscess size and even a small intraneural abscess can be associated with significant nerve function impairment depending on its location in the nerve.[4–6] Nerve function impairment occurs due to vascular damage caused by intra neural pressure secondary to inflammation and abscess formation, resulting in tissue anoxia. There would also be release of serotonin, which further increases the edema.

The abscess occurs usually within a swollen nerve as a fusiform swelling or it may rarely herniate like a pedunculated cyst which can be felt on the nerve (Fig. 22.1). Occasionally,

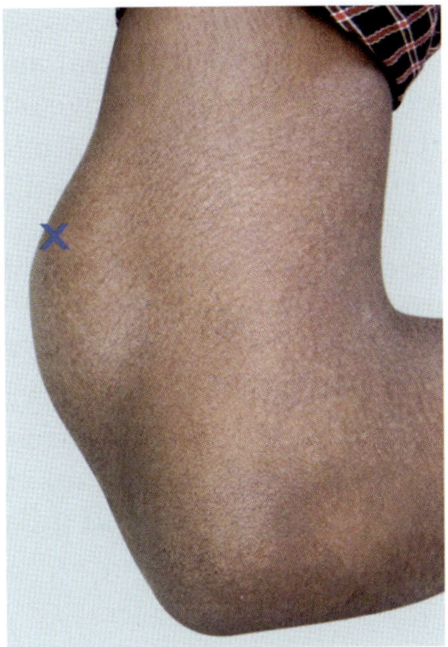

Fig. 22.1: Ulnar nerve abscess in a patient with BT Leprosy. The marked site indicates the point of insertion for drainage. Aspiration can be attempted with 19 or 20 G needle from the marked site (non-dependent) followed by medical decompression by injecting 20 mg/ml of triamcinolone acetonide. Maximum amount to be injected not to be more than 1 ml. The procedure can be repeated at 3 weeks. *Courtesy:* Dr Archana Singhal, Director Professor and head, GTB Hospital, Delhi.

pus may track through the epineurium and come out as a collar stud abscess to form a 'para-neural' abscess. It is characterized by necrosis of one or more fascicles within the nerve with pus production and a capsule formation. The swelling can be fluctuant and mobile transversally but not longitudinally.

DIAGNOSIS

In an otherwise healthy person, differential diagnosis mentioned in Box 22.1 should be ruled out for swelling along the course of nerve. In an individual with confirmed leprosy, diagnosis is relatively straightforward and made on clinical grounds. However, the diagnosis of an abscess should always be confirmed by imaging, either by high-resolution ultrasonography (HRUS) or magnetic resonance imaging (MRI). Aspiration of purulent material from the abscess can be of both diagnostic and therapeutic value. The fine-needle aspirate usually is sterile for bacteria on microbiological culture.[7] AFB can occasionally be detected by Fite stain.

Box 22.1: Differential diagnosis of nerve abscess

- Neurofibroma
- Plexiform neurofibroma
- Malignant peripheral nerve sheath tumor
- Neural lipoma
- Nontumor causes, such as intraneuronal ganglion cyst, pseudoneuroma can produce localized nerve swellings
- Non-neural conditions:
  - Lymph node swellings
  - Subcutaneous lipoma

HRUS has been found to be a very useful tool in the assessment of nerve enlargement in leprosy. It reveals heteroechoic collection, with central anechoic lesion suggestive of abscess fluid and peripheral hyperechoic shadow suggestive of the debris or organized pus. Serial HRUS following every percutaneous aspiration is extremely helpful in assessing the therapeutic response. On the whole, HRUS can be a useful tool for the diagnosis and follow-up of nerve pathology in leprosy patients, especially in diagnosing nerve abscess at very early stages.[8] Additionally, evidence of reaction can also be observed as increased neural vascular signals on color doppler imaging.

However, MRI neurography has a niche indication when it is difficult to differentiate nerve abscess from other pathologies like nodular neuropathies, soft tissue tumors and nerve sheath tumors, as it helps to provide the precise extent and type of involvement. Leprosy-associated nerve abscess usually reveals signal changes of an abscess with peripheral contrast enhancement of the abscess wall and inflammatory thickening of the whole nerve trunk.

TREATMENT

Medical Management

The first line of management must be directed towards control of the disease process with a course of steroids, anti-inflammatory medication and splinting if the nerve is painful. Multidrug therapy (MDT) should be continued and oral prednisolone in the dose of 1 mg/kg body weight has to be initiated. It has to be tapered by 5–10 mg at 4-week intervals.

Surgical Management

Decision on surgical management of the abscess depends primarily on the state of the nerve affected:

a. Significant NFI by way of anesthesia in its area or paralysis/weakness of the muscles supplied by that nerve.
b. Severe pain in the swelling along the nerve with a new deficit.
c. Abscess involves the overlying skin with an imminent danger of it bursting through. Of these, severe pain with new deficit and threatening rupture through skin need immediate expert surgical intervention.

Needle aspiration of pus: Nerve abscess can be decompressed under local anesthesia by antigravity percutaneous aspiration, using a 21 gauge wide-bored needle. At every 10–14 days interval, aspiration can be repeated. For reduction of inflammation, triamcinolone acetonide (20 mg/ml) can be injected perineurally post-aspiration. Physiotherapy can be advised to patients.

Surgical decompression: A chronic, or recurrent abscess can be surgically exposed under regional or general anesthesia, the abscess cavity opened and drained with longitudinal epi-neurotomy and very carefully cleaned of its pseudo-capsule wall, without avulsing nerve fascicles. The wound is then closed without drain with separate fascial layers to reduce the chance of a chronic wound sinus. Under no circumstances should the abscess be surgically excised as this might slice through nerve fascicles that might otherwise have recovered. It has to be performed by an expert under aseptic conditions. Excellent sensory recovery can be observed, earlier than motor recovery. Sensory recovery was seen more in younger than in older age group.[9] The patient should be followed up as needed till recovery.

SUMMARY

Nerve abscesses are an unusual presentation of leprosy. When found, they are particularly seen in paucibacillary spectrum of the disease and commonly involve the ulnar nerve. External (needle aspiration) and internal nerve trunk decompression is indicated when medical management of does not benefit the patient. When followed up, it was observed that these procedures relieve the the pain in nerves with significant sensory recovery. The sensory recovery restores protective sensation which prevents secondary injuries. The improvement of motor power will provide more functional hands and improved appearance.

REFERENCES

1. Siddalingaswamy MK, Rao KS. Nerve abscess in leprosy: a retrospective study. Leprosy review. 1993;64:357–61.
2. Fritschi EP. Surgical reconstruction and rehabilitation in leprosy. TLM New Delhi. 1984.
3. Virmond M, Joshua J, Solomon S, Duerksen F. Surgical aspects in leprosy. The International Textbook of Leprosy. Scollard DM, Gillis TP.
4. Thomas M., Emmanuel M. Facial nerve abscess in a case of leprosy—a case report. Neurol Asia. 2009;14: 41–2.
5. Rao PN, Suneetha S. Pure neuritic leprosy: Current status and relevance. Indian J Dermatol Venereol Leprol. 2016;82:252–61.
6. Arora A, Kaul B, Singh A. Multiple peroneal nerve abscesses: The first presentation of borderline tuberculoid leprosy Biomed Biotechnol Res J. 2018;2:159–60.
7. Kiran CM, Menon R. Fine needle aspiration cytology as an aid to diagnosis, categorization and treatment when pure neuritic leprosy presents as nerve abscess. J Cytol. 2013;30:237–40.
8. Sen D, Satija L, Chatterji S, Majumder A, Gupta A, Kumar A. Ultrasonography and magnetic resonance imaging of ulnar nerve abscess in leprosy. Med J Armed Forces India. 2016;72:78–81.
9. Bhagat KP, Wange HM, Tekani BU. Management of Nerve Abscesses in Leprosy. Indian Journal of Dermatology, Venereology and Leprology. 1980;46:110–2.

Chapter 23

Management of Type 1 Lepra Reaction with Emphasis on Neuritis

• Anupama Gopalan • Deepika Pandhi

INTRODUCTION

Type 1 reaction (T1R) in leprosy is a delayed hypersensitivity reaction characterized by swelling and redness of skin lesions.[1] Also known as "reversal reaction," it may occur in any form of leprosy, but borderline leprosy carries the highest risk as a result of its immunological instability. The importance of accurate diagnosis and early treatment of T1R is paramount as the resulting nerve function impairment (autonomic, sensory and/or motor) is the chief cause leading to disability among the leprosy affected persons.[2]

The occurrence of T1R indicates a shift in the immune status of the patient, which is usually observed either before or after initiation of multidrug therapy. Triggers like intercurrent infection, mental and/physical stress are also precipitate T1R among patients of unstable forms (borderline tuberculoid, mid-borderline and borderline lepromatous) of leprosy.[3]

CURRENT AVAILABLE KNOWLEDGE ON THE SUBJECT

A type 1 reaction limited to inflammation of existing skin lesions and characterised occasionally by the appearance of new lesions is considered a mild reaction. However, when it is associated with neuritis, it is considered severe T1R, as it can lead to impaired peripheral nerve function. Appearance of new skin lesions are in reality subclinical patches, now noticed due to inflammation. T1R may appear early within first year of initiation of MDT among borderline tuberculoid and late (post MDT) in patients of subpolar lepromatous group of patients. Reactions are also observed in untreated leprosy patients at the time of initial diagnosis; based on data from a study in three countries: Brazil, Nepal and the Philippines; around 22% of all new cases have some form of reaction.[3] In other words, T1R can be the first presenting sign of the disease in some patients. Recurrent T1R is defined as the reappearance of reactional signs or symptoms 6–12 weeks after the regression, following specific steroid or any other anti-inflammatory/immunosuppressive treatment.

Diagnosis is mainly clinical characterized by shiny, warm swelling and redness of pre-existing lesions. T1R affecting nerves manifest as severe neuritis, with inflammation of the peripheral nerves resulting in pain, paraesthesia, tenderness and nerve function impairment resulting in sensory and motor deficit, including acute nerve palsy. Presence of neuritis and ulceration within inflamed skin lesions indisputably classifies it as severe type of T1R. Neuritis can rarely be the only presenting feature of reaction without inflammation in the skin lesions. Intra ocular tissue is not affected in T1R but patient may develop corneal anaesthesia and lagophthalmos if neuritis involves trigeminal and facial nerves.

Histological features for diagnosis of T1R are: presence of epidermal erosion, spongiosis, dermal edema, edema within granuloma, and focal or diffuse immunostaining with histocompatibility complex DR antigen (HLA-DR).

TREATMENT

It is important to accurately classify T1R based on its severity into mild and severe type because if severe T1R is not treated adequately it is the single most important risk factor for development of disability. For assessing the severity and managing of T1R, the WHO technical guidance advocates (1) Nerve function assessment to identify any accompanying neuritis and (2) Laboratory tests to look for any contraindication for starting steroid therapy.[4] Any nerve function impairment of <6 months duration requires and known to respond to corticosteroid therapy. Assessment of nerve function impairment is detailed in Section 1, Chapter 5. If on assessment the limbs are found to be anesthetic, such patients should be counselled about how to take care of anesthetic hands and feet as described in Section 5, Chapter 29.

If the reaction is mild and there is no evidence of neuritis, nonsteroidal anti-inflammatory drugs (NSAIDs) such as acetyl salicylic acid, ibuprofen or paracetamol in required doses are usually sufficient to control symptoms. The healthcare provider should reassure the patient that T1R is not an adverse effect of MDT and on continuation of MDT uninterrupted and advice supporting measures. More important, however, is the severe T1R, wherein skin involvement is accompanied by inflammation in one or more nerves, known as neuritis. This can have serious consequences, including permanent nerve damage, impairment and disability. Nonetheless, it should also be noted that T1R involving only skin lesion can also be a possible pointer of impending neuritis of nerve supplying that segment of skin, which can happen over time.[5] Special attention should be paid to reactional lesions located over the face, because they are associated with a higher risk of facial nerve damage, resulting in lagophthalmos and its consequences.[6]

Corticosteroids

They remain the mainstay in the management of T1R. However, the ideal steroid regimen for treating reactions and neuritis, in terms of dose and duration, is still being debated. Prednisolone is the preferred corticosteroid molecule for the treatment. According to recently published technical guidance on management of T1R the starting dose should be between 0.5 and 1.0 mg per kg of body weight per day. In most settings 0.5 mg/kg daily would be an appropriate starting dose for a first course, meaning 40 mg daily for most adults. It may be given in single dose preferably in the morning after breakfast and the reaction is generally controlled within a few days.

Review the progress every two weeks. Attempt should be made to reduce the dose of steroid fortnightly by 5 mg and eventually stopped. If there is no response observed at end of that period, the same dose may be continued for further two weeks Alternatively, the reduction can be by 10 mg every 4 weeks, especially after reaching 20 mg/day dosage. Recent studies suggest that a course lasting 20 weeks gives the best results, starting at either 30 mg or 40 mg, depending on body weight.[7] Criteria for initiating and increasing the dose of corticosteroids are mentioned in Box 23.1.

Nonpharmacological Measures for Neuritis Accompanying Type 1 Reaction[2]

There are important nonpharmaceutical measures that should be employed in parallel to management of neuritis and NFI associated with it. Although this work is usually overseen

Box 23.1: Criteria for initiating and increasing the dose of corticosteroid[4]

- Type 1 reactions that are severe enough to cause skin ulceration or are
- Uncontrolled by paracetamol or NSAIDs (such as ibuprofen);
- Acute neuritis, as shown by the emergence of new nerve function impairment.
- Neuritis accompanying type 1 reaction, whether mild or severe, with pain in one or more nerves
- When silent neuritis is identified, i.e appearance of NFI without obvious symptoms of acute neuritis.

Criteria for additional prednisolone in recurrent T1R

Continued worsening of following symptoms while on treatment, for a period of at least two weeks:

- Progressing nerve function impairment (NFI)
- Continued neuritis and nerve pain
- Skin patches remain palpably swollen and/or appearance of new erythematous raised skin patches

by the physiotherapy department of referral centers, the basic measures mentioned below should ideally be undertaken wherever leprosy patients with neuritis and NFI are being managed.

- Resting of the affected limb in the acute phase can be aided by splinting, especially at night.
- Once the pain of the acute phase has reduced, passive stretching of any weakened muscles preserves joint mobility; active exercises then help to strengthen the weakened muscles.
- Soaking and oiling of dry skin helps to prevent cracking and preserves the integrity of the epidermis.
- As recovery begins, stretching and exercise therapy (outlined in Section 5, Chapters 28 to 30) can reduce pain and improve muscle function.

Sometimes nerve abscess can occur as a part of T1R, management of which is given in the preceding chapter (Section 4, Chapter 22). Rarely, surgery may be required to decompress the nerve in acute phase.

Management of T1R Not Responding Adequately to Conventional Dosage of Corticosteroids

Some patients do not respond adequately to corticosteroids or develop adverse effects to steroids requiring use of alternative drugs and adjuvants for steroid sparing effect and optimal control of T1R. When such a reactional episodes present as consecutive skin lesion flares or nerve impairments, precluding the patient's release from the corticosteroid treatment, some authors have termed it 'chronic T1R'[1].

Nevertheless, it should be noted that majority of T1R patients respond to 0.5 mg/kg of oral prednisolone therapy, but would rarely need to be put on higher dosages, up to 1 mg/kg bodyweight. It is only rarely that additional drugs like methotrexate, azathioprine, cyclosporine and other immunosuppressives are required to control neuritis during T1R, and there are anecdotal reports of benefit of their use. However, their use is not recommended by NLEP or WHO technical guidance on management of T1R and one should note that they need be used as adjuncts to the oral steroid therapy and not as substitutes.

Follow up of Patients with T1R

There are two important reasons for doing assessment for NFI regularly in all leprosy patients on treatment: (i) NFI may occur without any overt signs (e.g., pain) indicating a reaction;

Flowchart 23.1: Follow up of patients with type 1 reaction and neuritis

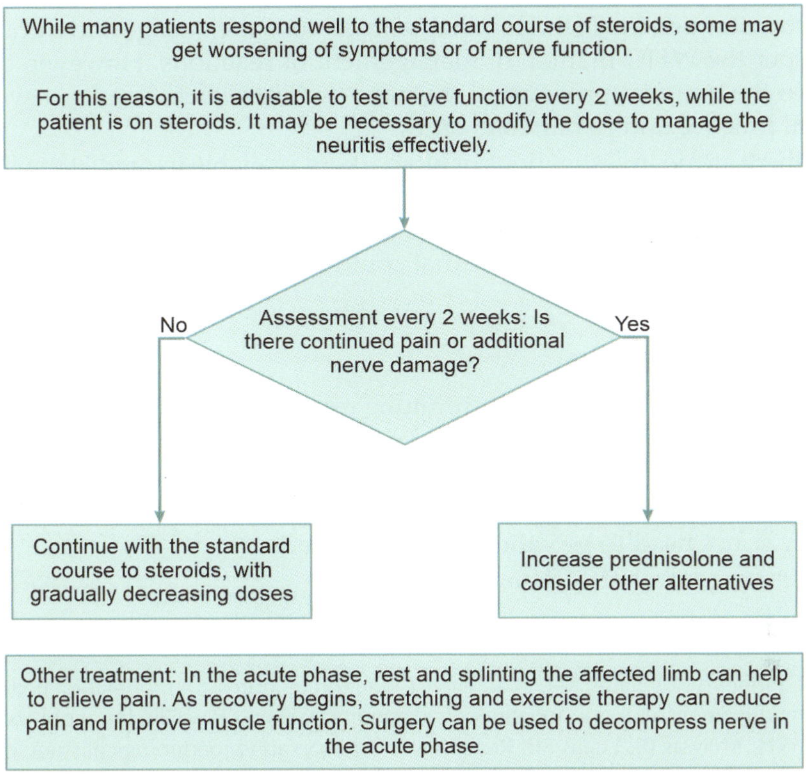

(ii) If NFI remains untreated for 6 months or more, recovery is unlikely. Patients' of T1R on corticosteroids should also be assessed every 2 weeks for worsening of nerve function or symptoms as mentioned in the Flowchart 23.1.[3]

Late Reversal Reactions

T1R are known to occur months and years after completion of MDT. Some workers label them as 'late reversal reactions'. By definition, reversal reactions observed within two years of completion of MDT have been labeled as late reversal reactions.[7] The principles of management of late T1R remain the same as of those occurring during the MDT. Moreover, occurrence/recurrence of T1R in post-RFT patient does not warrant reinitiation of MDT.[8] However it should be noted that clinically, it is often difficult to distinguish between relapse and late reversal reaction.

GAPS IN KNOWLEDGE

Some of the gaps in understanding of chronic/recurrent T1 are mentioned below.

- Nerve function impairment and neuritis overlap: A leprosy patient can have some nerve function impairment prior to development of T1R. Also, not all nerves undergo T1R simultaneously. When baseline nerve function assessment record of the patient is not available it becomes difficult to ascertain change in the NFI to plan steroid dosage and duration. Also, chronic neuropathic/nerve pain is now increasingly described entity in leprosy, which need to be differentiated from neuritis, at its management with neurotrophic drugs and not with steroids. A good understanding of such varied scenarios is required on the part of treating physician.

- Dose of corticosteroids for T1R: This chapter mentions the dosage and duration of steroid therapy as per the WHO manual of management of reactions. However, they may vary according to the national program of the native country, between leprosy care experts/ institutional practice and parameters used.
- At present there are no investigations or biomarkers available to predict the risk of chronic/ recurrent T1R at any stage of the disease. Identification of key pathogen molecules could also be helpful in differentiating between T1R and relapse. Identifying the key mediators would be an exciting field of research that could have a significant impact on future T1R therapies.

SCOPE FOR FURTHER RESEARCH

1. Identifying triggers for the excessive immune response leading to nerve damage during leprosy reactions remains a major challenge for management of T1R.
2. Evidence-based criteria for prescribing additional steroids to those with deteriorating NFI during T1R.
3. T1R severity scales need to be validated and utilized.
4. Newer drugs for control of T1R and nerve injury.

REFERENCES

1. Andrade PR, Pinheiro RO, Sales AM, et al. Type 1 reaction in leprosy: a model for a better understanding of tissue immunity under an immunopathological condition. Expert Rev Clin Immunol. 2015;11:391–407.
2. Van Brakel WH, Khawas IB, Lucas SB. Reactions in leprosy: an epidemiological study of 386 patients in west Nepal. Lepr Rev. 1994;65:190–203.
3. Scollard DM, Martelli CM, Stefani MM, et al. Risk factors for leprosy reactions in three endemic countries. Am J Trop Med Hyg. 2015;92:108–14.
4. van Brakel WH, Nicholls PG, Das L, et al. The INFIR Cohort Study: investigating prediction, detection and pathogenesis of neuropathy and reactions in leprosy. Methods and baseline results of a cohort of multibacillary leprosy patients in north India. Lepr Rev. 2005;76(1):14–34. Erratum in: Lepr Rev. 2005;76(3):264.
5. Nery JA, Bernardes Filho F, Quintanilha J, et al. Understanding the type 1 reactional state for early diagnosis and treatment: a way to avoid disability in leprosy. An Bras Dermatol. 2013;88:787–92.
6. Hogeweg M, Kiran KU, Suneetha S. The significance of facial patches and type I reaction for the development of facial nerve damage in leprosy. A retrospective study among 1226 paucibacillary leprosy patients. Lepr Rev. 1991;62:143–49.
7. Naafs B. Features of relapse in paucibacillary leprosy after multidrug therapy. Ind J Lepr 1995; 67: 61–8.
8. Available from: https://cltri.gov.in/MO%20Training%20Manual.pdf [Last assessed on 2024 Feb 22].

Chapter 24

Management of Recurrent Type 2 Reaction

• Neelakumari M Patel • Abhishek Bhardwaj

INTRODUCTION

The WHO Global Leprosy Strategy 2021–30 document acknowledges managing leprosy and its complications as the third strategic pillar and key component in the road toward zero leprosy.[1] Type 2 lepra reaction (T2R), commonly and rather incompletely referred to as erythema nodosum leprosum (ENL) is an immune complex syndrome (type III hypersensitivity reaction) that causes inflammatory reaction of any organ invaded by lepra bacilli or its products. It is characterized by subcutaneous nodules and at times accompanied by fever, lymphadenopathy, arthralgia and systemic involvement, that occur before, during or after treatment in patients of MB leprosy (BL leprosy and LL).

In this post-elimination era, especially in India, multibacillary cases outnumber paucibacillary ones, thereby keeping the pool of cases developing T2R intact and possibly increasing. It has been long perceived that both the incidence as well the severity of ENL is greater in patients treated with one year WHO MDT than MDT received for 2-year duration.[2] During last few years, number of MB cases with varied presentation of difficult-to-manage T2R are turning up for care in tertiary care centers.

DEFINITIONS

A patient diagnosed with leprosy has ENL if he/she develops crops of tender cutaneous or subcutaneous lesions, usually associated with systemic symptoms. In the absence of cutaneous signs ENL could also be diagnosed if a patient with leprosy had fever or malaise and histological features consistent with ENL in a tissue biopsy.

Other widely accepted useful definitions of ENL are:[3]

New ENL: Occurrence of ENL for the first time in a patient.

Acute ENL: A single episode lasting less than 24 weeks (6 months) while on corticosteroids treatment and in which treatment was slowly withdrawn with no recurrence of ENL whilst on treatment.

Recurrent ENL: When a patient experiences a second or subsequent episode of ENL occurring 28 days or more after stopping treatment for ENL.

Chronic ENL: When duration of ENL/T2R is more than 24 weeks (6 months)-And during which the patient was not treatment-free or when the treatment-free period for reaction was less than 4 weeks.

Steroid dependency in ENL: Recurrence of symptoms on tapering off the dose of systemic corticosteroids, which cause patient to either get new ENL or had a worsening of their pre-existing ENL.

CLINICAL SYMPTOMS AND SIGNS OF TYPE 2 LEPRA REACTION

This includes combination of any of the following:

1. Fever (with chills)#
2. Arthralgia or arthritis#
3. Erythema nodosum leprosum#
4. Neuritis#
5. Edema#
6. Myalgia and myositis
7. Episcleritis/iritis/iridocyclitis
8. Epididymo-orchitis
9. Dactylitis
10. Periosteitis
11. Glomerulonephritis
12. Lymphadenopathy
13. Organomegaly

CURRENT AVAILABLE KNOWLEDGE ON THE SUBJECT

T2R has been a focus of many studies. Researchers have identified many complex attributes in immunology and multitude of trigger factors are involved in the causation of T2R, which are summarized in Table 24.1.

The roles played by various components of immunity[7] are summarised in Table 24.2.

Table 24.1: Susceptibility and triggers related to type 2 lepra reaction

S.No	Factor (Susceptibility and trigger)	Role
1.	Genetic constitution	• IL-6 gene polymorphism as a possible biomarker (PROTECTIVE)[4] • Single nucleotide polymorphisms (SNPs) in nucleotide-binding oligomerization domain-containing protein 2 (NOD2) gene and six polymorphisms in IL-6 gene *(Increased susceptibility)*[5]
2.	Physiological states	• Gender: Male • Pregnancy • Lactation • Puberty • Vaccinations • Surgery • Psychological stress
3.	Disease state	• Intercurrent infections (e.g. Malaria, typhoid) • Bacteriological Index ≥4 • Coinfections[6] (oral mucosa, respiratory and urinary tract, liver infections)* • Immune reconstitution inflammatory syndrome (IRIS) • Helminthic infestation • Incomplete bacillary clearance, resistance

*role in maintenance of reactionary episode

#most common signs and symptoms

Table 24.2: Role of various components of immunity in type 2 lepra reaction

S.No.	Component	Role
1.	Neutrophils	Pivotal in pathogenesis (presence not overwhelming in biopsy though, dependent on timing of biopsy) Direct (CD64) and indirect (E-selectin) markers are demonstrable.
2.	Immune Complexes	Traditionally implicated pathogenesis, immune complexes against phenolic glycolipid-1 and major cytosolic protein of *M. leprae* 1 (MCP-1) found in circulation. Immune complex deposits now believed to be only an epiphenomenon.
3.	T-cells[7]	Increase in CD4+ cells and diminution in CD8+ cells. Diminution in T_{regs}
4.	Cytokines[7]	TNF-α, IFN-γ and IL-1β have been found to play an important role (evidence not uniformly consistent)
5.	Chemokines[7]	CCL-5 (Chemokine [C-C motif] ligand 5) followed by IFN-γ are the most important upstream regulator CCL-2, 3 and superoxide dismutase (SOD-2) may be potential biomarkers

CLASSIFICATION

Classification of T2R is required for: (a) better understanding of severity, (b) successful management, (c) Prognostication and research.

For grading of severity of T2R, the ENLIST ENL severity scale was devised and clinically validated recently. Initially the scale comprised of 16 items but subsequently it was pruned down to 10 items.[8] However, various ambiguities in terminology of this severity scale should be clarified, if the scale is intended to be ultimately used by health workers, physiotherapists or general duty medical officers involved in care of leprosy affected people.[9]

For straightforward management options, T2R can be broadly classified into mild and severe types (Table 24.3). Presence of neuritis is considered as a separate entity for management purposes. (NLEP Training Manual for Medical Officers 2019, CLTRI, Govt of India).

According to response to corticosteroids, T2R cases can be further classified into steroid responders, nonresponders and steroid dependent. Steroid-dependent cases are those for whom tapering the steroids results in flares. There is another small segment of 'steroid poor-responders' who require higher doses of steroids with each episode of ENL. All these patients, and those with serious comorbidities may require investigation for the diagnosis and management of underlying infections/infestations and comorbidities.

Table 24.3: Classification, features and treatment of type 2 lepra reaction

Type of ENL	Features	Treatment
Mild	Few nodules, mild fever	Analgesics
Severe	Severe pain over nodules, tendency for ulceration, high fever, involvement of internal organs	Steroid: Prednisolone course is given in the same dose as for type 1 reaction, but with faster tapering–given dose not exceeding 2–3 weeks.
Presence of neuritis	Accompanying new Neuritis or NFI of less than 6-month duration	Prednisolone regimen as for neuritis in type 1 reaction

KNOWLEDGE GAP

Leprosy reactions including T2R are distressing acute events with a potential of influencing the patient to give up on treatment. Studies have pointed out that these reactions negatively impact physical, psychological, and social well-being of patients.[10] There is ample scope for studying newer and convenient biomarkers for predictability, and as management tools.

DIAGNOSIS AND INVESTIGATIONS

Diagnostic tools: The diagnosis of ENL is predominantly clinical. Naaf's criteria based on clinical signs and symptoms can be used for diagnosis of T2R. Here a patient is considered to have a type 2 reaction if he/she has the major criterion or at least three minor criteria. (Box 24.1). The laboratory investigations and their significance is presented in Table 24.4.

Box 24.1: Diagnostic criteria for T2R

Major criteria

- A sudden eruption of tender (red) papules, nodules or plaques, which may ulcerate

Minor criteria

- Mild fever, the patient is unwell
- Tender enlarged nerves
- Increased loss of sensation or strength
- Arthritis
- Lymphadenitis
- Epididymo-orchitis
- Iridocyclitis or episcleritis
- Edema of extremities or face

Table 24.4A: Investigations in T2R

Investigation	*Significance*	*Significance during treatment*
CBC	Normocytic normochromic anemia, PMN leukocytosis	Thrombocytopenia due to Thalidomide
ESR	Raised (acute phase reactant)	
CRP	Raised	
RFT	Baseline	Caution: Increased creatinine and urea when on cyclosporine, Decreased creatinine clearance when on apremilast
LFT	Raised S. Bilirubin, AST, ALT, ALP, decreased total protein, albumin, increased globulin	
Urine analysis	Proteinuria	
USG abdomen, pelvis	To identify organomegaly	
Chest X-ray	To rule out pulmonary tuberculosis	
Others: FBS, PPBS Bone mineral densitometry		

Table 24.4B: Specific investigations in T2R

Investigations	*Expected alterations*
Slit skin smear	Fragmented and granular AFB
Biopsy from the ENL lesion	Intense perivascular neutrophilic infiltrate in dermis and subcutis, foamy macrophages containing lepra bacilli; special stains are Papanicolaou, May-Grunwald-Giemsa (MGG), modified Z-N stain
USG of peripheral nerves FNAC of nerves (only if required)	To confirm neuritis In case of suspected nerve abscess, etc.

MANAGEMENT

General Measures

1. Rest, splinting of limb in neuritis
2. Start/continue MDT
3. Identify/address triggers (infective foci, e.g. caries teeth/helminthic infestations/malaria, etc.)

Drug Treatment

Continue MDT MB in all patients who have not completed its duration. In addition, treatment of T2R can be initiated immediately after the diagnosis of ENL. The readers can follow Flowchart 24.1 as a management approach. **Mild ENL**/reaction is managed with

Flowchart 24.1: Algorithm for starting treatment for type 2 reaction

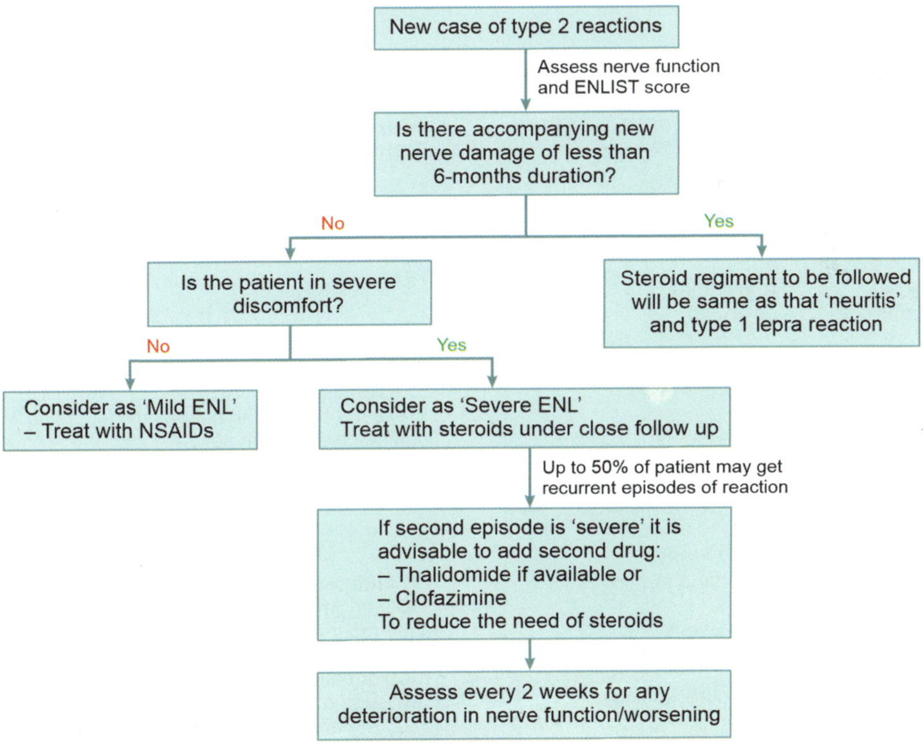

(Adapted from Leprosy/Hansen Disease: Management of reactions and prevention of disabilities. Technical guidance. New Delhi: World Health Organization, Regional Office for South-East Asia; 2017)

analgesics[11] (aspirin, indomethacin, ibuprofen, diclofenac, acetaminophen, tramadol) as per WHO recommendation. **Severe ENL**/reaction is initially best treated with moderate dose of 30-40 mg prednisolone per day.

1. If there is no worsening, gradually taper the steroids while maintaining patient on thalidomide/clofazimine
2. If there is worsening, make sure adequate dose of thalidomide or clofazimine is given, consider maintaining or increasing the dose of steroids.

Principles of Management of Recurrent ENL

The main focus of clinician managing recurrent ENL should lie in detecting and managing the triggering factors for recurring ENL, be it various physiological states as mentioned before or intercurrent infections. Adherence of the patient to the prescribed tapering schedule of the corticosteroids should be doubly checked as there is tendency to stop the drug once patient attains symptomatic relief which would trigger a flare of reaction leading to requirement of higher dose of steroid upon each ensuing episode of lepra reaction contributing to the steroid dependency. For a steroid dependent ENL patient; the key factor is to monitor and manage complication of long term steroid use. Prevention of osteoporosis guidelines should be instituted in such patients from the beginning. Addition of newer immunosuppressive has more defined role in such patients in order to reduce the dosage of the corticosteroids required to control the reactional episode (Flowchart 24.2).

Various drugs used in the management are described in the Table 24.5.

Flowchart 24.2: Algorithm for treatment of patients with recurrent/chronic type 2 reaction[12]

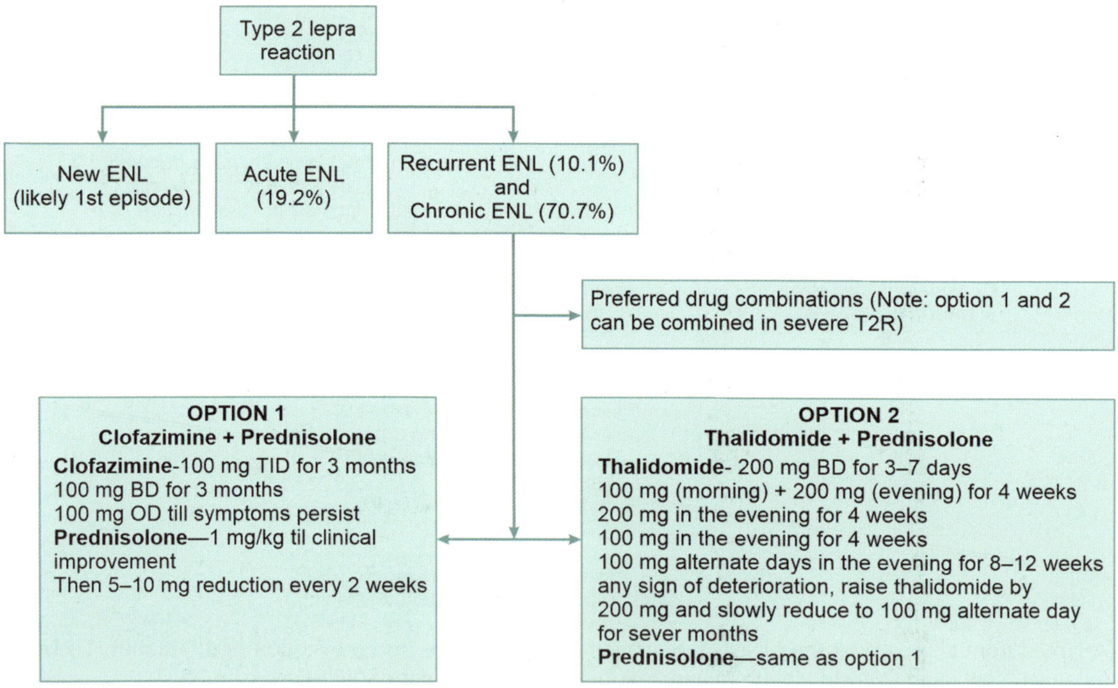

Table 24.5: Details of drugs use in the management of T2R

Drug group	***Molecule and dose***	***Mechanism of action***	***Specific information***	***Main adverse effects***
Anti-inflammatory				
NSAIDs	Acetylsalicylic acid (Aspirin): 600 mg 6 hourly with meals	Decrease prostaglandin synthesis, suppress Ag-Ab reaction and Ab production	Fewer side effects amongst all NSAIDs	Bleeding from stool, urine, cough, vomit. Purpura, ecchymosis
	Paracetamol: 1000 mg every 8 hours	Antipyretic and analgesic	Adjuvant to control pain and fever	
	Indomethacin 75 mg–150 mg in 3–4 divided doses		Mild ENL	Lower incidence of visual disturbances compared to other NSAIDs
Corticosteroids	Prednisolone 1 mg/kg/day till clinical improvement, then tapered every week by 10 mg up to 30 mg then every week by 5 mg up to 5 mg then 2.5 mg for 2 weeks for total 20 weeks.	Decrease cytokine production, i.e. IFN-gamma, IL-12, iNOS	To treat active reactions— not indicated to prevent recurrence of ENL	Major Adverse events include- Dependence, weight gain, pedal edema, steroid induced hypertension and hyperglycemia. Steroid induced osteoporosis– Baseline and repeated bone densitometry scan should be performed every 1–3 years depending on clinical risk factors
Thalidomide	100-400 mg daily, then tapered by 50 mg every 2–4 weeks. Maintain on lowest dose and dose reduction every 3–6 months	Decrease TNF alpha levels, increase IL10, decrease IL12 levels, decreases neutrophil numbers in lesions, reduces CD4 cells, increases CD8T, inhibits cyclo-oxygenase 2, IFN-gamma and NF-kB	Serendipitous discovery	In developing fetus: Phocomelia, cardiac and GI anomalies, ear deformity, ocular defects, facial paralysis, anomalies or absence of internal organs. In patients: Peripheral neuropathy (painful paresthesia and sensory loss)—dose dependent, SJS, TEN,seizures, hypertension, Bradycardia, Thromoboembolic complications-DVT and pulmonary embolism (risk increased if combined with dexamethasone), Drowsiness, somnolence and constipation, dizziness, fatigue. PREGNANCY TEST (in Females) is mandatory. Check and follow the protocol for pregnancy testing for women while on treatment with thalidomide (Note: Patient should be following double contraception methods)

(Contd.)

Table 24.5: Details of drugs use in the management of T2R *(Contd.)*

Drug group	*Molecule and dose*	*Mechanism of action*	*Specific information*	*Main adverse effects*
Clofazimine	100 mgTDS for 3 months, then BD for 3 month, then OD for over 20 weeks.	Antimicrobial activity, interference with ATP production	– Prevent new occurrence and reduce the dependence of corticosteroid – Effective in chronic ENL and no effect on acute episode	Abdominal side effects: Nausea, diarrhea, abdominal pain, anorexia, GI bleed, intestinal obstruction. headache, lymphadenopathy, red discoloration of body fluids, skin, xerosis,hair color changes.
Second-line drugs used in difficult to manage ENL: Immunosuppressives and Immunomodulators				
	Azathioprine 1 to 2.5mg/kg/day	Decrease DNA, RNA, protein synthesis; decrease B and T lymphocytes, IgM and IgG synthesis and IL 2 secretion, Has Anti TNF Alpha action	Good adjuvant as immuno-suppressive in patients with recurrent/ chronic ENL	Nausea,diarrhoea bone marrow suppression, leukopenia, thrombocytopenia
	Methotrexate 15 mg/week oral or sc for 48 weeks	Immunomodulating, anti-inflammatory. Increases adenosine levels, increases anti-inflammatory cytokines and reduces proinflammatory cytokines	Helpful in resistant ENL (adjuvant to corticosteroid and thalidomide)	Anorexia, nausea, vomit, diarrhoea, oral ulcers, hepatotoxicity, pancytopenia, flu-like symptoms, pneumonitis
	Cyclosporine 7.5 mg/kg	Immunomodulatory, inhibits transcription of IL2	Promising results but more studies are required	Renal toxicity, hypertension, nausea, diarrhoea
	Apremilast 30 mg/day	PDE4 inhibitor decreases TNF alpha, IL23,IL10,NO synthase Immunomodulatory and anti inflammatory action, decreases pro inflammatory cytokines	For resistant ENL Helpful in neuritis amd arthralgia	Nausea, vomiting, diarrhoea, weight loss
	Mycophenolate mofetil 500 mg BD upto a maximum of 2 g/day	Inhibits *de novo* purine synthesis		
Others				
Pentoxiphylline	400mg TDS	Decreases RBC aggregation and reduces plasma fibrinogen concentrations. Inhibits production of TNF Alpha	– Beneficial in vasculitis predominant episodes. – Can be used in patients in whom thalidomide is contraindicated. – indicated in HIV coinfected patients	Nausea, bloating belching, bruising, bleeding, bloody stool

(Contd.)

Table 24.5: Details of drugs use in the management of T2R ***(Contd.)***

Drug group	*Molecule and dose*	*Mechanism of action*	*Specific information*	*Main adverse effects*
Colchicine	0.5 mg TDS then taper gradually	Inhibits neutrophil chemotaxis thus inhibits vascular injury	More effective than aspirin in moderate ENL (neural and joint pain relief)	Diarrhea, myopathy, bone marrow suppression, peripheral neuritis, purpura.
Antibiotics	Minocycline 100 mg/day	Anti-inflammatory		AKI, hearing impairment, tinnitus
	Ofloxacin 400 mg/day			
Antimalarials	Hydroxychloroquine		Mild ENL	
Biologics				
Anti-TNF alpha inhibitors-used in difficult to treat cases of ENL despite being on standard therapy	Etanercept 50 mg/week		Can reduce corticosteroid and thalidomide requirement	Increase risk of fungal infections, tuberculosis, increased financial burden
	Infliximab 5 mg/kg On week 0,2,6		No further episode of ENL in 1 patient	
	Adalimumab			
Immuno-therapeutic Vaccines				
MIP vaccine	*Mycobacterium indicus pranni* (MIP) vaccine 0.5 x 10^9 cells per 0.1 mL 0.1 ml in right and left deltoid region intradermally followed by 0.1 ml in one deltoid area subsequently 4 doses repeated at 3 monthly intervals.	Upregulates host immune response	Reduction in frequency and severity of ENL	
Other agents:	High dose Zinc			

Situations Where Second-line Drugs can be Used in ENL

- Patients developing serious adverse effects of steroids like avascular necrosis of hip, cushingoid features with uncontrolled hypertension and hyperglycemia. This subset of patients need to use second line drugs as steroid sparing agents or to lower the dosage of corticosteroid required in steroid dependent ENL.
- There should not be a knee jerk response to introduce and withdraw second line drugs upon clinical nonresponsiveness withing few weeks of starting them. Individual drug may be given 6–8 weeks time minimum before they are replaced with another second line immunosuppressive and discarded as being ineffective.

FUTURE/NEWER DRUGS

A. Thalidomide analogs: Supidimide, lenalidomide (Revlimid) and pomalidomide (Actimid): Newer analogs of thalidomide have lesser side effects as compared to thalidomide. Supidimide (nonteratogenic analog) has been tried with success in ENL. They all inhibit TNF alpha and hence can be used in recurrent ENL.

B. Selective serotonin reuptake inhibitors (SSRIs) like citalopram, paroxetine, fluoxetine, sertraline have shown positive outcomes in recurrent ENL. These drugs act by suppressing microglial inflammation (TNF alpha) in response to inflammatory stimulus.

Management of Other Manifestations/Complications of T2R

Acute Iridocyclitis

- Oral/topical steroids (1% hydrocortisone, hourly eyedrops and eye ointment at night)
- Atropine eyedrops at night

Acute epididymo-orchitis

- Bed rest
- Oral corticosteroids
- Scrotal suspensory bandages

Neuritis, arthritis, arthralgia, myositis, dactylitis, lymphadenopathy, organomegaly, bone pain, etc. can be managed with routine anti-inflammatory agents and steroids. Multidisciplinary approach is required when extracutaneous manifestations occur.

Be Mindful of Atypical Presentations

Atypical ENL can present any time before, during or after MDT in leprosy. Various atypical presentations range from vesiculobullous, ulceronecrotic, erythema multiforme like lesions, Sweet's syndrome like lesions, to groups of pustules.[12]

However, they all have systemic manifestations similar to classic ENL, such as fever, malaise, arthralgia, nerve enlargement and neuritis. Atypical presentations may pose a diagnostic dilemma, and delay the diagnosis, especially when patient presents as hitherto undiagnosed leprosy. Though the clinical and histopathological presentations maybe atypical, the treatment remains the same as in classical ENL.

SUMMARY

- Managing a case of recurrent T2R requires identification, meticulous search for underlying causative factors and instituting appropriate treatment. The challenge is to establish long-lasting control over this reaction, initially with systemic steroids, later by addition of other agents as needed. The goal of management is to bring complete regression of ENL. The present armamentarium although suffices to manage most cases, however, few cases of chronic recurrent ENL or those with steroid dependence will need ingenuity on the part of the clinician to bring them under control.[14]
- Recent reports bring spotlight onto the phenomenon of resistance contributing to recurrent ENL[15] and benefit of second line anti-leprosy drugs like fluoroquinolones, clarithromycin and minocycline in such cases. Time is ripe for gathering more evidence and relooking at the existing treatment strategies and reorient the guidelines for encouraging testing for resistance in the event of recurrent ENL.

REFERENCES

1. World Health Organization. Towards zero leprosy. Global Leprosy (Hansen's disease) Strategy 2021–2030. New Delhi: WHO Regional Office for South-East Asia; 2021.
2. Balagon MV, Gelber RH, Abalos RM, Cellona RV. Reactions following completion of 1 and 2 year multidrug therapy (MDT). Am J Trop Med Hyg. 2010 Sep;83(3):637–44.

3. Narang T, Kamat D. Jopling's Handbook of leprosy. 6th ed. New Delhi: CBS Publishers and Distributors (P) Ltd; 2020. Reactions in leprosy. In: Sardana K, Khurana A, editors; pp. 211–6.
4. Sousa AL, Fava VM, Sampaio LH, Martelli CM, Costa MB, Mira MT, et al. Genetic and immunological evidence implicates interleukin-6 as a susceptibility gene for leprosy type 2 reaction. J Infect Dis 2012;205: 1417–24.
5. Sales-Marques C, Cardoso CC, Alvarado-Arnez LE, Illaramendi X, Sales AM, Hacker MA, et al. Genetic polymorphisms of the IL6 and NOD2 genes are risk factors for inflammatory reactions in leprosy. PLoS Negl Trop Dis. 2017;11:e0005754.
6. Motta AC, Pereira KJ, Tarquínio DC, Vieira MB, Miyake K, Foss NT. Leprosy reactions: coinfections as a possible risk factor. Clinics (Sao Paulo). 2012;67:1145–8.
7. Bhat RM, Vaidya TP. What is new in the pathogenesis and management of erythema nodosum leprosum. Indian Dermatol Online J. 2020;11:482–92.
8. Walker SL, Sales AM, Butlin CR, Shah M, Maghanoy A, Lambert SM, et al. A leprosy clinical severity scale for erythema nodosum leprosum: An international, multicentre validation study of the ENLIST ENL Severity Scale. PLoS Negl Trop Dis. 2017;11:e0005716.
9. Kumar B, Mehta H, Narang T, Dogra S. A critical appraisal of the ENLIST severity scale for erythema nodosum leprosum. PLoS Negl Trop Dis. 2022;16:e0010378.
10. Putri AI, de Sabbata K, Agusni RI, Alinda MD, Darlong J, de Barros B, et al. Understanding leprosy reactions and the impact on the lives of people affected: An exploration in two leprosy endemic countries. PLoS Negl Trop Dis. 2022;16:e0010476.
11. Kar HK, Sharma P. IAL textbook of leprosy. 2nd ed. New Delhi: JP Brothers Medical Publishers (P) Ltd; 2017. Management of leprosy reactions. In: Kar HK, Kumar B, editors; pp. 3465–77.
12. Alakad R, Nofal A, Assaf M. Atypical presentations of erythema nodosum leprosum: Diagnostic and therapeutic aspects. JDDG: Journal der Deutschen Dermatologischen Gesellschaft. 2021;19:1133–43.

Chapter 25

Neuropathic Pain and Management

• Neel Prabha • P Narasimha Rao

INTRODUCTION

Neuropathy and neuritis are two related conditions associated with nerve damage in leprosy. However, it is important to differentiate between neuritis and neuropathic pain (NP) in leprosy, as their pathology, sequelae, and management are significantly different.

Pain associated with neuropathy, otherwise called neuropathic pain (NP), occurs as one of the late complications of leprosy due to the damage to the peripheral nerves, which may clinically manifest continuously or intermittently. Neuritis, on the other hand, specifically refers to inflammation of a nerve or nerves. Intraneural bacilli and its products cause this inflammation or neuritis in leprosy. The main symptoms related to inflammation are tenderness and swelling of the affected nerve, commonly associated with lepra reactions. In addition, there may be similar symptoms to those of neuropathy, including pain, numbness, and weakness. In summary, while both neuropathy and neuritis involve nerve damage and may have similar symptoms, neuropathy is a more general term for nerve dysfunction and associated symptoms, whereas neuritis specifically refers to nerve inflammation. Undiagnosed neuritis can lead to severe nerve function impairment and disability as its sequel.

It should be noted that in general neuropathy is commonly associated with various underlying conditions, such as diabetes, multiple sclerosis, spinal cord injury, herpes zoster, and other conditions while leprosy is considered an uncommon cause of neuropathy in general. Nevertheless, it is important that NP in leprosy should be diagnosed and adequately treated since it is a distressing entity, which can hamper the quality of life of treated leprosy patients, leading them to believe that the disease is incurable. There is insufficient knowledge and a lack of training among leprosy healthcare personnel to manage neuropathic pain. Often steroids are misused for this pain, leading to iatrogenic steroid-induced side effects.[1]

DEFINITION

Neuropathic pain is defined by the International Association for the Study of Pain (IASP) as' pain caused by a lesion or disease of the somatosensory nervous system'.[2] The neuropathic pain in the context of leprosy is considered as the pain associated with peripheral neuropathy occurring in released-from-treatment (RFT) patients after completion of therapy, with no active nerve inflammation.

CURRENT KNOWLEDGE AND GAPS IN UNDERSTANDING

As NP is a subjective symptom which is difficult to measure or grade objectively, the diagnosis is often challenging, especially as there is yet to be a consensus on its definition.

This can be observed in the reports of its prevalence in leprosy being described as anything between 11 and 70% in various studies from different countries due to the use of different study models, clinical forms of the selected patients, and screening tools.[3]

The exact pathogenesis of neuropathic pain is unknown. One explanation could be the ongoing chronic inflammation even after MDT completion in and around the nerves. This may lead to sensitization and stimulation of nociceptors, their central synaptic targets, or both, resulting in persistent neuropathic pain.[4] NP is also believed to occur due to abnormal nerve signalling that transmits pain messages from the affected area to the brain. Unlike acute pain of neuritis, which serves as a warning signal of tissue damage, neuropathic pain often persists long after the initial injury has healed. It presents as chronic pain caused by damage or dysfunction of the nervous system. It is characterized by a sharp, shooting, burning, or electric shock-like pain that can be constant or intermittent. It can affect various body parts, including the hands, feet, and face. The pain may be accompanied by numbness or tingling in the affected area.

One observation incriminates vasculitis of small epineural vessels, leading to ischemic nerve injury and neuropathic pain.[5] Another study attributed it to small fiber neuropathy.[6] It is still poorly understood whether the clinical presentation of neuropathic pain in leprosy differs from neuropathic pain of other etiologies. In addition, there is currently no evidence-based treatment for managing neuropathic pain in leprosy.[7]

DIAGNOSIS

Neuropathic pain recognition requires a careful clinical history followed by meticulous physical examination. Characteristics of neuropathic pain[8] are mentioned in Table 25.1. It is essential to differentiate pure neuropathic pain from acute pain of lepra reaction. Without biomarkers or other gold standard investigation, the diagnosis is based on history, symptoms and clinical examination.[9]

Validated tools for neuropathic pain screening are Douleur neuropathique (DN4), NPSI, McGill Pain Questionnaire, and Leeds Assessment of Neuropathic Symptoms and Signs (LANSS). DN4 questionnaire is a simple and commonly used tool for diagnosing neuropathic pain.[10] It consists of four questions and a total of 10 items. The first two questions are based on the patient's interview, and the last 2 questions are based on the patient's physical examination. A score of ≥4 is an indicator of neuropathic pain. Some other quantitative assessment methods, like infrared thermography, can also be helpful in assessing neuropathic pain.[11] Infrared thermography allows the mapping of the skin surface temperature, capturing changes in the microcirculation blood flow.[11]

MANAGEMENT

It is only recently that NP of leprosy has gained prominence as an entity, while much attention is being given to managing leprosy and lepra reaction. At the same time, it is important to

Table 25.1: Characteristics of neuropathic pain

Quality	*Frequency*	*Distribution*
Burning, biting, pricking, cutting, electric-shock-like	Continuous or intermittent	Innervation territory of single or multiple peripheral nerves or glove and/or stocking

differentiate NP from pain associated with active neuritis, as their management principles differ. A dedicated questioning, as suggested above, should be asked to these patients suspected of NP. It should be noted that post-RFT patients who have completed adequate MDT do not require restarting the MDT to manage neuropathic pain.

Currently, there are no specific guidelines for managing neuropathic pain in leprosy. According to Brazilian Medical Association the treatment of neuropathic pain should involve the use of 3 classes of medication namely: tricyclic antidepressants (amitriptyline, nortriptyline, imipramine and clomipramine), phenothiazines neuroleptics (chlorpromazine, levomepromazine) and anticonvulsants (carbamazepine, gabapentin, oxcarbazepine, topiramate, pregabalin). They may be combined with analgesics and anti-inflammatories according to the needs of every patient.[12] These treatment options available for neuropathic pain of other etiologies are being tried for neuropathic pain in leprosy (Table 25.2).[13]

Drugs for Neuropathic Pain

Gabapentinoids: Gabapentin and its newer congener, pregabalin, are anti-seizure drugs. Gabapentin is GABA analog. Analgesia in neuropathic pain is achieved by binding to presynaptic calcium channels of primary nociceptive endings and reducing the central release of excitatory molecules.[14] Gabapentin is well absorbed orally. Side effects are mild sedation, dizziness, tiredness, tremor, and unsteadiness. The side effects are mild-to-moderate and usually resolve within two weeks of continued treatment.[14]

Dose: Start as 300 mg OD on the first day, increase the dose to 300 mg BD on the second day, and 300 mg TDS on the third day, with further increments every 2–3 days as needed to maximum of 3600 mg/day. A minimum of 600 mg or more is needed for optimal pain control. One needs to be mindful of severe drug hypersensitivity reactions which may occur with use of gabapentin.

Pregabalin is a newer congener of gabapentin with superior bioavailability. It is more potent than gabapentin; hence lower doses are required. It is tolerated well with mild-to-moderate, transient, dose-dependent side effects. Dizziness and somnolence are common side effects.[15]

Dose: Start with 150 mg/day; increase to 600 mg per day in 2 or 3 divided doses as required. As it is eliminated mainly by renal exertion in patients with reduced renal function, dose adjustment is needed.

Table 25.2: Drugs for neuropathic pain

	Group	*Drugs*
First-line therapy	Gabapentinoids	Gabapentin, pregabalin
	Tricyclic antidepressants	Amitriptyline, nortriptyline
	Serotonin-norepinephrine reuptake inhibitors	Duloxetine, venlafaxine
Second-line therapy	Opioids	Tramadol
Third-line therapy	Strong opioids	Morphine, oxycodone

Tricyclic antidepressants (TCAs): These drugs inhibit noradrenaline and serotonin presynaptic reuptake and have postsynaptic alpha-adrenergic, muscarinic cholinergic, and H_1 histaminergic receptor-blocking properties.

As norepinephrine and serotonin have a role in pain transmission, these drugs are commonly used to treat various pain conditions.[16] Amitriptyline and nortriptyline also block sodium channels, which may be responsible for their role in neuropathic pain.

Oral absorption of TCAs is good. Anticholinergic side effects are commonly seen with TCAs.[17] These anticholinergic side effects are more with amitriptyline and are dose-dependent.

Dose of amitriptyline and nortriptyline: Start as 10–25 mg in the evening to reduce sedative effects during the day, and increase the dose by 10–25 mg at a week's interval, with the maximum dose of 150 mg/day. The usual dose is 50–75 mg at night.[18]

Carbamazepine: It is the drug of choice for trigeminal neuralgia. It has been used in neuropathic pain in leprosy. Compared to trigeminal neuralgia, it is not so effective in diabetic, traumatic, and other forms of neuropathic pain.[19]

Side effects: Common side effects are sedation, vertigo, dizziness, diplopia, and ataxia. Adverse cutaneous reactions and agranulocytosis, although rare, are dangerous side effects.

Dose of carbamazepine: 200–400 mg, 2 times a day. Sustained release/continuous release formulations are preferred to avoid high peak and low troughs in plasma.

Serotonin and noradrenaline reuptake inhibitors (SNRIs): Venlafaxine and duloxetine are antidepressant drugs. Both inhibit the uptake of both noradrenaline and serotonin, and in contrast to old TCAs, these do not interact with adrenergic, cholinergic, or histaminergic receptors.[17]

Side effects: Both have a better side-effect profile than older TCAs. Common side effects are nausea, sweating, anxiety, dizziness, impotence, and hypertension.

Dose of venlafaxine: 75 to 225 mg/day. *Dose of Duloxetine:* 20–120 mg/day.

Opioids: Tramadol, an opioid agonist, has been proposed as the second-line treatment in neuropathic pain. It is a synthetic analogue of codeine with centrally acting analgesic action. Its analgesic effect may be attributed to serotonin and norepinephrine reuptake inhibition.[20] Oral bioavailability is good with $t^{1/2}$ of 5–6 hours, and effects last for 4–6 hours.

Side effects include nausea, vomiting, sedation, dizziness, xerostomia, urinary retention, constipation, and lowering seizure threshold (contraindicated in people with epilepsy). Like other opioids, tramadol is potentially subject to abuse.

Dose: Start with 100 mg/day and increase over one to two weeks to 400 mg/day in divided doses 6 hourly or maximum tolerated dose. Potent opioids (morphine and oxycodone) have been listed as third-line treatment. The risk of dependence and side effects are more as compared to tramadol.

Others: There are other treatments like transcutaneous electrical stimulation or peripheral nerve stimulation for patients whose pharmacological treatment options have failed. These are effective and not associated with drug-related side effects.[21] One major drawback is the availability of these facilities.

Salient Points about Drug Therapy for Neuropathic Pain

- Medication for neuropathic pain should be started with low doses and increased on a gradual basis as required.

- Tricyclic antidepressants and serotonin and noradrenaline reuptake inhibitors (SNRIs) should be trialled first. If they are ineffective, consider a trial of gabapentin/pregabalin, then tramadol.
- Tricyclic antidepressants are cost-effective options. Gabapentin and pregabalin are relatively safer drugs.
- Effective response in neuropathic pain is usually seen after 2–4 weeks of adequate dosage.
- To avoid sedation, ask the patient to take drugs early in the evening
- With a higher dose, divide the dose and keep the evening dose high.
- These drugs have a central analgesic action and do not affect the nerve damage process. It is essential to explain to the patient that complete pain relief with the treatment is unlikely, and approximately 50% pain reduction is realistic.[21]

Issues for attention: The main practical problem is lack of understanding about neuropathic pain and its management among leprosy healthcare personnel. In addition, the drugs for neuropathic pain are not provided under the leprosy program. Although amitriptyline is not costly, it is associated with side effects. The other effective drugs, such as gabapentin and pregabalin, with fewer side effects, are expensive.

SCOPE FOR FURTHER RESEARCH

Attention to NP in leprosy is relatively recent. Hence, literature on clinical-epidemiological profile, pathogenesis, and studies on treatment efficacy is scarce. Future research is required to address these important issues.

CONCLUSION

Neuropathic pain is an important entity in leprosy that needs attention as it can significantly hamper the quality of life of a patient. Currently, there are no recommended guidelines for its management in leprosy. Nonetheless, the existing knowledge should be put to best use for the benefit of leprosy patient with NP. At the same time, there is a need to identify evidence based drug therapy/options for its effective management.

REFERENCES

1. Gosling AP, Kenedi MD, Da Cunha AJ, et al. Characteristics of neuropathic pain after multidrug therapy in a tertiary referral centre for leprosy: A cross-sectional study in Rio de Janeiro, Brazil. Lepr Rev 2017;88:109–21.
2. Murnion BP. Neuropathic pain: current definition and review of drug treatment. AustPrescr 2018;41:60–3.
3. Tiago LMdP, Santos DFd, Antunes DE, et al. Assessment of neuropathic pain in leprosy patients with relapse or treatment failure by infrared thermography: A cross-sectional study. PLoSNegl Trop Dis 2021;15:e0009794.
4. Ellis A, Bennett DL. Neuroinflammation and the generation of neuropathic pain. Br J Anaesth 2013;111:26–37.
5. Bowen JRC, McDougall AC, Morris JH et al. Vasculitic neuropathy in a patient with inactive treated lepromatous leprosy. J NeurolNeurosurg Psychiatry2000;68:496–500.
6. Lund C, Koskinen M, Suneetha S, et al. Histopathological and clinical findings in leprosy patients with chronic neuropathic pain: a study from Hyderabad, India. Lepr Rev2007;78:369–80.
7. Raicher I, Stump PRNAG, Harnik SB, et al. Neuropathic pain in leprosy: symptom profile characterization and comparison with neuropathic pain of other etiologies. Pain Rep 2018;3:e638.
8. Lasry-Levy E, Hietaharju A, Pai V, et al. Neuropathic pain and psychological morbidity in patients with treated leprosy: a cross-sectional prevalence study in Mumbai. PLoSNegl Trop Dis2011;5(3):e981.
9. Mulvey MR, Boland EG, Bouhassira D, Freynhagen R, Hardy J, Hjermstad MJ, Mercadante S, Pérez C, Bennett MI. Neuropathic pain in cancer: systematic review, performance of screening tools and analysis of symptom profiles. Br J Anaesth. 2017;119:765–74.

10. Bouhassira D, Attal N, Alchaar H, et al. Comparison of pain syndromes associated with nervous or somatic lesions and development of a new neuropathic pain diagnostic questionnaire (DN4). Pain2005;114:29–6.
11. Chojnowski M. Infrared thermal imaging in connective tissue diseases. Reumatologia. 2017;55:38–43.
12. Arco RD, Nardi SM, Bassi TG, PaschoalVdel A. Diagnosis and medical treatment of neuropathic pain in leprosy. Rev Lat Am Enfermagem. 2016;24:e2731.
13. Cavalli E, Mammana S, Nicoletti F, et al. The neuropathic pain: An overview of the current treatment and future therapeutic approaches. Int J Immunopathol Pharmacol2019;33:2058738419838383.
14. McNamara JO. Pharmacotherapy of the epilepsies. In: Brunton, LL, Chabner BA, Knollmann BC, editors. Goodman and Gilman's pharmacological basis of therapeutics, 12th ed. New York: McGraw-Hill;2011.p.583–607.
15. Gajraj NM. Pregabalin: its pharmacology and use in pain management. AnesthAnalg. 2007;105:1805–15.
16. O'Donnell JM, Shelton RC. Drug Therapy of depression and anxiety disorders. In: Brunton, LL, Chabner BA, Knollmann BC, editors. Goodman and Gilman's pharmacological basis of therapeutics, 12th ed. New York: McGraw-Hill;2011.p.397–415.
17. Tripathi KD. Drugs Used in Mental Illness: Antidepressant and Antianxiety Drugs In:Tripathi KD, editor. Essentials of Medical Pharmacology. 8th ed. New Delhi, India: Jaypee Brothers Medical;2018.p.481–96.
18. Kalso E, Aldington DJ, Moore RA. Drugs for neuropathic pain. BMJ 2013 Dec;347:f7339.
19. Tripathi KD. Antiepiletic drugs. In:Tripathi KD, editor. Essentials of Medical Pharmacology. 8th ed. New Delhi, India: Jaypee Brothers Medical;2018.p.411–24.
20. Duehmke RM, Derry S, Wiffen PJ, et al. Tramadol for neuropathic pain in adults. Cochrane Database Syst Rev 2017;6:CD003726.
21. Gierthmühlen J, Baron R. Neuropathic Pain. Semin Neurol 2016;36:462–8.

Chapter

26 Management of Lepra Reactions in Pregnancy and Lactation

• Meghana Phiske • Smitha Prabhu

INTRODUCTION

Pregnancy and lactation are considered special events and when this happens in a leprosy patient it poses a different challenge to the care provider. Rarely, leprosy is diagnosed for the first-time during pregnancy, especially in countries where it is rife. Usually, these patients are referred to tertiary care centers/dermatologist by the obstetricians for an expert opinion to start or for modification of anti-leprosy treatment. It is important to know how the course of leprosy may be influenced by pregnancy and *vice versa*; and advice a leprosy patient of child bearing age on the expected course and complications that may arise during pregnancy due to altered immunological response.[1] In addition, during the postpartum period which is associated with recovery of immunological response in mother; there is an increased propensity for immune reactions. Neuritis, manifesting overtly or silently is also known to occur during this period.[2] In this chapter, we shall discuss the management of lepra reactions during pregnancy and lactation.

CURRENT KNOWLEDGE AND KNOWLEDGE GAP

Most epidemiological data on reaction/neuritis associated with pregnancy predates the MDT era. Annually out of 2000 globally detected leprosy patients, 2–3 are pregnant women, being diagnosed in third trimester.[3] However, there is not enough data about the epidemiology of leprosy during pregnancy or published evidence of natural history of leprosy during pregnancy and lactation or its impact on fetal outcomes.[4] Cesarean section is performed at times because of leprosy in mother, but it is not justified due to negligible risk of intrapartum infection it the child.

Appearance of new lesions/reactivation of old disease/relapse in treated patients can occur during pregnancy. In addition, the two types of immunologically mediated reactions: type I (T1R) and type II (T2R) or erythema nodosum leprosum (ENL), can be triggered during pregnancy due to variation in CMI and humoral immunity. Increased load of *M. leprae* is most frequently seen in third trimester.[3] In pregnancy, when CMI is low only surface antigens of *M. leprae* multiplying in skin are exposed, resulting in predominantly cutaneous lesions.[3] Increased susceptibility to reactions during and soon after pregnancy is associated with "Th1-Th2 shift" during pregnancy and rapid restoration of immune capacity after delivery.[4]

Type 1 reactions (T1R): They occur due to improvement in CMI, are less frequent during pregnancy (due to decreased CMI) and more frequent in lactation (due to improved CMI). When TIR occur in pregnancy cutaneous manifestations are more frequent and conspicuous than neuritis. Lesional erythema/edema is relatively subdued in comparison to those in nonpregnant state.

Type 2 reactions (T2R): Pregnancy is one of the risk factors for development of ENL. T2R have no clear temporal association with pregnancy but higher incidence is seen during first and third trimesters. ENL is type III, antigen antibody reaction, with systemic symptoms and with tender nodular lesions all over the body.[5] It is more commonly seen in lepromatous type of leprosy (seen in 50%), in those with high bacillary index, in untreated patients and in those harboring drug resistant *M. leprae*[6] (Figs 26.1 and 26.2). It can be severe and recurrent, but systemic symptoms are less marked in pregnancy, but conspicuous in lactation.

During lactation, T1R are more common due to Th2 to Th1 shift in the immunity of the patient that follows parturition.[2] BL patients are at greatest risk, followed by LL and BT patients. However, severe and recurrent ENL is also known to occur during lactation[3] as lactation is a known precipitating factor for ENL in up to 30–40% lactating women.[7]

Pregnancy and Neuritis

ENL in pregnancy is associated with nerve function impairment (NFI) and irrespective of treatment there is a deterioration in 50% of patients.[3] In BT/TT cases, neuritis is common, without relation to pregnancy or lactation.[3] ENL can occur in any trimester of pregnancy but most frequent, first and third) and can lead to new NFI. Continuation of both types of reactions long into lactation is possible making affected women vulnerable to sequelae of leprosy and lepra reactions.

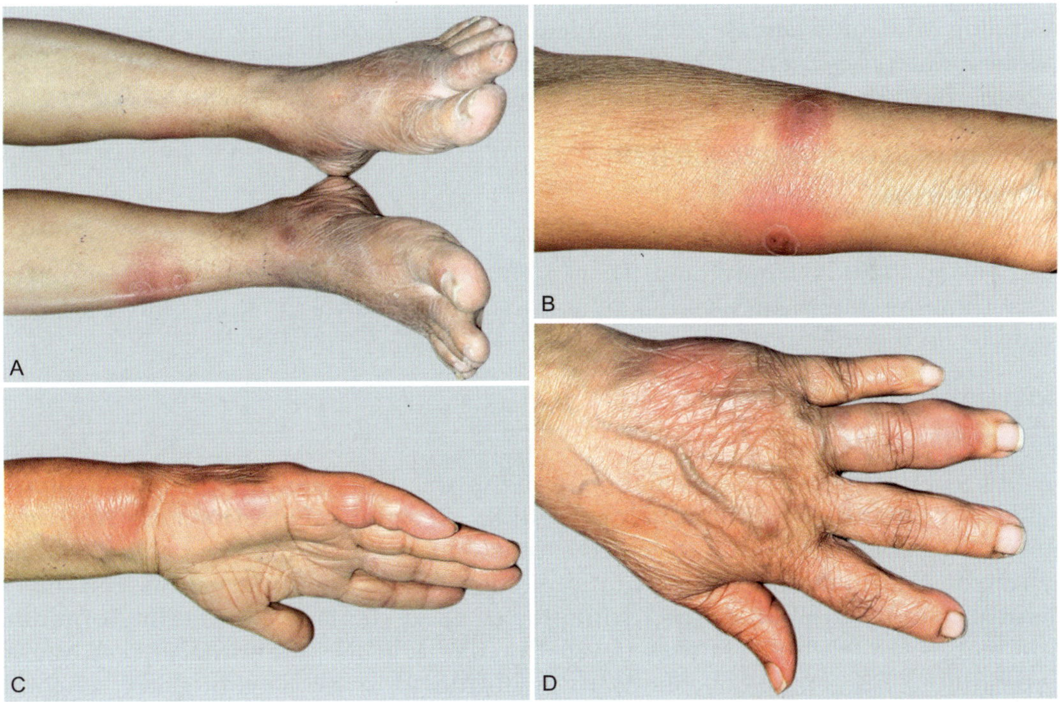

Fig. 26.1: (A) Ill-defined, erythematous plaques, on lower limbs; (B) Ill-defined, erythematous plaques with overlying central scaling on left upper extremity; (C) Ill-defined, erythematous plaque extending from right medial border of wrist to little finger with associated edema; (D) Ill-defined, erythematous plaque over left dorsal aspect of hand with dactylitis of ring finger

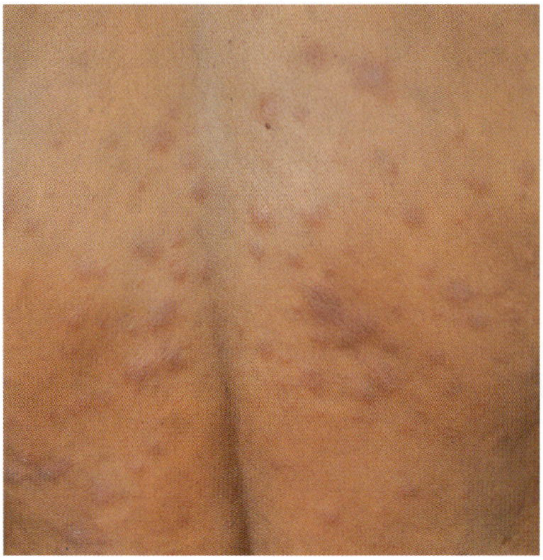

Fig. 26.2: Multiple erythematous papules, distributed bilaterally symmetrically over back

MANAGEMENT OF LEPRA REACTIONS IN PREGNANCY[4]

Diagnosis of type 1 lepra reactions and ENL is predominantly clinical and same as non-pregnant individual as described in Chapters 23 and 24, respectively. The common principle for both type of reaction is continuation of multidrug therapy during pregnancy as benefit of continuing MDT outweighs the risks. Adequate rest and counseling to avoid stress should be done for all pregnant patients. Salient aspects about usage of anti-leprosy drugs during pregnancy are described in the following Table 26.1.

Treatment of Reversal Reaction (T1R)

Corticosteroids

Steroids are relatively safe during pregnancy, but steroid-induced hyperglycemia or hypertension should be monitored. There is small increase in cleft palate incidence if given in first trimester and theoretical risk of hormonal disturbance in fetus.[4] Only Prednisolone should be used during pregnancy as oral corticosteroid preparation.[8]

Treatment of ENL in Pregnancy

General Principles

Principles of treatment include inflammation control, pain relief and prevention of further episodes. Rest and anti-inflammatory (mainly Aspirin) medications are treatment of choice for mild ENL. NSAIDs, colchicine, oral zinc, pentoxifylline and chloroquine have been used. Anti-inflammatory and immunomodulators are important as ENL has high potential to cause disabilities (occurring due to nerve damage). Counseling of mother is important as mental stress associated with the condition and infant concern can aggravate the condition. Triggers like alcohol, drug withdrawal, stress, lack of sleep, concomitant infection should be controlled.

Selection of mother's antimicrobial drug regimen must ensure adequate bacteria control while avoiding teratogenicity and in utero adverse effects. MDT is considered safe for mother and child. Anti-leprosy drugs are excreted into human milk but adverse effects are

Table 26.1: MDT in pregnancy

Constituent of MDT	*Applied aspects relevant to pregnancy and lactation*
Rifampicin	Pregnancy: Rifampicin can cross the placenta. No increased risk of birth defects has been reported (more than 300 reports) regarding rifampicin use during pregnancy. Neonatal bleeding related with use during the third trimester is reported. Lactation: About 5% of therapeutic dose can be transferred to human milk, without adverse effects in exposed neonates. It is compatible with breastfeeding.
Dapsone	Pregnancy: Successful pregnancies in women receiving dapsone during pregnancy are described. Dapsone-induced hemolytic anemia in mothers and their babies, with resolution of symptoms after dapsone discontinuation is reported. Patients are recommended to take 5 mg of folic acid daily with dapsone throughout pregnancy because of the potential for a small decrease in folate absorption. Testing for G6PD deficiency is recommended to identify and avoid severe hemolysis due to dapsone. Lactation: As nearly 15% of weight-related maternal dosage of dapsone can enter human milk, treatment should be decided on an individual basis. Dapsone has been associated with neonatal hemolysis and methemoglobinemia (rarely).
Clofazimine	Pregnancy: It can cross the placenta and pass into the milk, causing fetal skin discoloration. Lactation: Proportion transferred with the milk is approximately 22% of the maternal dose. Acute toxicity due to clofazimine secreted into the milk is unlikely.
Ofloxacin	Avoid in pregnancy and lactation due to risk of arthropathy (in animal studies).
Minocycline	Teratogenic in pregnancy and causes infant teeth discoloration and damage due to passage in breast milk.

not reported except for clofazimine induced skin discoloration in infants. MDT should be continued unchanged during pregnancy and breastfeeding. Accompanied MDT (AMDT) can be useful approach if it is difficult for woman to reach clinic in later stages of pregnancy or during postpartum period, but close observation is needed.

Corticosteroids

Same regimen as given to other patients with leprosy reactions (*see* Section 4, Chapters 23 and 24) is given as no published evidence for specific and effective steroid regimen for pregnant women and their outcomes is available. Prednisolone, first-line treatment, rapidly controls inflammation and pain. Dose is 40–60 mg/kg/day, maximum 1 mg/kg/day, with gradual tapering and stoppage.[8] At times high doses are required, increasing risk of adverse effects. In steroid dependency/complications, clofazimine is used in anti-reaction doses.[5,6]

Thalidomide

Due to its teratogenicity, (especially early in pregnancy) it should never be used for pregnant women or women of childbearing age group. Women of reproductive age group can only be prescribed thalidomide under supervision when have negative pregnancy tests and are using two different methods of contraception (STEPS program mandate), if at all, considering the benefit. Contraception should also be used when male partner is taking thalidomide.[9]

Clofazimine

Clofazimine is a dye, useful and inexpensive having anti-inflammatory and antimicrobial properties. It has antineutrophilic effect and inhibits prostaglandins. At a dose of 300 mg/day, serum concentration doubles. It is especially useful in managing recurrent and chronic ENL, acting as a steroid sparing agent. Disadvantage includes slow action (4–6 weeks to exert effects), gastrointestinal side effects and discoloration.

Other medications that can be used is mentioned in the Table 26.2.[10–11]

Cyclosporin use during pregnancy appears to be associated with premature delivery and low birthweight infants. Comorbidities such as hypertension, preeclampsia and gestational diabetes mellitus are also reported at higher incidences than the general population. The literature suggests that cyclosporin therapy during pregnancy should be carefully considered by the treating physician, but may be a safe alternative for patients' refractory to conventional treatment.[12]

Although, TNF inhibitors seem to be safe in pregnancy, some unfavorable pregnancy outcomes like low birth weight and preterm labor were reported with the use of biologics in pregnancy. Some studies have reported alterations in maternal and infant immune systems. Still, long-term data about children born to women treated with biologics in pregnancy are not attainable.[13]

Management of Lepra Reactions in Lactation

Principles of management are the same as in nonpregnant persons (*see* Section 4, Chapters 23 and 24). This involves starting MDT in a treatment naïve patient, and initiating anti-inflammatory therapy along with physical support or immobilization if there is active neuritis. MDT is imperative to reduce antigenic load, reducing recurrence and resistance. For mild T1R, NSAIDs can be used. However, oral steroids remain the mainstay of treatment for most cases.

Mild T2R can be managed with analgesics alone (Paracetamol, ibuprofen, diclofenac are relatively safer than aspirin and tramadol in lactation).

Moderate T2R: Prednisolone 30–40 mg/day can be started and tapered in the usual manner.

Recurrent T2R: Requires prolonged administration of oral steroids with slow tapering.

Chronic ENL: These patients may become steroid dependent; hence steroid sparing agents may have to be considered. Lactating mother with chronic ENL can opt for discontinuing lactation once the infant is 9–12 months old, after consultation with a pediatrician.

Though thalidomide is contraindicated in lactation, clofazimine is safe.[3] Limited data exist on pentoxifylline in lactation, but it is poorly secreted in breast milk and is considered safe in infants above 2 months of age.[14] Minocycline can stain breastmilk black, and there is

Table 26.2: Agents which have potential to be used for reactions during pregnancy

Drug	***Features***
Cyclosporine A	Provides a beneficial effect in ENL by increasing the number of T suppressor cells in lesions
TNFα inhibitors	TNFα plays a key role in the pathogenesis of ENL. Infliximab is a human murine chimeric monoclonal antibody against TNFα, Etanercept is a dimeric fusion protein of the extracellular portion of the p75 TNF receptor coupled to IgG1. Both of these effectively reduce TNFα levels and give good results in ENL.

theoretical risk of dental enamel staining and bone deposition of tetracyclines.[15] Long-term maternal use of colchicine (1.5 g daily) leads to less than 10% of maternal weight adjusted dose in infant, occurring at 2–4 hours after maternal intake. Hence, it is advisable not to breastfeed up to 4 hours of colchicine intake by mother.[16] Azathioprine is contraindicated. Cyclosporine, methotrexates are generally avoided, but can be given if benefits outweigh risks, with close monitoring of infant. Recommended daily dose of zinc sulpfate in lactating woman is 12 mg/day, and additional dose can lead to copper deficiency in infant, and hence should be avoided. MIP vaccine is avoided as there are no clinical studies to support its use.

Drugs used for lepra reaction in lactation is mentioned in Table 26.3.

PROGNOSIS AND FOLLOW-UP

For women still on MDT, or completed MDT, should be closely observed throughout pregnancy, and for 12 months postpartum. Each monthly visit should include history, physical examination, NF assessment, visual acuity assessment and enquiry about infant's welfare. Women who need MDT should be advised at each visit to continue treatment during pregnancy and to avoid treatment discontinuation due to maternal anxiety regarding fetal health.

CONCLUSION

Even the technical guidance documents of leprosy programs on management of reactions does not cover in detail the management leprosy and its reactional states during pregnancy

Table 26.3: Use of drugs for lepra reaction in lactation

Symptom	*Medications*	*Features*
Mild type of T1R: Pain and lesional inflammation	Paracetamol	Can be safely used in a lactating mother as levels secreted in breast milk are much less than the infant dose.
Pain and lesional inflammation	Aspirin	It is not safe in lactation as it is rapidly converted to salicylate in blood and is excreted considerably into breastmilk, and prolonged use can lead to complications like metabolic acidosis, thrombocytopenia, hemolysis in infants.
Pain and lesional inflammation	Other NSAIDs: Ibuprofen	It is a safe anti-inflammatory in nursing mothers due to its extremely low levels in breast milk and short half-life.
Pain and lesional inflammation	Indomethacin	It is also secreted negligibly into breastmilk and is considered safe.
Moderate-to-severe type:	Hydroxychloroquine	Pregnancy: Positive risk-benefit ratio for treating mild reactions in pregnancy has not been established; it is best avoided in first trimester Lactation: In doses upto 400 mg per day, it can be safely used in lactation as extremely low levels are excreted in breast milk.
	Cyclosporine	Cyclosporine levels in breastmilk vary considerably between studies, however only 1–2% of the mother's weight adjusted dose reaches the infant. Adverse effects have not been reported. For safety sake, infant serum levels of cyclosporine may be monitored during therapy.

and lactation. There is a need of formal recommendation for better outcome of pregnancy in patients with lepra reactions.[9] Pregnancy/lactation can affect clinical manifestations of leprosy, hence novel management strategies tailored to these situations are needed.[17] Women of childbearing age should be offered preemptive family planning advice, in case they suffer from severe form of leprosy or reactions. However, pregnancy termination due to leprosy is not justifiable on medical grounds.[3] Note that efficacy of contraceptive drugs may be reduced due to rifampin-associated induction of liver enzymes.[3] Referral to social services and counseling of family members to encourage and facilitate support is important.

REFERENCES

1. Vijay N, Sarma S. Leprosy with erythema nodosum leprosum in pregnancy: A rare phenomenon. J South Asian Feder Obst Gynae. 2019;11:329–30.
2. Lockwood DN , Sinha HH. Pregnancy and leprosy: a comprehensive literature review. Int J Lepr Other Mycobact Dis. 1999;67:6–12.
3. Bhatia R, Mehta S, Grover A, Dubey S. Leprosy in pregnancy: Obstetric diligence is the key. J Clin Diagn Res. 2017;11:QD01–QD02.
4. Butlin CR, Withington S. 4 March 2018, posting date. Mothers and children with leprosy, Chapter 3.2. In Scollard DM, Gillis TP (ed), International textbook of leprosy. www.internationaltextbookofleprosy.org.
5. Thangaraju P, Sajitha Venkatesan S, Gurunthalingam M, Babu S, and Tamilselvan T. Rationale use of Thalidomide in erythema nodosum leprosum-A non-systematic critical analysis of published case reports. Rev Soc Bras Med Trop. 2020; 53: e20190454.
6. Upputuri B, Pallapati MS, Tarwater P, Srikantam A. Thalidomide in the treatment of erythema nodosum leprosum (ENL) in an outpatient setting: A five-year retrospective analysis from a leprosy referral centre in India. PLoS Negl Trop Dis. 2020; 9:1–13.
7. Narang T, Kamat D. Reactions in Leprosy. Type 2 Lepra Reaction. In: Sardana K, Khurana A editors. Jopling's handbook of Leprosy. 6th ed. New Delhi: CBS Publishers and Distributors. 2020. P. 211–6.
8. Naafs B. Treatment duration of reversal reaction: A reappraisal. Back to the past. Lepr Rev. 2003;74:328–36.
9. Leprosy/Hansen Disease: Management of reactions and prevention of disabilities. Technical guidance. New Delhi: World Health Organization, Regional Office for South-East Asia; 2017. License: CC BY-NC-SA 3.0 IGO.
10. Christensen LA, Dahlerup JF, Nielsen MJ, Fallingborg JF, Schmiegelow K. Azathioprine treatment during lactation. Aliment Pharmacol Ther. 2008;28:1209–13.
11. Bethesda. Drugs and Lactation Database (LactMed) [Internet]. US: National Library of Medicine; 2006 Cyclosporine. [Updated 2021 Oct 18].
12. Paziana K, Del Monaco M, Cardonick E, *et al*. Ciclosporin use during pregnancy. Drug Saf. 2013;36:279–94.
13. Beltagy A, Aghamajidi A, Trespidi L, et al. Biologics during pregnancy and breastfeeding among women with rheumatic diseases: Safety clinical evidence on the road. Front. Pharmacol. 2021;12:621247.
14. Bethesda. Drugs and Lactation Database (LactMed) [Internet]. US: National Library of Medicine; 2006 Pentoxifylline. [Updated 2020 Jul 20].
15. Bethesda. Drugs and Lactation Database (LactMed) [Internet]. US: National Library of Medicine; 2006 Minocycline. [Updated 2021 Jan 18].
16. N. Herscovici T, Merlob P, Stahl B, Laron-Kenet T, Klinger G. Colchicine use during breastfeeding. Breastfeed Med. 2015;10(2):92–5.
17. Wankhade VH, Debnath P, Singh RP, Sawatkar G, Bhat DM. A retrospective study of the severe and uncommon variants of erythema nodosum leprosum at a tertiary health center in central India. Int J Mycobacteriol. 2019;8:29–34.

Chapter 27

Management of Leprosy in Children Including Reactions

• Bhumesh Kumar Katakam • Bikash Ranjan Kar

INTRODUCTION

Prevalence of leprosy in children is an indication of ongoing transmission of the disease in the community and also a target intervention of the enhanced strategy for leprosy control by WHO. Children with leprosy poses a variety of challenges to the healthcare provider. This is because with the general reduction in the expertise of leprosy management, the knowledge about the treatment options for leprosy in children is also decreasing. Furthermore, treating physicians need to be more aware about the dosing and pharmacology of drugs used for leprosy management in children. Unavailability of the blister packs of MDT for children of various age groups compounds the problem. This outlines the need of the practical manual for management of children with leprosy.

CURRENT KNOWLEDGE AND THE KNOWLEDGE GAP

With effective implementation of multidrug therapy decline in the prevalence of leprosy has been noticed throughout the world. However, child leprosy continues to be observed in new cases globally. For the year 2022, a total of 10,302 new child cases (5.9% of total new cases) was reported globally, corresponding to a rate of 5.1 per million child population. Most of the child cases were reported from South-East Asian Region (70.1%) with a child case detection rate of 14 per million child population.[1] For the same year, of the 9,554 new cases with grade 2 disabilities, 278 are children. The fact that child cases with G2D continue to be detected is a concern and indicates that early detection and timely treatment must be improved. However, treatment and drug usage information for management of lepra reactions in children are not yet standardized currently.

DIAGNOSING LEPROSY IN CHILDREN

The principle of diagnosis of leprosy in children remains the same as in adults. Diagnosing leprosy in children is not always straight forward, when they present with single hypopigmented patch, more so on the face, as it is difficult to assess sensory impairment in a child. In addition, pityriasis alba is a close mimic of indeterminate leprosy which is found more commonly in children than adults. Nonetheless, it should be noted that all clinical types of leprosy can occurs in children, although BL and LL leprosy are less common compared to adults.[2] Reactions, both type 1 and 2 can occur in children, with type 1 being more frequent. Hence, early diagnosis and treatment is paramount for prevention of deformity among leprosy affected children. Note that any deformity occurring in children leads to severe loss of self-esteem and stigmatisation. (Diagnosis of leprosy is described in Section 1; Chapter 1.)

TREATMENT GUIDELINES

1. **NLEP**-India guidelines of MDT for children: (NLEP training manual for medical officers, Govt of India 2019) (Table 27.1).
2. Most countries' national program follows guidelines issued by the WHO. However, it should be kept in mind that these guidelines can be modified by the countries as per their local needs. Current WHO recommendation (2018) for the treatment of child with leprosy is to treat all patients with a 3-drug regimen, only the duration is different, which is 12-month treatment for MB and 6-month treatment for PB (Table 27.2).
3. Guidelines for the Control of Leprosy. Brazilian Ministry of Health, 2002 differentiates children in the two age groups: 0–5 years of age and 6–14 years of age and suggest treatment as mentioned in Table 27.3.

Educating the parents regarding expected outcome and adverse effects is essential before starting MDT for the child. Majority of the children tolerate standard MDT very well. Available MDT blister packs (Fig. 27.1) though convenient and distributed free of cost they are not child friendly and hence reported treatment dropout rates in children ranges from 10 to 20% in some programs.[3,4] Non-availability of the anti-leprosy drugs in child friendly forms like dispersible tablet or syrup formulations is an issue, which is yet to be addressed by the national programme managers.

Investigations required with treatment are listed in Table 27.4.

Table 27.1: NLEP guidelines of MDT for children (10–14 years)

Type of leprosy	*Drugs used (Adult)*	*Dosage (mg)*	*Frequency of administration*	*Criteria for RFT*
MB Leprosy	Rifampicin	450	Once monthly	Completion of 12 monthly pulses
	Dapsone	50	Daily	
	Clofazimine	150	Monthly	
	Clofazimine	50	Alternate day	
PB Leprosy	Rifampicin	450	Once monthly	Completion of 6 monthly pulses
	Dapsone	50	Daily	

The Appropriate dose for children under 10 years of age can be decided on the basis of body weight Rifampicin: 10 mg/kg/month. Clofazimine: 6 mg/kg/month and 1 mg/kg/day (to be given weekly capsule as the lowest available dose is 50 mg). Dapsone: 2 mg/kg/day.

Table 27.2: WHO guidelines of MDT for children

Age group	*Drug*	*Dosage and frequency*	*Duration*
Children <10 years old or <40 kg	Rifampicin Clofazimine Dapsone	10 mg/kg once month 100 mg once a month, 50 mg twice weekly 2 mg/kg daily	12 months for MB and 6 months for PB
Children (10–14 years)	Rifampicin Clofazimine Dapsone	450 mg once a month 150 mg once a month, 50 mg on alternate days 50 mg daily	12 months for MB and 6 months for PB

Table 27.3A: MDT for MB leprosy in children- Guidelines of Brazil

Age in years	*Daily*	*Supervised*	*Supervised*	*Weekly*	*Supervised*
	Dapsone (mg)	*Dapsone (mg)*	*Rifampicin (mg)*	*Clofazimine (mg)*	*Clofazimine (mg)*
0–5	25	25	150–300	100	100
6–14	50–100	50–100	300–450	150	150–200

Table 27.3B: MDT for PB leprosy in children- Guidelines of Brazil

Age in years	*Daily dapsone (mg)*	*Supervised dapsone (mg)*	*Supervised rifampicin (mg)*
0–5	25	25	150–300
6–14	50–100	50–100	300–450

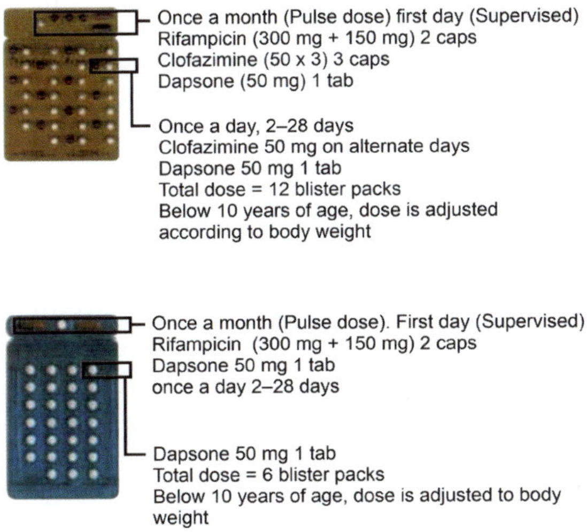

Fig. 27.1: MDT blister packs for children (pediatric dose: 10–14 years). (A) Multibacillary leprosy; (B) Pauclbacillary leprosy

Table 27.4: Recommended laboratory tests and frequency

	Initial visit	*2nd visit (1–2 months)*	*3 m*	*6 m*	*12 m*
CBC + platelets	X	X	X	X	X
AST	X		X	X	X
ALT	X		X	X	X
Ca	X				
BUN	X				
Creatinine	X				
Bilirubin	X				
G6PD	X				

Alternative Anti-leprosy Drugs for Use in Children

Children who do not tolerate dapsone or develop dapsone hypersensitivity syndrome while on MDT PB, it should be substituted with clofazimine. Ideally ofloxacin should be avoided and used with caution if at all in children and growing adolescents.[5] Minocycline is also relatively contraindicated in children. Any child with rifampicin resistance need to be given a customised regimen as per recommendations from the WHO expert committee under supervision.[6] Fortunately, alternative anti-leprosy drugs are not usually needed in children.

Reactions

Reported frequency of reactions in children varies from 3.1 to 33.9%.[7–9] Risk factors for the reactions in children are borderline unstable disease and older age.[10,11] Higher incidence of reactions have been reported with or without deformities in children mostly from hospital based studies where children with severe form of disease are likely to be seen. Clinical presentation and the diagnosis of type 1 lepra reactions (Fig. 27.2) and type 2 lepra (ENL) reactions (Fig. 27.3) are same as that of adults. Though in children reactional episodes in leprosy and disabilities are less frequently seen, but when they do occur it is particularly difficult to manage them due to lack of consensus guidelines by the health agencies. Even the technical guidance document prepared by WHO does not provide guidance on management of reaction in children.[12] Same flowcharts as mentioned in Section 4; Chapters 23 and 24 should be followed, with dosages adjusted to the weight of the child patient.

Treatment of Reactions

Early identification and optimal use of systemic corticosteroids remains the main stay of treatment for both type of lepra reaction in children. It is important to recognize and manage leprosy reactions and neuritis effectively, so that nerve function is preserved.

Drug regimen for lepra reactions: It is imperative that ongoing MDT must never be stopped due to fear of exacerbation of lepra reaction and should be continued. For mild

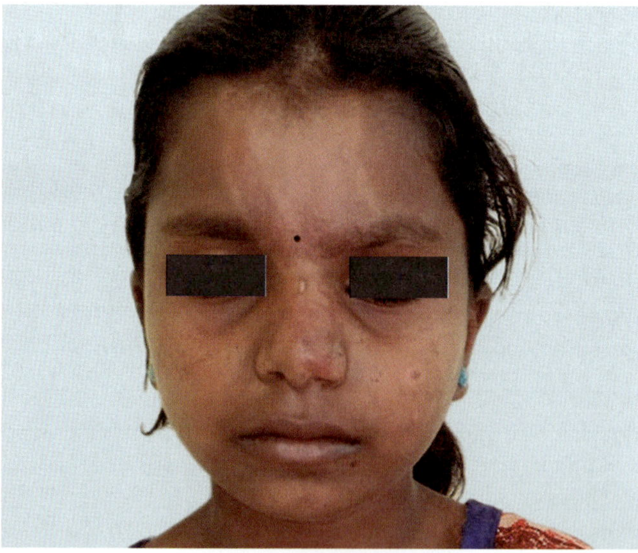

Fig. 27.2: Type 1 reaction in a 10-year-old girl child (*Courtesy:* Dr Subodh Patjoshi)

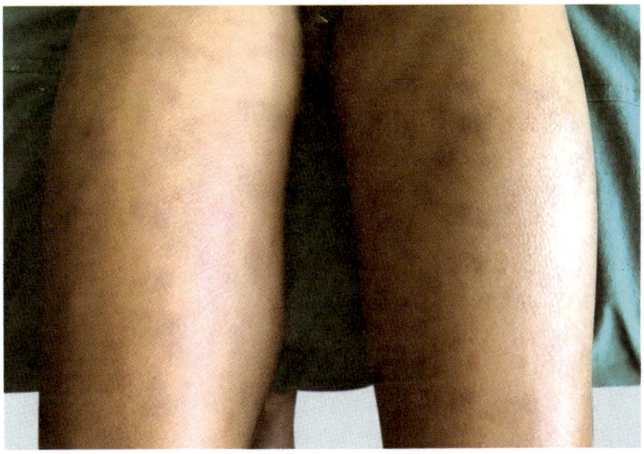

Fig. 27.3: Type 2 reaction in an 8-year-old female child (*Courtesy:* Dr Krupa Sindhu Pradhan)

type of lepra reactions, NSAIDs are sufficient to control the pain and inflammation. In case of severe reaction and presence of neuritis, use of systemic corticosteroids is indicated. Unfortunately, there is a scant published evidence on steroid dosages and regimens in children for the management of reactions. Hence, the steroid regimen similar to adult regimen, with modification for the child's weight is used[13] (Box 27.1).

Growth retardation, HPA axis suppression and cushingoid features are the chief adverse effects noticed in children when corticosteroids are used for more than 3 months duration. One way to reduce above adverse effects is to limit the use of corticosteroids to less than 1 mg/kg body weight or giving them on alternate days. Children's growth should be charted during the follow-up.

Type 2 reaction in children: For mild type of ENL reactions, NSAIDs are indicated to control the pain and inflammation. For severe type 2 reactions, regimen similar to adult patient should be used, adjusted to patient's weight.

Prednisolone

Tapering principles are slightly different for T1R compared to T2R, with a more slower taper in case of severe T1R. Tendency to rapid taper should be avoided and patient to be maintained on lower effective dose of corticosteroid. Starting dose can be 1 mg/kg in severe T1R. Every month 5 mg should be tapered and duration of complete course will last up to 4–6 months.

Clofazimine can be added for more severe T2R in the dosing range of 1.5–2 mg per kg thrice a day for first month and subsequently reducing by one dose per day each month.[13] It is a slow acting drug and onset of action builds up over 4–6 weeks.

Box 27.1: Steroid regimen for children with severe reaction/neuritis

- Start with 1mg/kg of prednisolone for one week
- Then taper by 5 mg/week till 20 mg
- Then 20 mg/day for 28 days
- Then 15 mg/day for 14 days
- Then 10 mg/day for 14 days
- Then 5 mg/day for 14 days

Thalidomide is contraindicated for use in children below 12 years as safety is not established. However, it may be given to adolescent boys. For patients below 35 kg body weight, thalidomide can be given in a dose of 6 mg/kg/day.[14]

Other drugs that can be used as steroid sparing agents or adjuvants are hydroxychloroquine, methotrexate, azathioprine, cyclosporine and paracetamol.[2] Nerve function assessment should be done periodically while children are on treatment and dosage of corticosteroids need to be modified accordingly.

Response and Follow-up

The patient and the parents should be educated to monitor the progress of nerve impairment by looking at their hands and feet regularly and they should be advised to report to the healthcare provider at the earliest. Patients with sensory loss over feet should use protective MCR shoes with soft insoles. Reconstructive surgery is considered for those patients with motor loss resulting in deformities once the patient is completely treated and is reaction and neuritis free. RCS is mostly recommended above the age of 15 years. It has been found in various studies that the skin lesions of leprosy can undergo self-healing in children.[15] Nevertheless, it will not be possible to predict in which group of patients such self-healing occurs. Hence, we must provide full course of MDT for the recommended duration to all child leprosy patients.

Preventive Measures

Annual examination of children and household/neighbourhood contacts of index case of leprosy remains the mainstay for early identification and management of leprosy.

CONCLUSION

Childhood leprosy is the strong indicator of disease transmission in the community and performance indicator of the NLEP. Clinical diagnosis still remains the mainstay for the detection of leprosy in childrens; however, in certain situations, histopathological examination can be helpful in confirming the diagnosis of leprosy in children. Correct labeling of PB and MB cases is a prerequisite. No MB case should be treated as PB case. Reactions in children require urgent treatment as they can lead to irreversible deformities.

REFERENCES

1. WHO Weekly epidemiological record, 37, 2023; 98,409–30.
2. Narang T, Kumar B. Leprosy in children. Indian J Paediatr Dermatol 2019;20:12–24.
3. Singal A, Sonthalia S, Pandhi D. Childhood leprosy in a tertiary-care hospital in Delhi, India: A reappraisal in the post-elimination era. Lepr Rev. 2011;82:259–69.
4. Chaitra P, Bhat RM. Post elimination status of childhood leprosy: Report from a tertiary-care hospital in South India. Biomed Res Int. 2013;2013:328673.
5. Kar HK, Gupta R. Treatment of leprosy. Clin Dermatol 2015;33:55–65.
6. World Health Organisation.WHO expert committee on leprosy.World Health Org Tech Rep Ser. 2012;968:1–61.
7. Selvasekar A, Geetha J, Nisha K, Manimozhi N, Jesudasan K, Rao PS, et al. Childhood leprosy in an endemic area. Lepr Rev. 1999;70:21–7.
8. Dogra S, Narang T, Khullar G, Kumar R, Saikia UN. Childhood leprosy through the post-leprosy-elimination era: A retrospective analysis of epidemiological and clinical characteristics of disease over eleven years from a tertiary care hospital in North India. Lepr Rev. 2014;85:296–310.

9. Palit A, Inamadar AC. Childhood leprosy in India over the past two decades. Lepr Rev. 2014;85:93–9.
10. Oliveira MB, Diniz LM. Leprosy among children under 15 years of age: Literature review. An Bras Dermatol. 2016;91:196–203.
11. Pandhi D, Mehta S, Agrawal S, Singal A. Erythema nodosum leprosum necroticans in a child--an unusual manifestation. Int J Lepr Other Mycobact Dis. 2005;73:122–6.
12. Leprosy/Hansen Disease: Management of reactions and prevention of disabilities. Technical guidance. New Delhi: World Health Organization, Regional Office for South-East Asia; 2017. Licence: CC BY-NC-SA 3.0 IGO.
13. Butlin CR, Withington S. 4 March 2018, posting date. Mothers and children with leprosy, Chapter 3.2. In Scollard DM, Gillis TP (ed), International textbook of leprosy. www.internationaltextbookofleprosy.org.
14. Shanbhag PS, Viswanath V, Torsekar RG. Thalidomide: Current status. Indian J Dermatol Venereol Leprol 2006;72:75–80.
15. Pradhan S, Nayak BP, Dash G. Childhood Leprosy: A Review. Indian J PaediatrDermatol. 2019;20:112–6.

Section 5

Role of Physiotherapy

Chapter 28

Principles of Physiotherapy

• Sathish Kumar Paul • David Prakash Kumar • Delicia Roshini

INTRODUCTION

Physiotherapy plays a vital role in the rehabilitation of a person affected by Leprosy. It helps in the identification and management of the impairments and thus improving the quality of life of patients. Importance of providing optimal physiotherapy for a patient with leprosy and lepra reactions have been stressed time and again and is the need of the hour in achieving the target of reduction in the grade 2 disability as suggested by the WHO. The Dermlep Survey showed that only 33.28% patients were advised physiotherapy as a part of management by dermatologists.[1] This shows that there is a need for all heath care providers to realise the importance and learn principles of physiotherapy for prevention of disabilities in leprosy. Physiotherapy is an integral part of management of leprosy and if physiotherapeutic measures are added to MDT and other management, affected persons can be managed better. The need for physiotherapy is mentioned in Table 28.1.

Commonly used physiotherapeutic methods are simple and can be organized with very little inputs. Various techniques of physiotherapy are listed in Table 28.2.

CLINICAL APPROACH TO IMPLEMENT OPTIMAL PHYSIOTHERAPY

This includes following: (a) Baseline assessment, (b) Goal setting based on the assessment (c) Physiotherapy intervention, followed by reassessment. These are the major principles of physiotherapy[3] to achieve optimal outcomes as depicted in Fig. 28.1.

Baseline Assessment

The baseline nerve function assessment of the person affected by leprosy which includes sensory testing and motor testing is very important to identify existing impairments. Touch/ pressure, temperature and vibration are assessed in sensory testing. Testing for presence of

Table 28.1: Need for physiotherapy in leprosy[2]
• Prevent the onset of disabilities and deformities
• Arrest the progression of disabilities and deformities if already developed
• Relieve nerve pain and keep limb functional
• Maintain integrity of muscle intact till they are reinnervated, if palsy has set in
• Help in resolution of inflammation and edema of the extremities in leprosy reactions
• Keep joints mobile
• Essential for reconstructive surgery, both before and after the operation

Table 28.2: Various techniques of physiotherapy	
Physiotherapeutic methods	**Practical implication**
Hydro-oleo therapy	Soaking in water, followed by oil application to make the skin supple and soft. To be practiced at least twice a day but is not advised if affected part is inflamed or infected
Exercises	Exercises are performed to increase muscle strength and retain their tone 1. Active exercises are most useful in cases with early and incomplete motor paralysis. 2. Assisted active exercises are performed to prevent damage to the anatomical structures by adaptive postures. These exercises are called assisted because external support is used to stabilize the joints rendered unstable by muscle palsies. 3. Passive exercises, where joint movements are carried out with full outside support (instead of by the muscles which normally perform that movement), are aimed to put the joint through full range of movement so that contractures do not develop in opposite group of muscles and also in the joints.
Heat therapy	1. Superficial heating modalities like heating pads, hydrotherapy and paraffin baths heat by conduction. 2. Wax bath is most commonly used. The physiologic effects of heat application are increased collagen extensibility, decreased joint stiffness, relief of pain and muscle spasm, increased blood flow and resolution of inflammatory infiltrates, edema and exudates.
Electrical stimulation	Electrical stimulating currents have low frequency and long wavelengths and easily penetrate human tissues. Electrical stimulation has been used for reduction of pain, stimulation of neuromuscular function and to stimulate the bone and soft tissue healing.

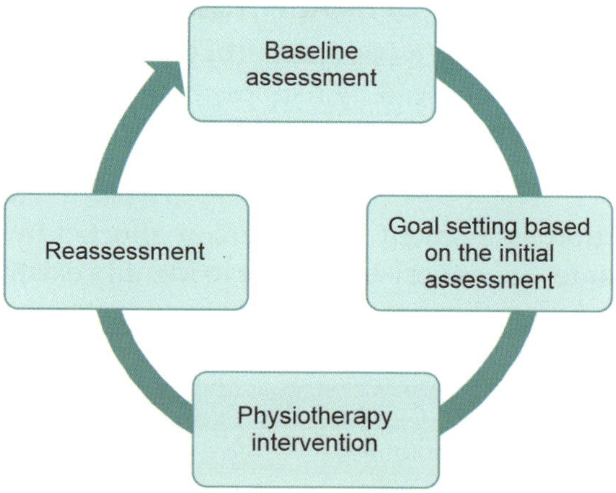

Fig. 28.1: Principles of physiotherapy

touch/pressure sensation is the one that is most commonly performed. Semmes-Weinstein (SW) filaments are used to test sensation of the palmar surface of hands and plantar aspect of the feet, on specific points. A minimum of 4 points and a maximum of 10 points are tested. Any impairment identified in the assessment forms the basis of planning treatment that will help in preventing deterioration and improving function. Persons identified to have nerve function impairment should religiously follow self-care regime as described in detail in next chapter.

Principles of Passive and Active Exercises[3]

Muscle strength can be defined as the ability of a muscle to perform its action with adequate tensile force. In addition, the muscles also need to remain elastic to contract through the range of movement without restriction. Muscles with good strength can help to prevent disability and retain good functional efficiency. Strengthening helps in increasing muscle bulk and maintains strength of the muscles. Strengthening is indicated in all weak muscles. It will prevent muscle from getting paralyzed.

Passive exercises: When a muscle is paralyzed and cannot move a joint, passive exercises are needed to prevent that joint from becoming stiff and maintain the joint range of motion and also to prevent muscle wasting or atrophy. They can also be performed to improve the range of motion of a joint that is stiff or having contractures.

Passive exercises can be performed by the patient using the unaffected hand or the exercises can be done with help from the health worker or assistive aids. Example of passive exercise is using a towel placed over forefoot and held by hand to dorsiflex the ankle joints in those patients suffering from foot drop. Ideally, these exercises can be performed with the help/under supervision of a trained leprosy physiotherapist for first few weeks.

Active exercises: Active exercises are performed by the patient with their own muscle power. Active exercises are possible even when there is muscle weakness and limited range of joint motion. The patient is encouraged to actively move the joint through the freely available range of movement. This helps to maintain the joint movement and function. When the patient tries to actively move the joint repetitively to the extreme range possible, this effort can help to improve the range of motion by breaking down adhesions and stiffness. Active movement can also help to increase muscle relaxation and improves coordination and functional activity.

Active 'assisted' exercises are performed when an external assistance is provided to the joint movement by the physiotherapist or an external appliance or even gravity.

Active 'resisted' exercises are a progression from active exercises and help in providing resistance to the active movement. This helps in strengthening the muscle that is being exercised.

Principles of Physiotherapy Assessments for Tendon Transfer Surgeries

The muscle to be transferred in tendon transfer surgery needs to be isolated and strengthened. Tibialis posterior muscle isolation and strengthening is commonly done before a 'tibialis posterior tendon transfer surgery'. Providing resistance to the movement of the muscle when it is performing its action is the best method of strengthening it. Resistance can be provided manually by the patient or by the therapist. External appliances like springs, sandbags and other weights can also provide mechanical resistance. Even moving the muscle against gravity can help in strengthening it. First step in tendon transfer surgery is to identify a muscle-tendon that can be transferred. The strength of the muscle to be transferred is assessed using VMT and the power should be 5, which means that the muscle should be strong, even against resistance. The excursion of the muscle chosen should be adequate so that it can move the joint even when it is transferred. The ideal muscle chosen for tendon transfer surgery should not be a prime mover of a joint.

Range of Motion Assessment

The passive range of motion of the joint where the muscle tendon transfer is being done should be assessed. If there is any restriction of the range of motion in the joint where the tendon transfer is being targeted, surgery will not be successful. Hence, assessment of the passive range of motion of the interphalangeal joints of the fingers is important before selecting a patient, e.g, for claw hand correction. Similarly, the thumb interphalangeal joint range and thumb web range should be assessed before ape thumb (loss of thumb abduction) correction. The ankle dorsiflexion range should be assessed before tibialis posterior transfer surgery. If any restriction in the range of motion is identified during assessment, passive exercises and other manual or surgical interventions have to be performed to overcome the stiffness or contracture.

Functional Assessment

A functional assessment of the hand function should be performed before tendon transfer surgery. This can be compared with the postoperative results to identify the functional benefits of surgery. Some of the components of the functional assessment are grasp contact, pinch contact, grasp power, pinch power, picking up objects using fingers and hand as a whole, buttoning, unbuttoning, opening and fastening a zip and counting paper sheets.

Goal Setting

Once the initial baseline assessment is completed, the next step is to set long-term goals for the holistic rehabilitation of the patient. For the long-term goal to be achieved, the physiotherapist has to set several short-term goals based on the impairments that are identified through the assessment.

Short-term Goals to Prevent and Manage Impairments

- Providing sufficient rest to the nerves that are painful due to acute neuritis
- Passive exercises for the paralysed muscle to keep them pliable and prevent atrophy
- Active exercises for the weak muscles to improve their strength and endurance
- Maintaining and improving the range of motion of joints with strengthening and stretching exercises, thus preventing them from becoming stiff due to muscle weakness or paralysis
- Principles of self-care/lifestyle modifications to be practiced by the patient
- Offloading of the ulcers to enhance healing
- Gait training
- Splinting and providing assistive devices
- Pre and postoperative physiotherapy to improve outcome of tendon transfer surgeries
- Use of physiotherapy adjuncts to improve treatment outcome.

Physiotherapy Interventions to Achieve the Above Goals

1. Providing rest to painful nerves is essential, as acute neuritis can lead to progressive nerve damage.
   - The affected limb with a acutely inflamed nerve must be splinted to provide rest.
   - Splinting with plaster of Paris (POP) casts will help to prevent excessive movement in the joint over which the affected nerve is passing. This prevents worsening of symptoms and also helps in enhancing the healing process.
   - Splints like ulnar neuritis slab for ulnar neuritis and median neuritis slab for median neuritis are commonly used.

2. Stretching exercises
   - The principle behind stretching exercises is to make the soft tissues mobile and increase the range of motion in the joints.
   - Stretching is performed when soft tissues are stiff or if there is adhesion formation in the tissues.
   - Static stretching method is used to stretch tissues in the hand or legs of a leprosy affected person. This entails a gentle and slow but sustained stretching for a period of 30 seconds to one minute.
   - Such stretching can be performed by the therapist or the patient can be taught to stretch their tissues that have already become tight or could become tight or stiff due to muscle paralysis.
   - Examples of stretching in leprosy affected individual are stretching of the Tendo Achilles in patients with foot drop, stretching of thumb web in those with median nerve damage and resultant ape thumb deformity, stretching of the interphalangeal joints in those with ulnar nerve damage and resultant claw hand deformity.
3. Offloading of the ulcers to enhance healing
   - Patients with nerve damage in leprosy are likely to suffer from insensitive feet. Walking and other activities with the insensitive feet lead to occurrence of peak plantar pressures. Offloading is the redistribution of this peak plantar pressure by using modified footwear, aids, appliances and other devices.
   - In leprosy affected individuals with plantar anesthesia, cost effective tactile sensors were used to design and develop bio feedback system that can help and prevent peak plantar pressures.[4]
   - Computer simulation studies have helped in the identification of peak plantar pressures and in fabricating offloading devices as well as customized insoles for leprosy affected patients.[5,6]
   - The insoles and the offloading devices facilitate the healing and prevent the worsening of plantar ulcers. Simulation studies have helped in identifying the ideal material for dissipating the peak plantar pressure in a footwear[7] used by a person with anesthetic foot.
   - The use of advanced computer technologies is available to help identify and provide feedback on the progression of ulcer care in leprosy.[8]
   - The mobile based technology is useful to access health care from the comfort of their homes for patients. The urban leprosy project in Kolkata has utilized the mobile based technology for early detection and in prevention and management of impairments in leprosy.[9]
   - Accommodative and functional orthosis have helped in the reduction of peak plantar pressures. However, there is a need to find the ideal ways to mass produce these orthoses cost effectively for all patients who need them.
4. Principles of gait training
   - A pre-evaluation will help to identify existing status of the patient before gait training is initiated. Lower limb rehabilitation usually involves gait training in front of a mirror within a parallel bar. The visual feedback in the mirror corrects posture and corrects gait abnormalities.
   - Foot drop, amputation, tendon transfer surgeries, use of lower limb orthotic devices are some of the indications for gait training.

- Gait training improves balance, increases lower limb muscle strength and improves general endurance of patient as well as confidence of patient.
- Progression from slow conscious walking with conscious use of the correct gait pattern to normal functional gait is achieved in gait training.

5. Principles of splinting and providing assistive devices
   - The use of an ideal assistive device would help the leprosy affected individual to overcome deformities by becoming functional and gain socioeconomic independence. This will improve the self-esteem of the individual by making the person an active contributor in the society. Therefore, it is essential to promote the use of assistive devices in preventing and managing impairments of leprosy.
   - The need of the hour is on using assistive devices and including the people with disabilities for their participation in achieving the sustainable development goals by 2030.[10]
   - Any lack of movements (stiffness or contractures), abnormal movements, reduced movements can all be corrected with the help of splints and assistive devices. Note that certain splints are designed to provide complete or selective immobilization.
   - Splints and assistive devices can also help in assisting certain movements and alter other movements.
   - If there is any abnormal alignment of the anatomical structure, splints can correct them and improve biomechanical efficiency.
   - Comfort in using the splint will help in better outcome and reduce risk of pressure injuries on the skin.
   - The materials with which splints are made should be skin friendly, light weight and comfortable to wear.
6. Pre- and post-physiotherapy to improve outcome of tendon transfer surgeries
   - Physiotherapy is an essential component in isolating, preparing and re-educating the individual muscles of the eye, hand and feet of the leprosy affected individual before and after the corrective surgery.
   - The simplified selection criteria developed by Govindasamy et al. can be used as a guideline and help therapists working in the field of leprosy to identify and carry out pre and postoperative physiotherapy in individuals waiting for corrective surgeries of their hands.[11]
   - Isolation and strengthening of the tendon to be transferred should be carried out for individuals identified to undergo eye, hand or foot surgeries.
   - A minimum of 3-week postoperative physiotherapy would help the patient learn the re-education of the muscle.
   - Daily monitoring, provision of isolation exercises, splints and exercises are essential in a successful post-operative physiotherapy.
   - Functional training following the re-education will help the patient become functionally independent.
   - The indications, process followed in identifying appropriate tendon to be transferred, the pre and post-operative physiotherapy techniques would help the therapists make the patients functionally active early.
7. Principles of using physiotherapy adjuncts to improve treatment outcome

   Electrical muscle stimulation: If the muscles are weak or completely paralysed, electrical muscle stimulation of the affected nerve or the muscles will keep the neuromuscular junctions active.

Paraffin wax therapy: The paraffin wax baths are a useful adjunct used in the rehabilitation. The dip and wrap method or the dip and re-immerse methods can be used. Adequate precautions need to be taken because of the anaesthetic limbs in many patients. The temperature of the wax bath needs to be checked to prevent burns and infection of the skin.

Ultrasound therapy: Ultrasound therapy is provided to post-operative stiffness and contractures.

Physiotherapy adjuncts are not to be prescribed in case the patient has any contra-indications.

Reassessment

The reassessment is necessary in any physiotherapy program, more so in a leprosy, to monitor the progress in the rehabilitation of the patient. The reassessment status of the patient needs to be compared with the baseline values to check the progress of the patient. Positive outcome and response to the interventions can mean that the same interventions can be continued and if not, the goals and interventions need to be modified as needed.

CONCLUSION

Physiotherapy plays a very important role in the identification of impairments in leprosy. Physiotherapy assessments are used as the important method to check the disease progression in the affected individual. Any improvement and deterioration can be identified with the data from these periodic assessments. The physiotherapy interventions help in the management and correction of deformities. Use of Plaster cast in healing ulcers, use of exercises to overcome stiffness in joints and strengthening weak or paralysed muscles are examples of effective physiotherapy interventions in leprosy. Pre- and postoperative physiotherapy are the cornerstone of the success of reconstructive surgeries.

REFERENCES

1. Rao PN, Rathod S, Suneetha S, Dogra S, Gupta SK, Vora R, Kamoji S, Tambe S. The DermLep Study I: Results of Prospective Nation-Wide Survey of the Number and Profile of Leprosy Patients seen by Dermatologists in India. Indian Dermatol Online J. 2020;11:701–11.
2. Central Leprosy Division, Directorate General of Health Services, Training Manual for Physiotherapists 2020.
3. Paul MSK, Kumar DP, Govindasamy K. 26 January 2019, posting date. Physical rehabilitation in leprosy, Chapter 4.3. In Scollard DM, Gillis TP (ed), International textbook of leprosy. www.internationaltextbookofleprosy.org.
4. Paul MS, Siva B. Peak plantar pressure analysis using customized tactile sensory feedback system—A short report; Lepr Rev. 2021; 92:82–7.
5. Kumar MD, Paul MS, Siva B. Computer designed orthotic device for offloading plantar ulcers—Technical paper. Lepr Rev. 2021; 92:152–61.
6. Kumar Paul, S., Vijayakumar, R., and Sivarasu, S. "Customized insole fabrication for foot deformities in leprosy patients." ASME. J Med Devices.2014; 8: 020950.
7. Paul S, Kumar DP, Siva B. Material analysis for therapeutic insoles—A short report. Lepr Rev. 2021;92:75–81.
8. Shah P, Mahajan S, Nageswaran S, Paul SK, Ebenzer M. Non-contact ulcer area calculation system for neuropathic foot ulcer. Foot Ankle Surg. 2019;25:47–50
9. Lal V, Das S, Pal S. Improving quality of care using Mobile Technology: experiences from urban leprosy project in Kolkata, India. Lepr Rev. 2017;88:270–3.
10. Tebbutt E, Brodmann R, Borg J, MacLachlan M, Khasnabis C, Horvath R. Assistive products and the Sustainable Development Goals (SDGs). Global Health. 2016;12:79.
11. Govindasamy K, Das P, Paul VJ, Kumar J. Selection criteria for reconstructive surgery to correct mobile hand deformities in leprosy. Lepr Rev. 2015;86:278–82.

Chapter

29 Self-care of Anesthetic Limb

• Shivani Ranjan • Santoshdev P Rathod • P Narasimha Rao

INTRODUCTION

Self-care is defined as 'the ability of individuals, families and communities to promote health, prevent disease, maintain health, and cope with illness and disability with or without the support of a healthcare provider'.[1] Effective self-care of anesthetic limbs is the key in the management and prevention of disabilities and deformities for people living with leprosy. Patient and the family members should be made aware about the need for optimal self-care in order to prevent deformities of the limbs as a result of anesthesia by the healthcare professional (HCP). Anesthesia/hypoesthesia is defined as 'complete or partial impairment of sensation over the skin to touch, pain and temperature'. Details of assessment of nerve function impairment (NFI) and medical management of the same has been discussed in other chapters of this book. This chapter shall focus on how to teach the 'self-care aspects' to the patients and their close relatives.

For the care of anesthetic limb in a leprosy patient the following steps are needed: (a) Identifying NFI. This comes first and has to be done by the HCP and explaining the same to the patient. Note that the care patient needs to take depends on the type and extent of NFI. (b) Monitoring impairments. Here there is a role for both HCP and the patient. (c) Preventing further deterioration of impairments. Here, the patient affected and the care giver have major role and their active participation is vital to reverse and/or prevent progression of disability. Of course, the HCP has to continue to monitor periodically as an advisor and counselor.

While the prevention and treatment of primary impairment such as NFI falls within the responsibility of health professionals, once NFI develops the person affected need to take up the responsibility to protect the limb and contribute by monitoring themselves. The two arms of prevention of disability by self-care by the patient are: (i) care of existing impairments to prevent worsening of disabilities and (ii) risk reduction methods to prevent new secondary impairments.[2]

PATIENT EDUCATION

The practice of self-care consists of procedures, techniques, and exercises all of which can be performed at home or at work.[3] To enable oneself to benefit from this, patients need to be educated and counseled on importance of protection of an anesthetic limb. This will help them, not only in developing attitudes and abilities that favor the protection of limbs with NFI, but also their mental, and social functions.

It is important that patient should first be informed in their own language that, due to anesthesia/hypoesthesia resulting from NFI, they do not have the 'normal protective sensation' in their affected limbs. Hence, they will not feel any trauma; like a cut or burn on a finger, injury to foot on stepping on something sharp or a shoe bite on wearing tight footwear. As the painless injuries tend to remain un-attended and further injured, it leads to continued tissue damage and increased pressures on injuries, progressing to ulceration, secondary infection and finally to deformities. *The only way to find out whether an insensitive hand or foot has been injured is to examine it daily in good light*. Hence, it is important that patients look after their anesthetic limbs by following a daily routine of self-care. It should also be informed, with required sensitivity and firmness, that such a self-care procedures need to be followed till return to normalcy, which may take many months to years, or indefinitely in case of established NFI of a limb. The time spent by HCP with the patient, initially and at every visit, emphasizing the importance of care of anesthetic limb and methods to prevent disability (and possible stigma associated with it), is the most valuable and useful time spent both by the HCP and the patient. The success of prevention of grade 2 disability and deformity rests squarely on the this important aspect of making patient understand and motivated to take-up the self-care routine and measures regularly and diligently. In addition, the patient must and wherever possible with the help of the family members, should carry out these checks systematically and regularly (Table 29.1). It is also ideal to keep a record of the results, e.g. once a month.[4]

PRINCIPLES OF SELF-CARE

The main principles guiding practice of self-care would best be described under the subheadings.

Inspect, Prevent, Intervene and Maintain

Inspection of the affected limb regularly will help in identifying any new unknown injuries, prevent worsening and promote care for those body parts already injured, and maintain the status quo of the impairment and do not allow further damage. Hence, the person affected should be taught to inspect hands and feet daily, to identify at the earliest any injury, burn or ulcer and to protect them from new injury, ultimately to prevent occurrence of future

Table 29.1: Checks to be carried out regularly by the patients or by the care-giver and record the observations (ideally once a month).[4]
• To check, by looking and feeling, whether there are any areas in the palms and soles that do not sweat and, if so, whether they are increasing in size.
• To notice any abnormal sensations (e.g. numbness or burning) confined to one area in the palms or soles.
• To check whether there is any loss of feeling of pain, heat or touch in any areas of skin in the palms and fingers (this must be done with care and due diligence) and, if so, whether they are increasing in size.
• To check that all the fingers can open out fully and be kept together in that position; and that the thumbs can move freely in all directions.
• To check that the toes can be raised off the ground and held up for at least 30 seconds without drooping down; and that the feet can be held up for the same time without drooping.
• To check that the eyes are in good condition and the eyelids can close tight.

disabilities. Family members/caretaker are also encouraged to learn and practice the dressing of ulcers and care of patient.

Inspection and Care of Hands and Feet (Boxes 29.1 and 29.2)

- Examine the hands and feet daily.
- Set aside a definite time each day for this hand and foot-care routine. Inspect the hands and feet for redness, swelling, hot-spots, blisters, cracks, or wounds. To soften the hard skin of hands and feet, soak them in water about 15–20 minutes. For feet it should be followed by cleaning between toes and removal of any foreign material.
- Scrape off hard skin around cracks and old wound sites with the help of a hard cloth, coconut coir or scrubber, without damaging the skin. Rub in oil on the wet skin immediately after soaking and scraping. In addition it is ideal to keep the limbs soft and moist by applying oil/moisturizers at least twice daily, more so if there is dryness/ichthyosis, cracks and deep fissures.
- Check for new wounds every day and attend to them. Always cover wounds with a clean cloth or bandage to protect them against injury, dirt, and infection. Look for and treat wound infections. If the wounds are getting bigger, or if the skin around the wound is red and swollen, or if there is any pus or bad smell, then report immediately to the nearest healthcare center. If the wounds are smaller and clean, and if there is no pus, then continue with self-care activities. Rest the limb with ulcer as much as possible.

Prevent Injuries and Protect the Anesthetic Limb

- Protect the hands, while cooking food, always hold hot items/utensils from the sides with the help of a thick cloth to protect against heat and fire. Use of tongs or handling cooking appliances with thick cotton cloth or cotton gloves while cooking is desirable.
- *Patient with NFI should be advised to consider all cups/mugs with beverages as hot!* For drinking tea or coffee, put the hot glass inside a cup or simply use a protective padding of cloth to hold the hot glass, as hot liquids can burn anesthetic hands. While eating, allow the food to cool and eat with a spoon.

Box 29.1: Message for person with Insensitive hands

- Think before you use them. And Use them with extra care!
- Protect them from burns and injuries.
- Consider all vessels and tumblers/cups hot!
- Check them daily for fissures and ulcers!
- Soak in water and massage with oil daily.

Box 29.2: Message for person with insensitive feet

- Main cause of disability in insensitive feet is ulceration.
- Ulcers develop when injuries to insensitive feet are often neglected. Hence, these injuries can be infected easily and get further damaged.
- Insensitive feet may be injured by brisk walking (internal injury) or by contact with sharp or hot objects (external injury).
- Never walk barefoot.
- Always inspect feet every night! Massage with oil/paraffin wax daily.

- Use of vessels and appliances with protective handles at home and at workplace, to avoid friction, pressure and burns is recommended. Cover the handles of tool used regularly with a pad or soft cloth to prevent friction induced wounds and blisters on hands.
- Protect the feet; patient should always sit away from heat and fire. They should avoid squatting or sitting cross-legged to avoid pressure injury (at bony prominences like malleoli) to feet. They should be advised not to wear tight strapped footwear or shoes and to never walk barefoot. Walking barefoot in summer, even for short distances especially on a paved road or tiled surface, is one of the most common causes of blistering/ulceration of insensitive feet in persons affected. They should wear footwear with protective padding, preferably made with microcellular rubber. Even with special footwear they should avoid walking long distances at a stretch, which can lead to blistering and ulceration.

Intervene and Maintain Integrity of Hands and Feet

Prevention of disability (POD) is an important component of 'quality leprosy services' emphasized in the WHO's Global Strategy. WHO has come out with a self-care booklet titled *'I can do it myself'* which with the help of text and pictures teaches the many ways in which complications of leprosy can be minimized by practizing good self-care at home. The booklet is intended for 'persons affected by leprosy', their close family members and friends who can help them practice self-care at home and can be downloaded free from https://apps.who.int/iris/handle/10665/205317. *It will be ideal if the HCP provides the printed copies of the self-care booklets to all the persons affected.*

In addition, there are number of booklets with detailed instructions on how to prevent disability for free download for HCPs too. Some of them are 'How to prevent disability in leprosy' by ILEP[5] and 'Disability prevention and Medical rehabilitation, Guidelines for primary, secondary and tertiary care'. NLEP, Govt of India.[6] These are very informative and useful instruction manuals providing details of how to care for anesthetic limbs, including basic exercises, supported through pictorial representation.

Exercises for Hands and Feet

For hands and feet with no motor deficit, the above mentioned daily self-care methods would usually suffice. However, when a person develops any grade of motor deficit or deformity, both *passive* and *active* exercises are needed, based on the type of deficit. In addition, splinting and orthotic support is needed as necessary (refer to Section 5, Chapter 30). It is beyond the scope of this chapter to detail all those exercises. Nonetheless, few basic passive exercises are mentioned in the Table 29.2.

Inputs needed for self-care:

- Self-care kit/ulcer dressing kit should be provided to the patient with an ulcer[5] and educated about its use. It should contain a scraper, an antiseptic cream, antiseptic solution to be diluted with water for soaking the feet, sterile gauze to cover the ulcer, Vaseline/moisturizer for hydration of skin, bandage, scissors, sticking plaster (Fig. 29.1). In addition, guidance as how homemade materials can be used for dressing of wounds may be given.
- In case of simple ulcers, as already mentioned, management by good wound care and protection from further injury by self-care measures and rest would usually suffice. Nevertheless, for complicated and chronic ulcers and if the patient is unable to rest, HCP should provide splints to immobilize the injured part to relieve oedema and promote healing.

Table 29.2: Basic passive exercises for hands and feet
For stiff fingers: After oiling the hands, a weak hand is placed with palm up on a soft flat surface (e.g. the thigh of the patient). The ulnar border of the palm of the other hand is placed firmly on the wrist of the weak hand. It is then gently pushed forward to the edge of the hand along the palm of the weak hand, to straighten the fingers. Hold and count to ten before you relax the other hand. The exercise should be repeated ten times in each session and should be done at least three times a day.
For weakness of thumb: The thumb of other hand is placed in the space between the thumb and first finger of the weak hand and then press gently in the space and count to ten whilst drawing the thumb away from the hand. The exercise should be repeated ten times, and should be done at least three times a day.
Exercise for the foot drop: It is very important that person with foot drop should do stretching exercises to prevent the foot from being pulled into a plantar flexion position by the stiffness/contracture of muscles at the back of the leg. The cloth is placed around the weak foot. The cloth is pulled to force the foot up. The foot is held in position, while the person counts slowly to ten, then the foot is allowed to relax. The person repeats this passive exercise ten times, and should be done three times a day.

Note: These basic passive exercises should be supplemented by drug therapy, splinting and active exercises as needed, under the guidance of trained leprosy HCP and physiotherapist to regain full function of the limb.

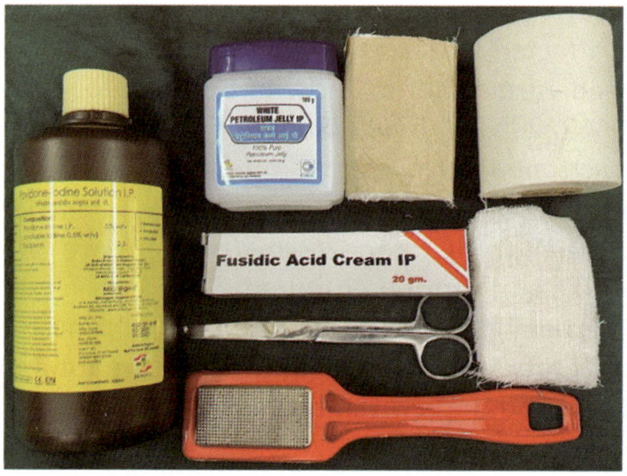

Fig. 29.1: Self-care kit

- Material support: Many patients require aids and appliances, such as protective footwear made of MCR, gloves, splints, spectacles and modified tools with protective handles, instant grip-aid kits (Fig. 29.2) to practice disability prevention. While some of these aids and appliances can be improvised, others are available to patients as a part of disability prevention programme of NLEP. Many NGOs working for leprosy also provide these aids free of cost to the patients.

CONCLUSION

Self-care guidelines and interventions support and promote a comprehensive, people-centerd and occupation-oriented approach to self-awareness and mental well-being, leading to prevention of further disability.[1] Promoting self-care interventions will provide opportunities for active participation of persons affected in their own health needs, by empowering them with knowledge and understanding about their disability. It is important for the HCP to communicate with the patient and provide specific information about the care of anesthetic

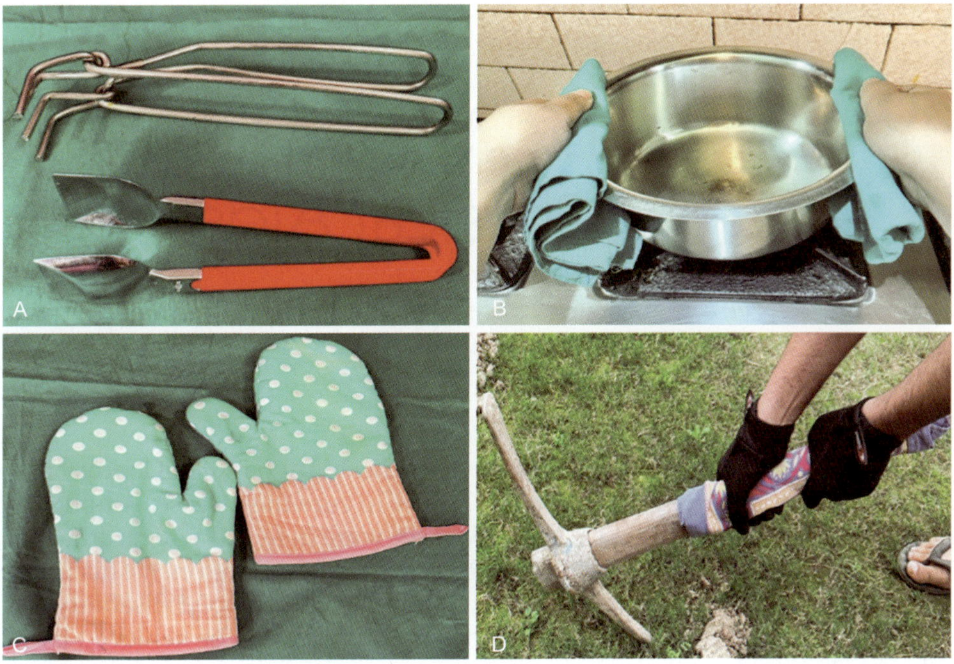

Fig. 29.2: (A) Tongs; (B) Use of cotton cloth to handle hot objects; (C) Cotton gloves; (D) Use of protective gloves and cotton cloth while working in fields

limb and instruct on how to prevent disabilities. In addition, it would also be helpful if training is provided to the patient to become competent in carrying out the tasks necessary for preventing the onset or worsening of disabilities and deformities. While instruction is largely theoretical, training is highly practical. Instructions may be given through various channels, including discussions (formal and informal), books and e-manuals, audiovisual aids, through social media platforms and demonstrations on volunteers (usually the most effective method). The use of digital health platforms to support the use of self-care interventions must also be considered.[7] Training should be carried out by first demonstrating a task to patients and then letting them practise it under supervision until they can do it properly. Emphasis should also be on education of patients with anesthetic limbs about lifestyle modifications to protect their limbs from injuries based on their disabilities and occupation.

REFERENCES

1. World Health Organization. Self-care in the Context of Primary Health Care (No. SEA-HSD-320). Bangkok; 2009.
2. Darlong J. Self-care in leprosy at the front line. Lepr Rev. 2021;92:356–65.
3. Bhuyan KK. Health promotion through self-care and community participation: elements of a proposed programme in the developing countries. BMC Pub. Health. 2004;4:11.
4. H Srinivasan. Prevention of disabilities in patients with leprosy, A practical guide, WHO Geneva 1993.
5. Available from: https://ilepfederation.org/wp-content/uploads/2020/02/LG4.pdf.
6. Available from: http://www.clinicalestablishments.gov.in/WriteReadData/516.pdf.
7. NelsonL A, Williamson SE, Nigg A. Implementation of technology-delivered diabetes self-care interventions in clinical care: a narrative review. Curr Diab Rep. 2020;20:71.

Chapter

30 Splints, Supports and Physical Aids

• Meghana Phiske • Shylaja Someshwar

INTRODUCTION

Leprosy is commonly identified with deformity and disability. Failure of leprosy programs to prevent disability in patients is considered as failure to cure the disease. Among the 127,558 new cases detected globally in 2020, 7,198 new cases were detected with grade 2 disabilities (G2D) and new G2D rate was recorded at 0.9 per million population.[1,2] This is in addition to burden of large number of patients already treated but developed disability or those on treatment. Effective management of this mammoth problem can be achieved by providing splints, physical aids and psychological support as an essential part of rehabilitation. States are given the responsibility to ensure the development and supply of assistive devices for people with disabilities with an objective of assisting them 'to increase their level of independence in their daily living and to exercise their rights'.[1] This responsibility goes further and states are to promote not only the availability of assistive devices but also their use. Priority should be given to technologies at an affordable cost. This chapter outlines available splints and physical aids for the leprosy affected person and give practical guidance on how to use them.

DEFORMITY AND DISABILITY

In leprosy patient's "disability" and "deformity" have been used interchangeably. 'Disability' is an incapability of patient to perform normal work, and it may exist even without any obvious disfigurement.[3] According to WHO, leprosy disabilities can be classified into 0,1 and 2 grades considering eye, hand and foot impairments (Table 30.1). 'Deformity' is defined as any deviation from normal appearance of any part/parts of body which may or may not be accompanied by disability. Deformities can develop due to factors which operate singly or in combination (Box 30.1) [1] and are of different types (Table 30.2).[1,2]

Table 30.1: Classification of disability in leprosy[3]

Disability grade	*Eyes*	*Hands and feet*
0	No eye impairment due to leprosy; no evidence of visual loss	No sensory impairment, no visible impairment
1	Eye problems due to leprosy present (irregular blink), but no vision impaired (can read fingers at six-meter distance)	Anesthesia present, but no visible deformity or damage, including muscle weakness without clawing
2	Severe visual impairments (cannot read fingers at 6-meter distance), lagophthalmos, uveitis, corneal opacities	Visible impairments present, including ulcers and atrophy

Box 30.1: Causes of deformity
1. Direct result of infiltration of tissues by *M. leprae* (e.g. as observed in face in LL patients)
2 Muscle imbalance secondary to motor paralysis
3. Secondary effects of impaired sensations and anesthesia

Table 30.2: Types of deformities[1,2]		
Type	***Cause***	***Example***
Primary deformity due to the disease	Occurs due to bacterial load and is direct result of disease process and infiltration with *M. leprae* with local damaging effect on tissues	Leonine facies, sagging of ear lobules, loss of eyebrows, gynco-mastia, saddle nose deformity.
Paralytic deformities	They are produced due to indirect effects of disease. These are difficult to prevent and are amenable to treatment at least partially if not totally.	Motor paralysis Claw hand and toes Foot and wrist drop
Anesthetic deformities (Also called secondary deformity)	Occurs as a result of damage to the anesthetic parts of the body. They can be easily prevented. However, they are difficult to treat if little attention is paid.	Plantar ulcers, loss of toes and fingers, corneal ulcers and Charcot joints

ROLE OF PHYSIOTHERAPY IN LEPROSY

Physiotherapy[3,4] is the system of treatment using physical energies like heat, light, electricity and mechanical forces and its principles are introduced in Chapter 28 of this section. This chapter will focus on the use of various splints in the management of leprosy patient with disability and/or deformity.

Splints

Splints are external appliances which are worn over affected part of body to hold it in a desired position.

Objectives of Splinting

Splinting is done to achieve different objectives, individually or in combination (Box 30.2).

Materials Used to Make Splints

Splints can be made from different materials like wood, aluminum, polythene, leather, steel wire, plaster of Paris, polyvinyl tubes or thermoplastic materials.[1] Of these plaster of Paris

Box 30.2: Objectives of doing splinting
• To relieve pain • To stabilize a joint • To retain the joint/part after release of contracture in a particular position • To immobilize a part • To prevent its movement in a particular direction • To provide continuous gradual stretching

splints are most popular for temporary use because they can be directly molded on the body. Some commonly used splints are illustrated in Figs 30.1 to 30.4.[5] Prefabricated splints are now available, made of organic polymer with screw mechanism incorporated. Screw can be manually tightened to stretch contracture especially of proximal interphalangeal (PIP) joints. Their use in leprosy is risky as affected hands are anesthetic; hence these are not routinely recommended. Methods of using splints for above purpose are described below

1. **Splinting to rest the part:** When a body part is injured or inflamed it can be rested in a splint, in such cases splinting is done in such a way that even if part becomes stiff, limb still remains useful. Acute neuritis, reaction hand, minor infection/injury of hand are conditions which would require resting part temporarily in splint (plaster slab). Plantar casts for healing plantar ulcer serves same purpose. When foot swelling subsides and ulcer is clean with granulation tissue, below-knee walking plaster is applied for 4–5 weeks[4] (Fig. 30.5).

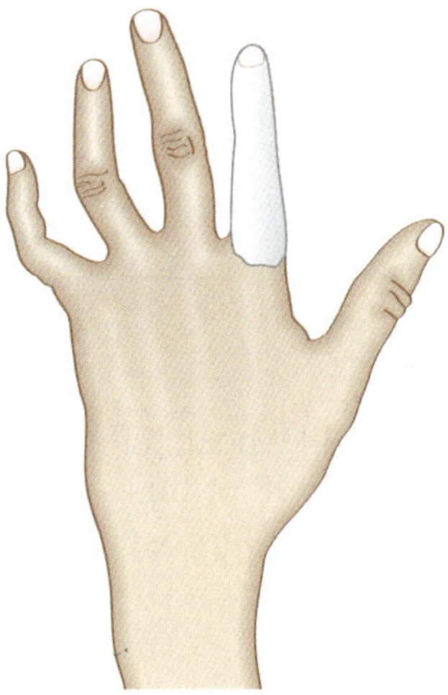

Fig. 30.1: Cylindrical finger splint

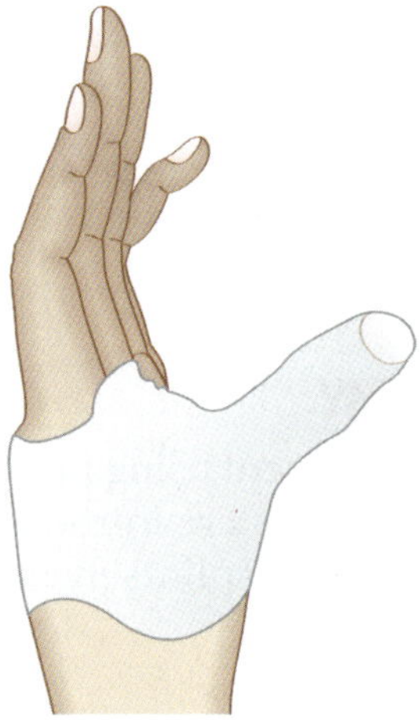

Fig. 30.2: Serial splinting for thumb web contracture, one sitting shown

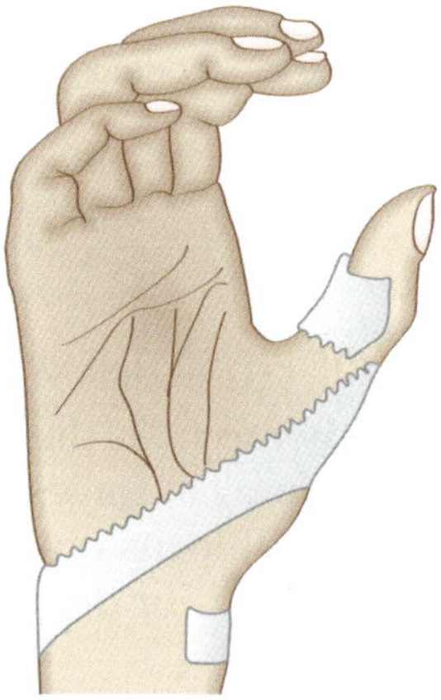

Fig. 30.3: Strapping of thumb for early thenar paralysis

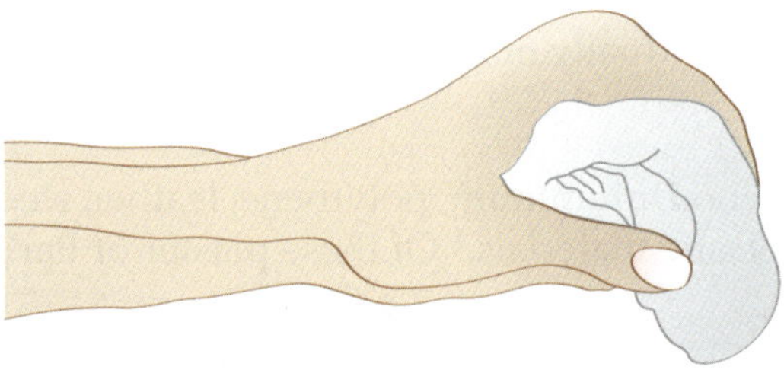

Fig. 30.4: Hand fixed in functional position during reaction with help of plaster of Paris

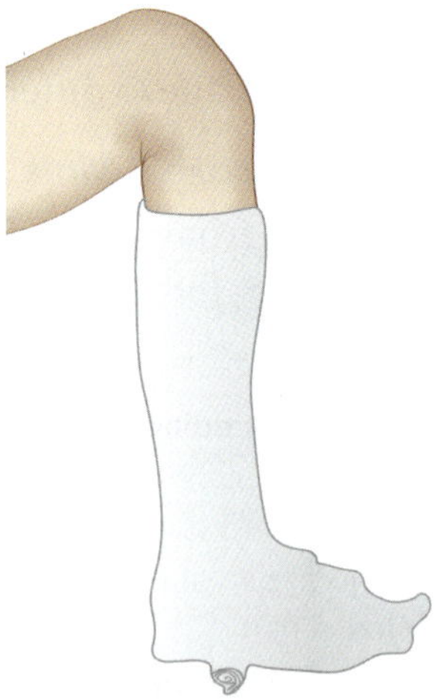

Fig. 30.5: Below knee plaster cast for treatment of ulcers

2. **Splinting for immobilization:** Immobilization in leprosy is required after corrective operations like, arthrodesis, tendon transfer/grafting. In later cases immobilization is done in such a position that will put least strain on sites of tendon suture, to protect these sites and prevent disruption of tendon anastomosis during immediate postoperative period. Plaster swab and cast are used for this.[5]

3. **Splinting to prevent specific movement:** At times total immobilization is not required and only some movements are to be prevented. This is needed when an appliance is worn as permanent/long-term measure for correcting deformity. These are therefore made of leather and metal and movements in unwanted directions are prevented by springs, strap or stop cork, e.g. cock-up splint for wrist drop, drop-foot appliances and knuckle-duster type of finger splint for clawing deformity.[5]

   Namasivayan has devised simple method of keeping paralyzed fingers extended when hand is not in use, protecting paralyzed intrinsic muscles from stretching while in stage of recovery and preventing flexion contracture at first interphalangeal joint. Galvanized iron wire 8–10 gauze, 29 cm long, inserted into rubber tubing with an internal diameter of 2–3 mm and 30 cm long, bent to form an S-shaped spiral is used for make this splint.[4] (Fig. 30.6).[5]

4. **Splinting to provide continuous traction:** Sometimes, splinting is done to provide continuous traction, helpful to overcome spasm of muscle, seen after major injuries to limbs or disease of major joint. Continuous traction can be used to overcome contractures and can be tried in finger contracture of leprosy patients. Continuous traction can be obtained by incorporating circular or semicircular wire frame to forearm plaster cast and pulling on fingers continuously by means of leather loops which are fixed at other end to the wire frame through elastic cords. These splints must be used carefully in leprosy patients due to risk of ulceration due to continuous pressure on anaesthetic fingers, hence may not be essential.[5]

5. **Splints to stabilize joints:** Splinting for joint stabilization is not needed in leprosy, but some patients after tendon transfer operations for correction of claw fingers find it difficult to use transferred tendon in early postoperative period until wrist joint is stabilized in plaster cast.[5]

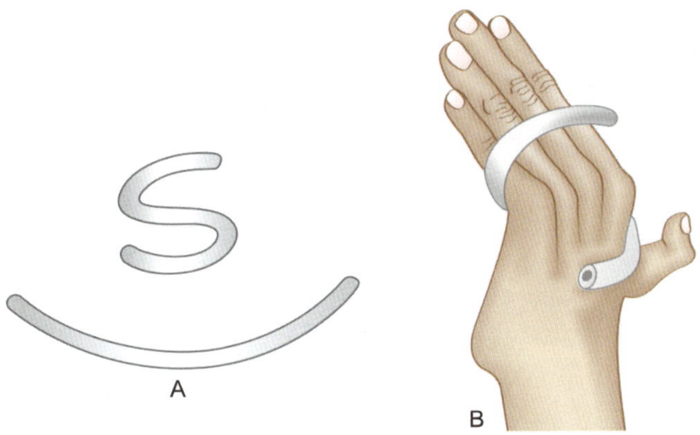

Fig. 30.6: (A) Thick-walled rubber tube (bottom) and spiral splint (top); (B) Claw hand with splint, so the finger can be held straight

6. **Serial splinting:** It is a method of repeated splinting at regular intervals and is used when contractures are to be released (especially for severe contractures).[5]

   Varieties of splints have been developed to serve specific purpose. These are easy to carry, simple to apply and effective in preventing deformity progression.

Types of Splints[5]

1. Static, to maintain joint position.
2. Dynamic where some form of mechanism is incorporated to exercise fingers. Table 30.3 gives types of splints and their place of use.

Common Splints in Use for Hand Deformities

These are easily fabricated at local level and include

1. **Gutter splint:** It is static splint in which half cut tube (made of thick, firm polyvinyl material) is lined with felt and provided with Velcro fasteners at its either ends (Fig. 30.7).
2. **Loop splint:** It consists of loop of rexin/other suitable soft material having an eyelet at its end through which rubber band is threaded and tied to itself, other end of rubber band is

Table 30.3: Types of splints and place of their use[1,5]

Type of splint	*Place of use*
1. Adductor band splint	Used when the palsy is just begun and little finger is not able to adduct.
2. Loop splint	It is used for a hand with mobile finger clawing. If the thumb is also paralyzed then opponens splint is used in addition.
3. Gutter splint	It is used for fingers with obvious contractures and for the thumb interphalangeal (IP) joint.
4. Loop and gutter splint	If the fingers have mild stiffness, then loop splints are used during day time to exercise the fingers and gutter splints are used during night to maintain the stretched position of the fingers.
5. Opponens splint	It is used if thumb web has mild contracture
6. Plaster of Paris wedges	In the leprosy hand with paralysis of the ulnar and median nerves contractures are likely to develop at 1. Proximal interphalangeal joints of the fingers 2. Interphalangeal joint of the thumb 3. Thumb web. These contractures are corrected by the use of cylindrical plaster of Paris splints (Plaster of Paris bandage 5 cm wide and 30–35 cm long) that provide a passive stretching force. They are applied on alternate days, following wax baths, oil massage and exercises. No padding is used and no pressure is applied over the dorsum of the fingers. It is important to avoid excessive stretching force when applying these plasters.

tied to wrist band at appropriate tension. This is dynamic splint and is used for exercising fingers. It helps in strengthening extensor systems of fingers (Fig. 30.8).

3. **Opponens splint:** It is similar to loop splint, but loop is wider to accommodate for diagonal movement of thumb (Fig. 30.9).
4. **Adductor band:** It consists of straight band of appropriate dimensions, at either end of which Velcro fasteners are stitched (Fig. 30.10).

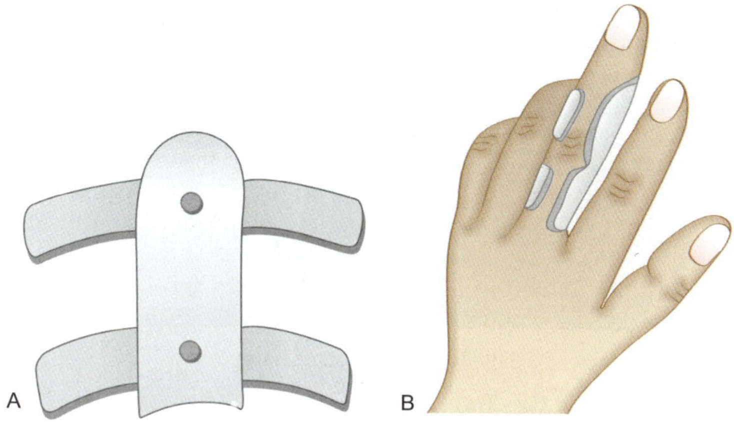

Fig. 30.7: (A) Gutter splint with velcro fasteners; (B) Gutter splint with V cut to accommodate PIP joints in case of Boutonniere deformity

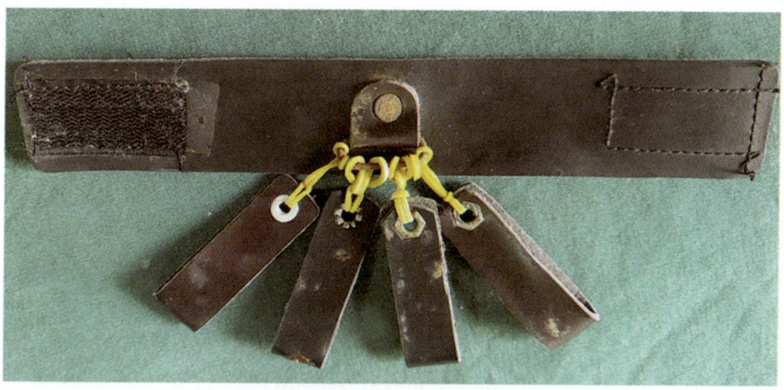

Fig. 30.8: Loop splint

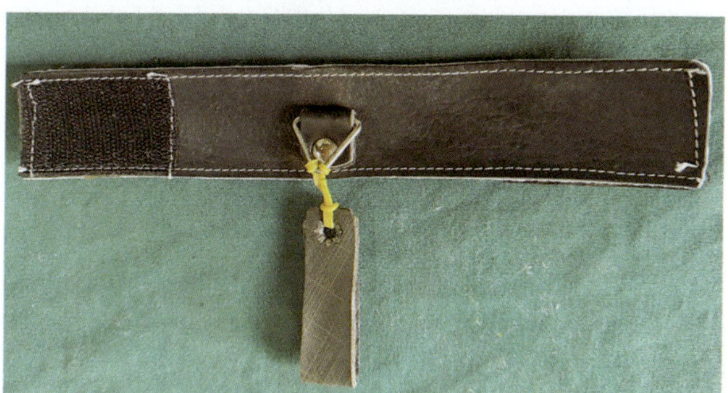

Fig. 30.9: Opponens splint

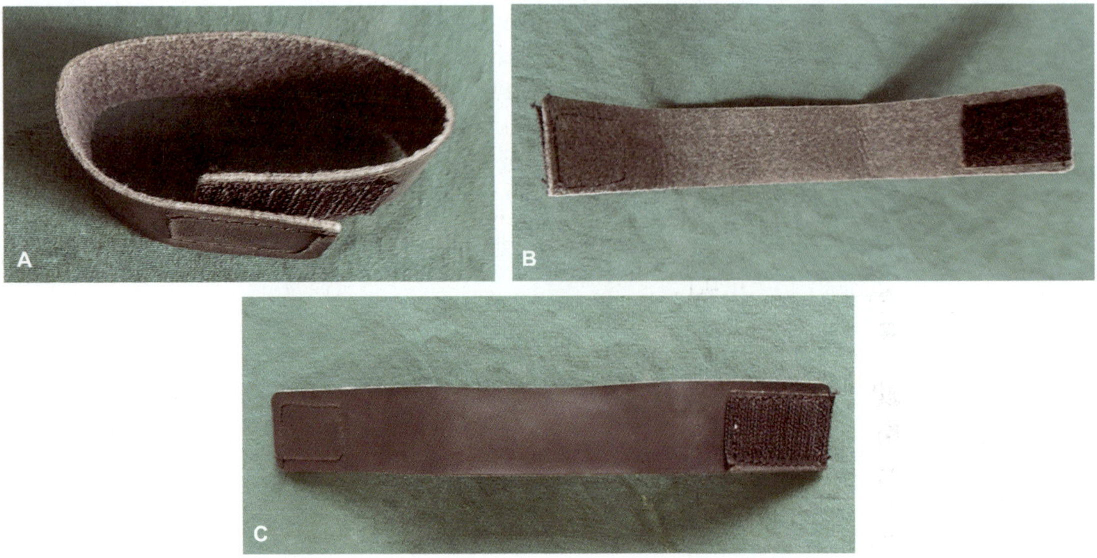

Fig. 30.10: Adductor band

Flowchart 30.1: Method of serial splinting

Contracted finger is passively stretched and held in that position by plaster of Paris cast

⇩

Plaster cast is made by wrapping wet plaster of Paris bandage, 45 cm long and 5 cm wide, to form 4–5 layers around PIP joint

⇩

Layers are made with moderate tightness so as not to impair blood circulation and not to press on knuckles as it can cause skin necrosis

⇩

PIP joint is held in desired position till cast is dry

⇩

Fingertip is left exposed to monitor circulation

⇩

This cast is retained for a week and then removed

⇩

Wax therapy is given and cast is reapplied with some more stretching. Minimum force is used while stretching so that circulation is not compromised and soft tissues are not injured.

⇩

The process is repeated till the contracture is overcome.

⇩

The release so obtained, is then maintained by gutter splints.

5. **Simple spiral splint**: It is made out of 10 SWG galvanized steel wire sheathed with thick rubber sleeve is easy to fabricate and can be used anytime. It stabilizes all four fingers.
6. **Serial splinting**: It involves repeated application of plaster of Paris casts to PIP joint of fingers at regular intervals to overcome contractures gradually. (Flowchart 30.1). For stretching thumb, web wedges of increasing angles, made of plaster of Paris, are applied

at regular intervals as above (Fig. 30.11). Large arm slings can be used for upper limb and long gutter splints for lower limb. Types of splints and place of their use are mentioned in Table 30.3.

Duration of Splinting

It is difficult to predict duration of splinting but majority of case improve in 8–12 weeks. Splints are used till improvement reaches a plateau and continued thereafter to keep fingers mobile till surgery is performed. If patient is unwilling for undergo surgery, he can continue using static splints during night.

Precautions to be Taken While Splinting the Fingers and thumb[1]

Before applying splints to fingers, adjustment of tension is critical. Steps to be followed during splinting are mentioned in Table 30.4.

Foot-drop splints: Splinting for foot drop (Fig. 30.12A) is aimed to prevent stretching of dorsiflexor muscles of foot and prevent contracture of tendo-Achilles.[1] They are worn to maintain foot in dorsiflexion.[1] A below knee slab of plaster of Paris, to keep foot in neutral

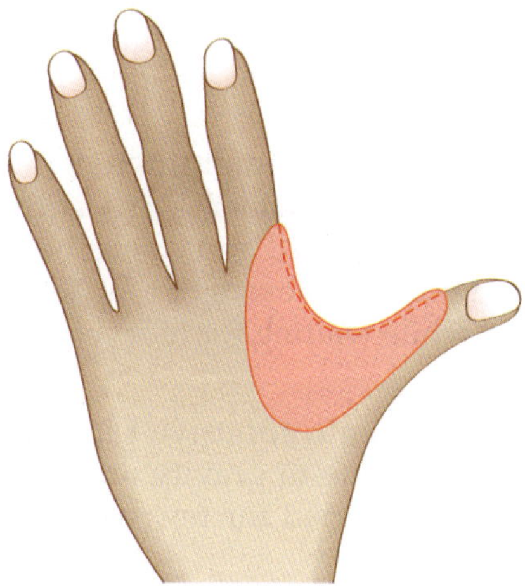

Fig. 30.11: Plaster of Paris thumb web splint

Table 30.4: Steps to be followed during splinting[1]
In contracted fingers, there should be no attempt to open up the fingers fully on first day itself
Gradual stretching of fingers should be done
If redness or blisters develop on the dorsal aspect of the finger, use of splints should be discontinued
Immediate removal of the splint is advised if patient complains of pain, swelling or bluish discoloration of nail or pulp and its use should be discontinued till the condition is settled. Reapplication should be done at a lower tension.
For loop splints the tension in the rubber bands is adjusted in such a way that metacarpophalangeal (MCP) joint is kept in 70–90° flexion. The rubber bands should not be over stretchable (beyond 10°) to prevent full MCP joint extension.
The splints are ineffective in cases where the contracture has become fixed, i.e. it cannot be passively stretched by force. Such cases require a prior surgical release.

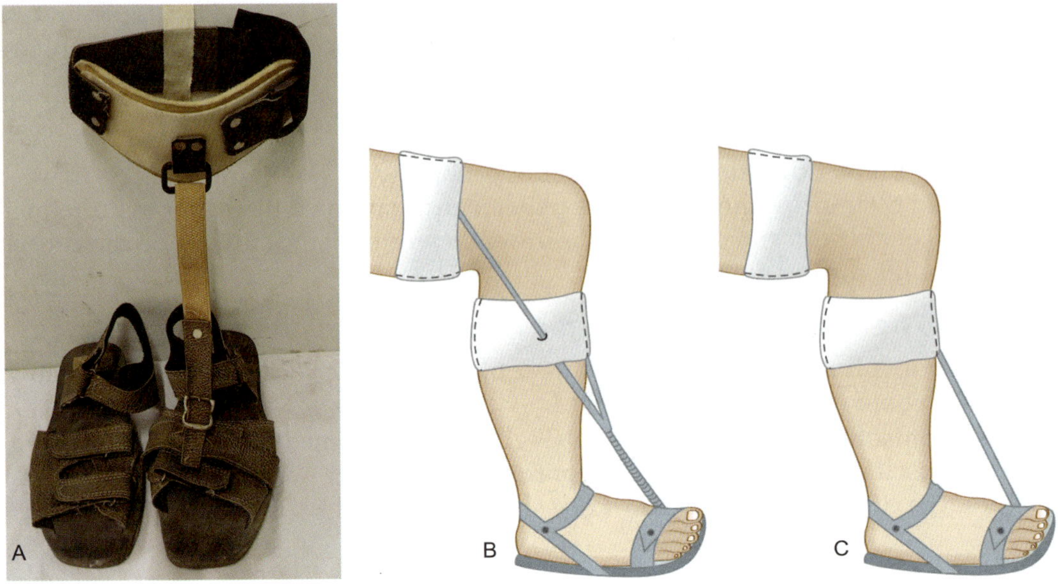

Fig. 30.12: (A) Drop foot splints; (B) Drop foot splints-'Y' strap with spring; (C) Drop foot splints—single elastic strap

position, is adequate. Splint should be worn at night, as foot muscles can be unduly stretched by foot movements during sleep or while maneuvering sheet to cover oneself. A 'Y' strap with spring or single elastic strap (Fig. 30.12B and C) can be used to provide lift to forefoot while walking, prevent stretching of dorsiflexors of foot and prevent contracture of tendo-Achilles. This splint can be used while waiting for recovery of muscles and also if patient is unwilling for surgery.

Splints for facial palsy: Hypoallergenic adhesive tape strips are used to splint facial skin so that lower lid is not sagging due to gravity and angle of mouth is not deviated. It is a temporary measure and can be tried for few weeks after its occurrence, while on treatment.

Splinting for Nerve Pain

Splint made of suitable and easily available material is used and affected limb is placed in it to prevent nerve movement and provide rest to nerve. Joint is immobilized in such a position that nerve is relaxed. Splint should be padded so that there is no pressure on inflamed nerve.

Splint Used in Neuritis

Splints are used in neuritis management, to immobilize joint, to prevent stretching and to provide rest to inflamed nerve in resting position, e.g long arm posterior slab, long leg posterior slab etc[4] (Fig. 30.13).

Table 30.5 mentions purpose of splinting for neuritis, its method and level. Neuritis slab could be fabricated either using plaster of Paris or thermoplastic material.[5,6] Splints for deformity correction/maintenance of joints in optimal position mentioned in Table 30.6A. Offloading measures for plantar ulcers mentioned in Table 30.6B.[6] Position of nerves before splinting is mentioned in Table 30.7 [1] and following precautions after splinting should be taken (Box 30.3).[1]

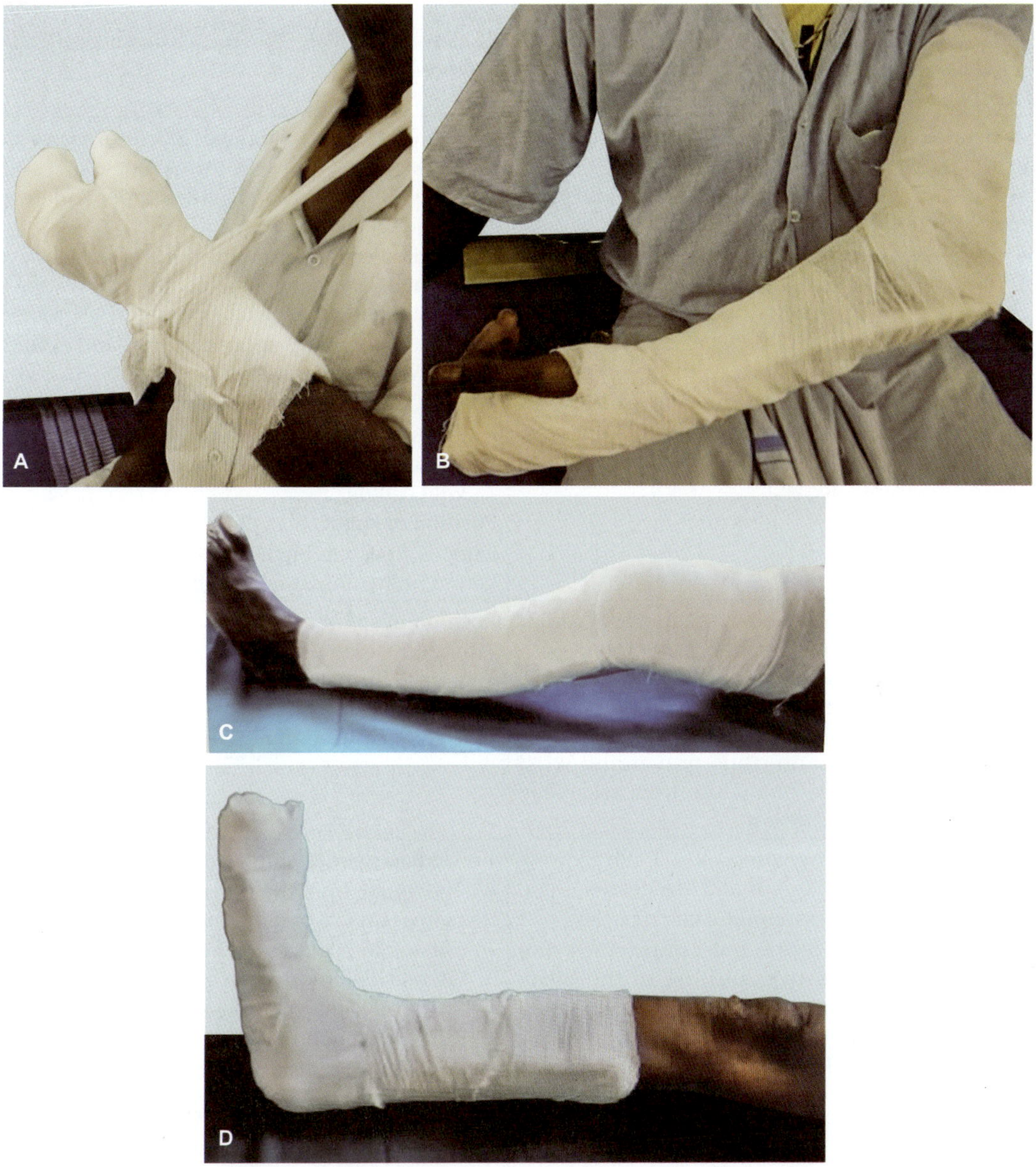

Fig. 30.13: (A) Median neuritis slab including thumb; (B) Ulnar neuritis long arm posterior slab; (C) Lateral popliteal neuritis slab; (D) Posterior tibial neuritis slab

Physical Aids and Assistive Technology

Physical aids or Assistive Technology is composed of resources and services that aid in providing/improving functional skills.[7] It can be considered an indispensable tool to provide inclusion and integration of people with deficiency in to society.[8] They also assist by safeguarding user's body from likely injuries sustained during daily routine or at work place. They range from simple, basic devices like cups with wooden handles, walking sticks, wheel chair/crutches to computer assisted devices or motorized wheel chairs (Table 30.8).

Table 30.5: Purpose of splinting for neuritis and its method[5,6]

Affected nerve and its splint	*Purpose of splinting*	*Method*
Ulnar neuritis splint	1. To rest and give warmth to the nerve. 2. To support weak/paralyzed muscles. 3. To prevent contracture due to over pulling of the weak muscles by the opposite group muscles. 4. To relieve pain. 5. To help maintain elbow in flexion of about 60 degrees, providing adequate rest to nerve.	• The length from the lower 2/3rds of upper arm to the palmar crease is measured. • The width is measured at the upper and lower ends of the slab. • Padding is done from the back of the elbow at about 3″ above to 5″ below the elbow joint and is extended up to ulnar side of the wrist joint. • The ulnar neuritis splint can be made excluding the wrist joint or including it. • Upper end should be wider than the lower end. • The slab should be secured by firm bandaging and the elbow position should be supported with a sling. **Position of splint** Extends from the back of the elbow to the palmar crease, if the fingers are not included.
Cock up slab	Indicated when there is radial nerve damage associated with paralysis or weakness of the wrist extensors. To stretch and maintain the extensors in their optimal position, thus preventing wrist joint contracture from excessive wrist flexion.	**Position of splint** The splint extends from the upper 2/3rd of the forearm to the palmar crease. The wrist is maintained in extension. The fingers are included in the splint if they are paralyzed; if not, they are excluded.
Median neuritis splint (Palmar slab/ Anterior slab)	1. To give rest and warmth allowing it to heal and regenerate. 2. To support weak muscles. 3. To prevent contracture due to over pulling of the weak muscles by the opposite group muscles 4. To help prevent thumb web contracture (if the thumb is included).	• Median neuritis splint excluding the thumb • The length from the upper 2/3rd of forearm to palmar crease of hand measured. • The width is measured from the medial to the lateral side of forearm. • The POP roll is measured accordingly and the space for the thumb is cut out. • Padding is applied over the area where the slab is to be placed. • The POP roll is then placed in water. Excessive water is squeezed out and placed in position. • The hand is fully supported in supinated position (Palm facing up). • The slab is placed on the palmar aspect of the forearm and the edges are folded back at the base of the thumb. • The thumb and the MCP joints of the fingers must be free. • Median neuritis splint including the thumb • The length from the upper 2/3rd of forearm to palmar crease of hand is measured • The width is measured from the medial to the lateral side of forearm.

(Contd.)

Table 30.5: Purpose of splinting for neuritis and its method[5,6] *(Contd.)*

Affected nerve and its splint	*Purpose of splinting*	*Method*
		• The POP roll is measured and the space for the thumb is not cut out. • After application of padding, the POP is placed in position. • The thumb is held in full abduction and some opposition till the plaster becomes hard. **Position of splint** • Extends from the upper 2/3rd of forearm to palmar crease. • Usually thumb is excluded from splint, unless thumb needs to be in functional position or thumb web contracture needs to be prevented.
Lateral popliteal neuritis slab	1. To give rest and allow the nerve to heal and regenerate. 2. To support weak/paralyzed muscles. 3. To prevent contracture due to over pulling of the weak muscles by the opposite group muscles. 4. To relieve pain	• Padding is done from the back of the mid-calf to mid-thigh at about 6″ above to 5″ below the popliteal fossa. • The upper end should be wider than the lower end. • The position of the knee joint is at 20 degree flexion. • The patient is made to lie in prone position and the slab is moulded properly **Position of splint** Splint should extend up to lower third of thigh
Posterior tibial neuritis slab	1. To give rest and allow the nerve to heal and regenerate. 2. To support weak/paralyzed muscles. 3. To prevent contracture due to over pulling of the weak muscles by the opposite group muscles. 4. To relieve pain.	• Padding is done from the back of the neck of fibula to the toes. • The position of the ankle should be in 90°. • The patient is made to lie in prone position and the slab is molded properly keeping the ankle in 90° **Position of splint** Splint should extend up to middle of the leg

Table 30.6A: Splints for deformity correction/maintenance of joints in optimal position[6]

Splint	*Indication*	*Purpose*	*Level*
Cylindrical splint	1. Interphalangeal joint stiffness or contracture 2. Finger wounds and cracks	• To prevent contracture. • To correct existing contracture. • To provide rest or encourage healing.	• Extends from the tip to the base of the finger. • Wound healing cylindrical splints can have a window over the wound.
Thumb web spica/ tuck-in splint	1.Thumb web contracture	• To prevent and treat thumb web contracture, such as by maintaining the thumb in an abducted position. • To protect transferred tendon after reconstructive surgery to correct ape thumb deformity.	

(Contd.)

Table 30.6A: Splints for deformity correction/maintenance of joints in optimal position[6] *(Contd.)*

Splint	*Indication*	*Purpose*	*Level*
Functional slab for hand	1. Reaction or wound infection that causes swelling in the hand.	To help rest the hand in a functional position. To relieve pain To assist in healing	Applied with the metacarpophalangeal joint at 45° the proximal interphalangeal joints at 25 degrees, and the distal interphalangeal joint at 15°
Lumbrical slab	1. Need to maintain the hand in the lumbrical position after surgery.	Need to maintain the hand in the lumbrical position after surgery.	
Non-weight bearing cast	1. After Tibialis Posterior Transfer (TPT) surgery (The patient is not allowed to bear weight on this cast, but instead must use crutches for locomotion)	To heal simple ulcers.	From the neck of fibula to the tip of the toes, with the ankle joint maintained at 90° of dorsiflexion.

Table 30.6B: Offloading measures for plantar ulcers[6]

Splint	*Indication*	*Purpose*	*Level*
Below knee (BK) cast with Bohler iron	Simple heel ulcer in a foot, whether or not the foot is deformed. If an ulcer needs dressing, a window can be left in the cast over the ulcer area to enable dressings.	Helps transmit weight and pressure to the calf area, preventing weight bearing on the foot, helping ulcers heal more quickly	Extends from the neck of the fibula to the tip of the toes
Molded double rocker shoe (MDRS)/boot (Name is a misnomer, as there is no proper rocker, but the cast provides an effect similar to that of a rocker)	Heal plantar ulcers on the forefoot. It is contraindicated in the presence of foot drop, stiff claw toes, or heel ulcers.	Provides an effect similar to that of a rocker. It is shaped like a boot	Applied below the malleoli, but covers the entire foot, just like a boot.

Table 30.7: Position of nerves before splinting[1]

Nerve	*Level of splinting*
Ulnar nerve	For ulnar nerve (behind the elbow) joint is kept at 110°
Median nerve	For median nerve wrist is rested in neutral position
Common peroneal nerve	For common peroneal nerve knee is kept in 35–40° flexion
Posterior tibial nerve	For posterior tibial nerve pain, foot is kept in 15–20° plantar flexion.

Box 30.3: Precautions after splinting

1. Splinting is continued till pain subsides.
2. On subsidence of pain, joint position is gradually altered to gently stretch nerve trunk so that it gains some freedom to move with joint movements.
3. Total duration of splinting may vary from 3–4 weeks, i.e. until tenderness subsides.
4. If heat therapy is given alongside, then splint is removed for heat application and then reapplied.

Table 30.8: Household tools and their possible modifications for anaesthetic hands [8]

Household item	*Modification*
Tumbler	Attached wooden handle of about 20 cm length (Fig. 30.14) or wooden cups
Spoon	Attached wooden or rubber handle
Ladle	Attached long handles of about 45cm (to prevent injury from fire) of which the farther 20cm fitted with wooden covering (to prevent injury to hands while cooking) Wooden handles should be broad and preferably hexagonal in cross section to improve grip (Fig. 30.15) A wooden ladle made of coconut shell and bamboo handle (Fig. 30.16)
Tong	The handle covered with wooden material (Fig. 30.17)
Cooking gloves	Made of thick cloth

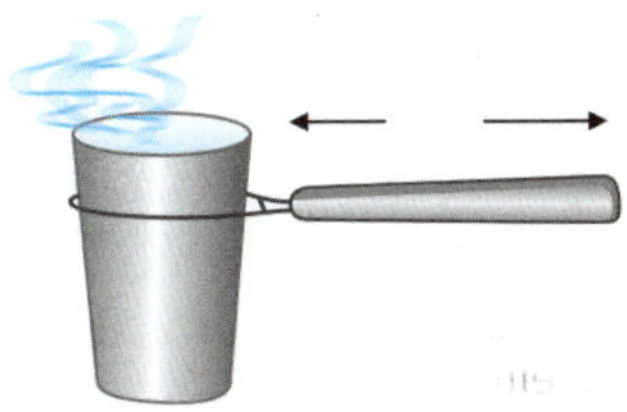

Fig. 30.14: Attached wooden handle for cups

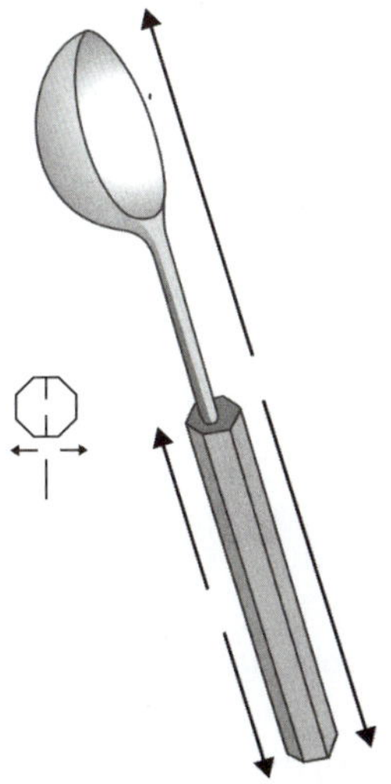

Fig. 30.15: Long wooden handle with a hexagonal cross section for ladle

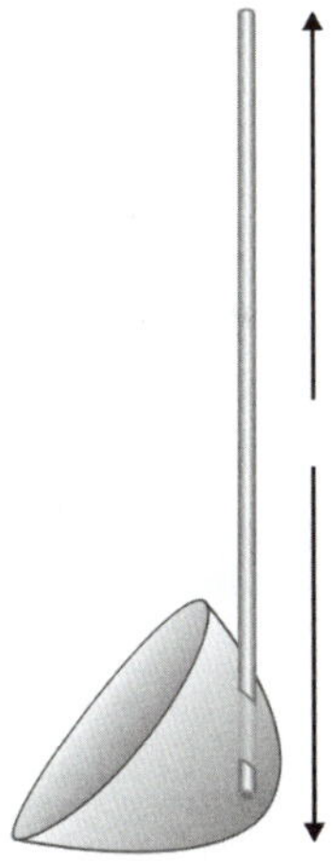

Fig. 30.16: Ladle made of coconut shell with long bamboo handle

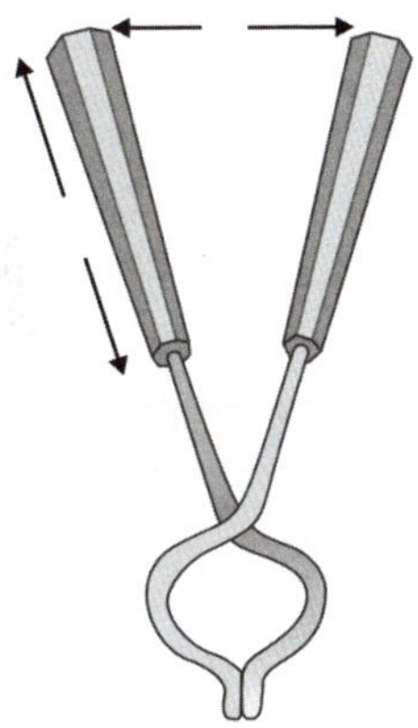

Fig. 30.17: Tong with wooden covering

Necessity of Physical aids in the Management of Leprosy

Physical aids assist leprosy patients to preserve and improve functional capabilities/skills thus helping them to become confident, self-dependent and also promote their social inclusion (Box 30.4).

Box 30.4: Requirement of physical aids
• Prevent deformities in a patient with loss of sensation without overt deformities. • To improve existing deformities and prevent their further progression. • To help the patient live a near normal life with the help of various aids making him independent both in the personal and the professional front.

Evaluation for Physical Aids

Initial Assessment

Physical aids or assistive technology is composed of resources and services that aid in providing/improving functional skills.[9] It can be considered an indispensable tool to provide inclusion and integration of people with deficiency in to society.[8] Patient needs to be properly examined and evaluated before tailored scheme for his rehabilitation can be worked out.[9] Treating physician needs to assess deformities by grading them. Health care provider and occupational therapist should assess and understand patient's daily needs enabling them to customize required products. It is important that tools need to be made aesthetically acceptable and be made in a undifferentiating/inconspicuous manner to prevent unnecessary attention and stigmatization.[10] Education, counseling and training is required both for patient and relatives/caretakers to use devices effectively.

Footwear (Table 30.9) *and Physical Aids* (Table 30.10)

Physical aids can be incorporated in simple daily tasks like brushing teeth, combing, eating, doing house hold chores and mobility to complex works like cooking, washing utensils, writing, driving, etc.

They may be divided into; (a) For facilitating day to day activities. (b) For use at work place. (c) To protect anesthetic tissue thus preventing secondary deformities (d) Those to make deformities less evident to escape social embarrassment.

Grip Aids

Grip aids made of an epoxy resin by Ciba Geigy, called 'Modulan' was developed in 1980s which is chemically inert the grip-aid and ready to use.[11] However, there is a paucity of

Table 30.9: Prerequisites for footwear
Prerequisites for footwear
• They should preferably be made of microcellular rubber (MCR) as it gives a cushioning effect due to the bubbles of air enclosed in a rubber matrix.
• They should be free of nails or metal fasteners and all the components should either glued together or stitched.
• Should be of a comfortable size so that there is no excessive compression on toes or other parts of the feet.
• Should be comfortable enough to be worn all the time
• A padding effect to be provided in a foot with loss of fat pads of feet preferably with MCR (Fig. 30.18)
• Plastazote moulding should be used in a foot with loss of contours (Fig. 30.19)
• A rigid material like tyre to be provided wherever needed.
• Should be aesthetically acceptable

data regarding its present availability. It is durable and adheres well to almost any surface; wood, metal, plastic, glass, etc. It is washable, autoclavable and does not shrink. There is a need to identify and develop a similar material which can be used as grip-aid for protective purposes. Advantages of grip aids in general are described in the Box 30.5.

Table 30.10: Various physical aids

Aids for feet	Patients with anesthesia and clawing	These require above modifications but with thinner handles for better grip
	Patients with mutilated hands	Here all items used for daily essential activities like brushing teeth, combing hair, eating, drinking, bathing, etc need an attachment with wrist cuffs with holder.
	Protective Footwear is the most important physical aid for patient with anesthetic feet.	It should be made with such a material and design so as to prevent ulceration and further damage to feet,
Aids for eye	Goggles, eyeshades, hats with rim, eyepads	To protect eye and prevent damage to eye with motor and sensory NFI

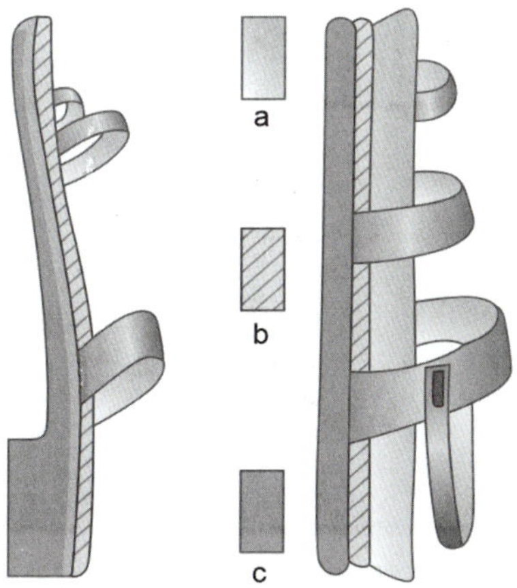

Fig. 30.18: MCR footwear:
(a) Microcellular rubber; (b) Leather; (c) Tyre

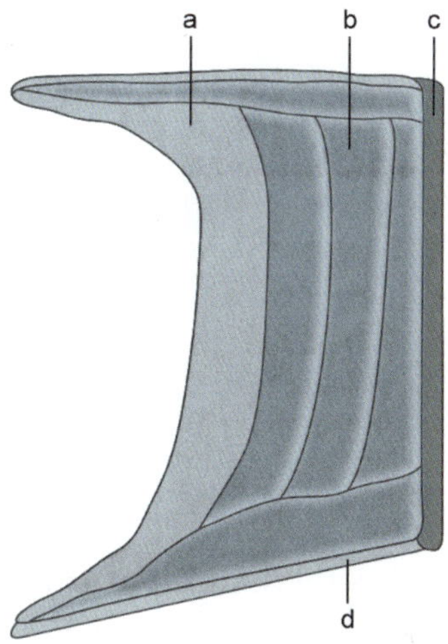

Fig. 30.19: Plastazote moulded footwear:
(a) Plastazote; (b) MCR; (c) Hard rubber;
(d) Covering rexine

Box 30.5: Advantages of grip aids in general

a. It not only facilitates normal grip with crippled hands but also protects from pressure, heat and abrasion
b. Helps in even distribution of pressure during its use.
c. It prevents slippage of hand thus avoiding accidental injuries.
d. Insulates the handle of the tool or utensil and gives protection against heat.
e. They can be incorporated into the utensils used for day to day life, like cups, spoons, pens, keys or for various occupational tools like spanners, screw driver, tools used in carpentry. (Fig. 30.20 and 30.21)

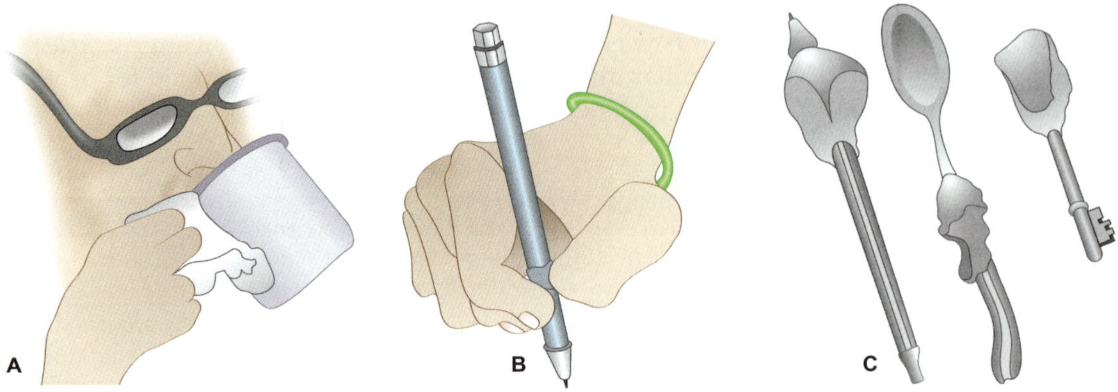

Fig. 30.20: (A) Grip aid for cup handle; (B) Grip aids for tools of daily activities; (D) Grip aids for tools of daily activities

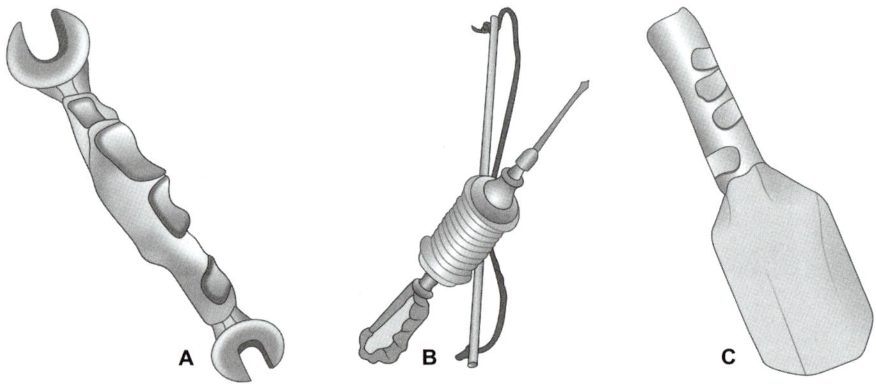

Fig. 30.21: (A) Grip aid for spanne; (B) Grip aid for hand drill; (C) Grip aid attached to tools used in carpentry

CONCLUSION

Physiotherapy methods for deformity prevention are widely and effectively used.[3] With innovative approaches, variety of splints and physical aids have been developed which are easy to carry, simple to apply and effective in deformity prevention and progression.[1]

REFERENCES

1. Malaviya GN. Deformity and Disability Prevention. In: Kumar B, Kar HK, editors. IAL textbook of leprosy. 2nd ed. New Delhi: Jaypee Brothers Medical Publishers (P) Ltd; 2017.p. 541–61.
2. Deformity and their management. In: Thangaraj RH, Yawalkar SJ editors. Leprosy for medical practioners and paramedical workers. 4th revised ed. Switzerland: Ciba-Geigy limited Basle;1989. p. 85–96.
3. Dharmendra S. Physiotherapy. In: Khotari D. editors. Leprosy. Bombay: Kothari Medical Publishing House; 1978.p. 575–98.
4. Furness M. Physiotherapy in leprosy. The Australian Journal of Physiotherapy. 1982;6:9–12.
5. Management of reactions and neuritis. Training manual for physiotherapist. National Leprosy Eradication Programme. 2020. p. 31–44.

6. Paul MSK, Kumar DP, Govindasamy K. Physical rehabilitation in leprosy. In: Scollard DM, Gillis TP, editors. International Textbook of Leprosy. p. 1–42.
7. Maia FB, Teixeira ER, Silva GV, Gomes MK. The Use of Assistive Technology to Promote Care of the Self and Social Inclusion in Patients with Sequels of Leprosy. PLoS Negl Trop Dis. 2016;10(4): e0004644.
8. Rocha E, Castiglioni M. Reflections on technological resources: technical aids, assistive technology, assistive technology and assistive technology. Rev Ter Ocup Univ São Paulo.2005;16:97–104.
9. Malaviya GN. Rehabilitation of insensitive hands. Indian J Lepr.2002;74: 151–7.
10. Reeder GD, Pryor JB. Dual psychological processes underlying public stigma and the implications for reducing stigma. Mens Sana Monogr. 2008;6:175–86.
11. Yawalkar S, Shah A, Ganapati R, Lian-Bin Y, Guo-Chen Z, Hong C, et al. Modulan® grip-aids for leprosy patients. Int. J. Lepr. 1992;60:250–4.

ACKNOWLEDGEMENTS

For Diagrams/illustrations

1. Mr Shridhar Tambatkar, Artist, Community Medicine, MGM Institute of Health Sciences, Kamothe, Navi Mumbai.
2. Mrs Bhavana Patil, Teacher, North Point School, (ICSE), Koperkhairane, Navi, Mumbai.

Chapter

31 Management of Trophic Ulcers in Leprosy

• Brahmaiah Upputuri • Sugat Jawade

INTRODUCTION

The trophic ulcer is one of the common leprosy related complications leading to grade 2 disability.[1] They occur secondary to an injury to a site affected due to sensory loss due to the disease and compounded by vascular insufficiency and the tissue breakdown from within due to paralysis of the intrinsic muscle.[2] Plantar anesthesia is the key to pathogenesis of ulcers and an anaesthetic foot is considered to be "ulcer-liable." These so-called trophic (tropho: Nutrition) ulcers in leprosy are essentially 'neuropathic ulcers' arising commonly on pressure bearing bony prominences of insensitive feet during ambulation. Due to the lack of sensation in the area, the patient is much less likely to feel pain or tenderness even after ulceration. The moment ulceration develops, this foot becomes "ulcer-prone" and a vicious cycle of scar-ulcer-scar sets in.[3] Most trophic ulcers occur in the forefoot. It was found that the majority of trophic ulcers in leprosy were chronic and recurrent. Ulcers recur due to anesthesia of the foot, formation of poor-quality scar from previous ulceration, increased pressure on the scar, aggravated especially by secondary infection and walking barefoot.[1]

DEFINITIONS

Stages of Trophic Ulcer[4]

Trophic ulcers are classified according to ulcer stage. These include:

- *Threatened ulcer*: It presents with edema, warmth, deep plantar tenderness with an increased interdigital gap. This is also considered as preulcerative aseptic inflammations.
- *Concealed ulcer*: It presents as a necrotic blister. The inflamed area undergoes necrosis due to continuous pressure of walking but they are covered with overlying skin.
- *Open or frank ulcer*: Blister breaks down and the site of tissue damage gets exposed.

Open ulcers are can be further divided into acute, chronic, and chronic complicated ulcers.

- *Acute ulcer:* These ulcers are manifesting with signs of acute inflammation.
- *Chronic ulcer:* Ulcers develop when the signs of acute inflammation have disappeared and patients continue to walk, becoming nonhealing ulcers.
- *Complicated ulcer:* This ulcer involves deeper tissues such as tendons, ligaments, or joints. Rarely, long-standing plantar ulcers undergo malignant changes and have a cauliflower-like appearance (Fig. 31.1).

Grading of Plantar Ulcers

National Pressure Ulcer Advisory Panel (NPUAP) staging:[5] NPUAP staging can be employed in clinical settings to define the evolutionary stages of the ulcers, denoted in grades I (intact skin with non-blanching erythema), II (partial-thickness loss of skin with exposure of the dermis), III (full-thickness loss of skin) and IV (full-thickness loss of skin and loss of tissue) (Fig. 31.2).

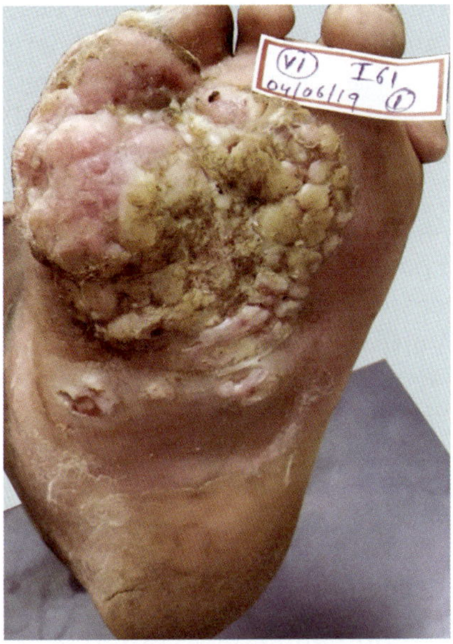

Fig. 31.1: Showing cauliflower growth arising from a chronic plantar ulcer

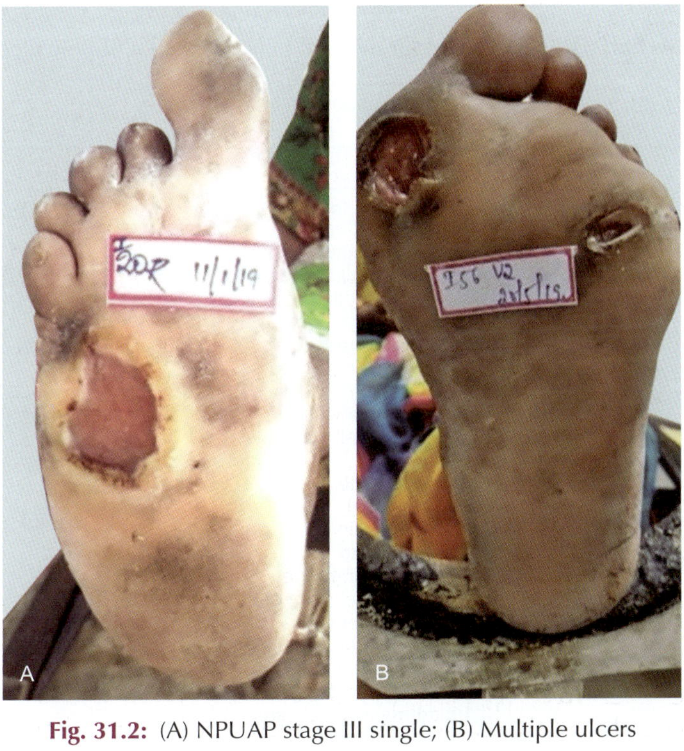

Fig. 31.2: (A) NPUAP stage III single; (B) Multiple ulcers

MANAGEMENT

Neuropathic ulcers are caused due to the presence of hypo/anesthesia of a limb (WHO grade 1 disability) leading to the inability to withdraw the area from painful stimuli such as friction, shear forces, or traumatic processes leading to the fissuring of skin and ulceration (categorized as WHO grade 2 disability). Patients should be educated on role of numbness or anaesthesia in the causation and persistence of ulcers in leprosy. The principles of trophic ulcer treatment include elimination of abnormal pressure, injuries, adequate rest, treatment of secondary infection, antiseptic dressings, maintenance of nutrition, in addition to the effective treatment of the underlying disease to restore or prevent further deterioration of sensations (Flowchart 31.1).

The management of trophic/neuropathic ulcers require a twofold approach: (a) Treatment of ulcer itself, (b) Counseling of patient about the reasons for development of fissures/ulcers in an anesthetic limb, so that measures may be adopted to prevent its occurrence/recurrence and promote healing. Further, understanding of the biomechanics behind the structures at risk by the healthcare provider would help in effective advise on clinical practice guidelines, including orthotic prescriptions and modifications to decrease the chances of disability and deformity. In addition, it would also help in planning possible surgical intervention and reconstruction. Of course, full drug treatment of leprosy and neuritis, including reactions should be provided simultaneously to all these patients.

Clinical Examination and Investigations

Detailed history, sensory-motor examinations and comprehensive clinical assessment should be performed along with screening for comorbid conditions including hypertension and diabetes. Patients are advised to quit smoking. X-ray, CT scan and MRI are recommended

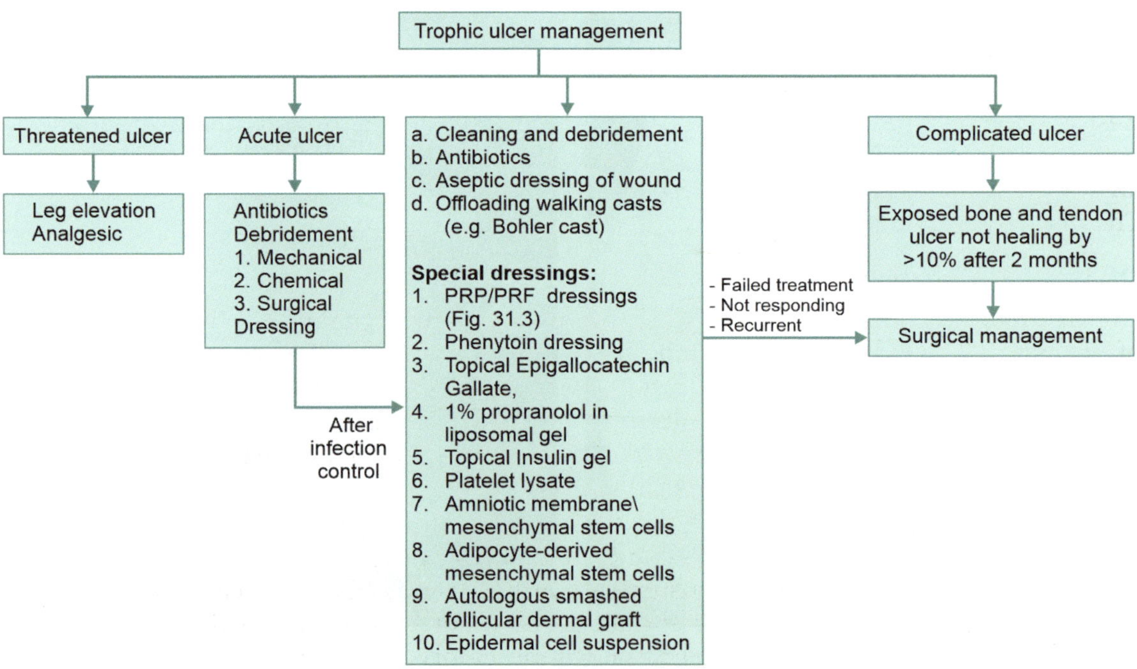

Flowchart 31.1: Algorithm for medical management of trophic ulcer

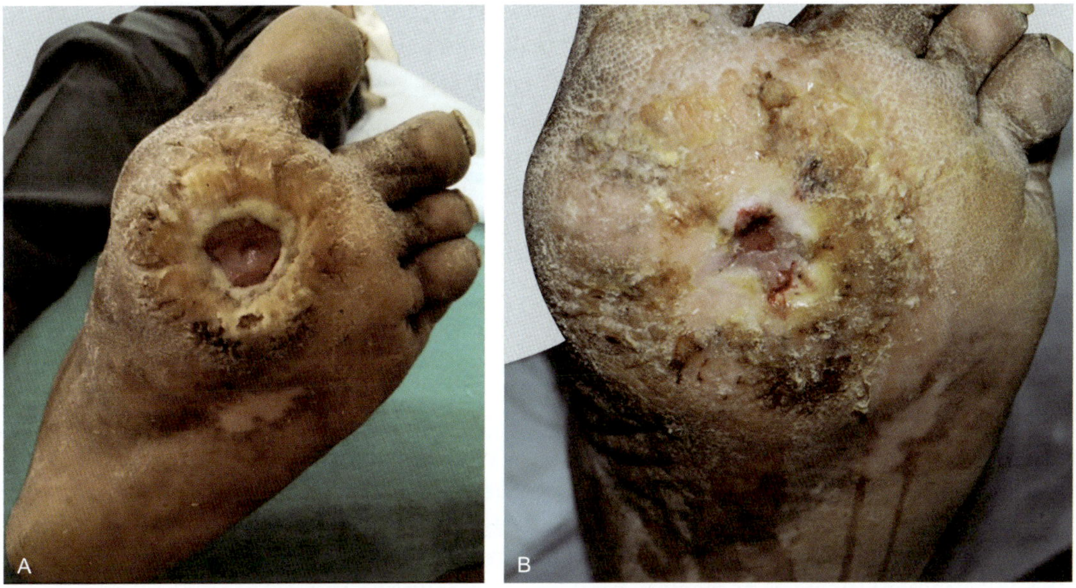

Fig. 31.3: Improvement of trophic ulcer after 6 week of PRF treatment

as necessary, to exclude involvement of underlying structures. Ankle brachial index (ABI), Doppler study and digital subtraction angiography of limbs are advised when vascular insufficiently is suspected.

Treatment of Ulcer

Ulcer treatment in leprosy includes a multimodal approach, based on the physical examination, clinical evaluation, and laboratory findings. The general principles of ulcer management in leprosy are detailed below.

Rest

Rest is necessary for all acute and complicated ulcers of anaesthetic limb as pain is not perceived by the patient. It includes complete restriction from weight-bearing; elevation of affected foot and use of splints. This enables a reduction in edema and improves blood flow. The majority of ulcers considerably heal in 3–4 weeks.[4]

Off-loading Measures

Off-loading pressure from the ulcer is of profound importance in the effective management of a trophic ulcer in an neuropathic limb. It works on the principle of reduction of pressure at ulcerated area and redistribute forces to the surrounding tissues. Hence off-loading has shown to help promote healing in current ulcers as well as prevent the recurrence of neuropathic ulcers. Upon healing, in the early phase, the re-epithelialized/scar tissue is still liable to breakdown (6–8 weeks), and hence stringent off-loading devices are necessary before the patient can progress to appropriate footwear.

The offloading measures include: complete bed rest, use of axillary crutches, walkers, wheelchairs, total contact casting, customized orthoses and MCR footwear. The shift from one offloading measure to the other should be slow. For instance, if a patient has been on strict bed rest and leg elevation, moving on to ambulatory offloading should be performed in a graded manner.[6] In addition to proper offloading, wound care should be based on the size, depth, moisture, drainage and type of tissues involved.

***Total contact casting*:** Total contact casting (TCC) is a special casting technique proven to eliminate the excess pressure that impairs ulcer healing and it has been considered one of the best offloading interventions[6] (Fig. 31.4). After wound debridement, a sterile dressing is applied over the ulcer followed by the application of a bandage over the whole foot and part of the leg. Roller cotton is applied on top of it and TCC is performed by moulding a Plaster of Paris (POP) casts over the entire surface of the roller cotton.[7] TCC has an advantage, that the patient could not remove it easily thus restricting the activity leading to ulcer healing. However, proper care must be taken during the procedure as the wrong application could lead to the development of more ulcers.

Ulcer Management Principles

In most clinical settings in the field, infected trophic ulcers are treated with empirical antibiotic therapy. However, it is ideal to perform wound swabbing for bacterial culture and sensitivity, before initiating antimicrobial agents.[8] Secondary bacterial infection with pathogens (*S. aureus* and *Pseudomonas* species) are one of the important contributing factors to the chronicity of ulcers; if neglected, may result in cellulitis and osteomyelitis, necessitating surgical interventions including foot amputation.[8] If the bone is reached during ulcer probing, an X-ray of the affected foot should be done to rule out osteomyelitis.[6] Clinical manifestations suggesting infection include erythema, warmth, pain, tenderness, induration, purulence; foul odour and presence of necrotic tissue.[9] Swabs from ulcer are found to be equally effective as deep tissue cultures for microbial assessment.[10] Note that there measures are in addition to rest and offloading of pressure from the ulcer.

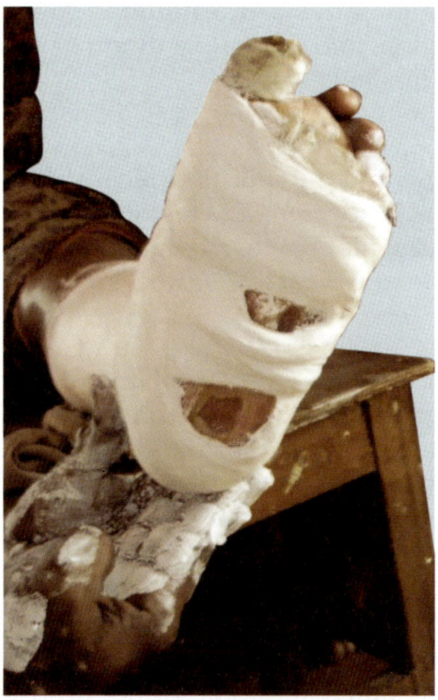

Fig. 31.4: Total contact casting

Dressings for Chronic Simple/uncomplicated Ulcer

Moist wound dressings: A moist wound environment enables the keratinocyte migration across the ulcer bed thus facilitating healing. However, care must be taken to keep the wound moist and to prevent maceration of the surrounding tissues. Saline or collagen dressings are tried to improve ulcer healing. Similarly, infected ulcers can be treated with antimicrobial dressings using silver to destroy bacteria.[6] Many different ulcer care products and grafts are available in the market may be made use of to promote the healing of wounds with different characteristics.

Special Dressings

Platelet-rich plasma (PRP)/platelet-rich fibrin (PRF): Growth factor dressings have been found to be viable treatment alternatives for non-healing ulcers.[11] Platelet-derived autologous products such as PRP/PRF are a rich source of growth factors and cytokines that are proven to expedite wound healing via tissue regeneration in non-healing ulcers, including trophic ulcers.[12,13]

Phenytoin sodium dressings: Phenytoin-sodium zinc oxide paste dressings are found to be a good alternative treatment option in trophic ulcers. These dressings led to the formation of granulation tissue in 4–6 weeks time in the majority of ulcers.[14]

In addition, topical Epigallocatechin Gallate,[15] 1% propranolol in liposomal gel[16] and insulin application[17] were also reported to have achieved faster ulcer healing.

Surgical Management of Trophic Ulcer

Surgical management is indicated when ulcers with exposed bone, tendon, and ulcer area not reduced by more than 10% despite continued medical management for about 2 months.[6] Surgical management aims at eradication of deep seated infection and removal of necrotic tissues to promote wound healing, reconstitution of normal skin and sensation, and deformity correction. Various surgical methods including surgical debridement, skin grafting, flap microvascular surgeries and rarely amputation can be tried in isolation or in combination.

Surgical Debridement

The main intention of surgical debridement is to decrease inflammation at the site and to promote granulation tissue and healing of the wound.[18] It is done to remove callus, debris, surrounding fibrous tissue, infected and necrotic tissue, bone, fascia, capsules, tendons, and sequestrum as required, resulting in soft nonkeratotic edge with well vascularized tissue bed.[3] During debridement activation of platelets leads to the release of growth factors that help in healing process. Patients undergoing regular debridement facilitate better wound healing when compared to those who never or seldom had debridement. Extensive surgical debridement needs to be done under anaesthesia in OT taking all aseptic precautions. Methylene blue is used to demarcate granulation tissue.[19] During surgical debridement, if osteomyelitis is found, management differs as perfused vascular tissue is essential to cover necrotic area to foster healing.[20] In addition, mechanical, enzymatic and autolytic debridement can also be done by using wet-to-dry dressing, collagenase and papain, and occlusive dressing respectively to help healing process and promote tissue growth.

Reconstructive Surgeries

The purpose of reconstructive surgery is to correct soft tissue defects, sustain weight bearing and independent ambulation.[21] Reconstructive surgeries are planned in cases of associated osteomyelitis, failed previous attempts, a large sized defect, insensate and friable local tissue, and to conserve non–weight-bearing regions of affected leg for offloading. The choice of reconstructive surgery depends on the site, depth and extent of ulcer, underlying tissue structures involved, neurovascular status, adjacent tissue quality and associated co-morbidities.[20] However, evaluation for vascularity of the affected limb is indispensable which can be clinically assessed by palpation of distal arterial pulsations and confirmed by Doppler study as required.

PREVENTION OF TROPHIC ULCERS IN LEPROSY

For a patient of leprosy with an anaesthetic limb, the care of the effected part and prevention of ulcers and disability is a life-long process, as absence of pain makes limb highly prone to trauma and ulceration. Trophic ulcers due to leprosy are known to cause significant physical, psychological and financial disability to the affected patients. The aim of preventive measures is to relieve and/or distribute pressure evenly from pressure point areas of the feet and to avoid repetitive trauma at the anaesthetic site. Maintaining local hygiene of hands and feet followed by daily application of oils, creams/gel is recommended to make the skin and nails soft, supple and free of fissures. Patients are advised to refrain from smoking as nicotine can inhibit normal cellular metabolism and its vasoconstrictive properties can delay the wound healing. Strict glycemic control and treatment in diabetic patients will prevent further vascular, sensory-motor compromise complicating the healing of ulcers.

The care of anesthetic hand or foot needs both focus and attention by the leprosy affected, as the avoidance of occupational trauma and damage to pressure bearing areas needs be done daily, over years and decades, which needs high levels of motivation. Health education of the affected and caretakers to identify early signs of inflammation suggestive of threatening ulcers and regular care of the anesthetic limb plays a very significant role improving the quality of life of these patients.

REFERENCES

1. Upputuri B, Srikantam A, Mamidi RS. Comorbidities associated with non-healing of plantar ulcers in leprosy patients. PLoS Negl Trop Dis. 2020;14:e0008393.
2. Viswanath V, Vasani R. Viva questions from the IJDVL. Indian J Dermatol Venereol Leprol. 2016;82:468–73.
3. Riyaz N, Sehgal VN. Leprosy: Trophic Skin Ulcers. Skinmed. 2017;15:45–51.
4. Chauhan VS, Pandey SS, Shukla VK. Management of plantar ulcers in Hansen's disease. Int J Low Extrem Wounds. 2003;2:164–7.
5. Edsberg LE, Black JM, Goldberg M, et al. Revised national pressure ulcer advisory panel pressure injury staging system: Revised pressure injury staging system. J Wound Ostomy Continence Nurs. 2016;43: 585–97.
6. Puri V, Venkateshwaran N, Khare N. Trophic ulcers-Practical management guidelines. Indian J Plast Surg. 2012;45:340–51.
7. Saha S, Patra AC, Gowda SP, et al. Effectiveness and safety of autologous platelet-rich plasma therapy with total contact casting versus total contact casting alone in treatment of trophic ulcer in leprosy: An observer-blind, randomized controlled trial. Indian J Dermatol Venereol Leprol. 2020;86:262–71.
8. Ebineshan K, Pallapati M, Srikantam A. Occurrence of bacterial biofilm in leprosy plantar ulcers; Lepr Rev. 2020;91:130–8.
9. Hay R. Trophic leprosy ulcers–what is a secondary infection?; Lepr Rev. 2020;91:126–9.
10. Pellizzer G, Strazzabosco M, Presi S, et al. Deep tissue biopsy vs. superficial swab culture monitoring in the microbiological assessment of limb-threatening diabetic foot infection. Diabet Med. 2001;18:822–7.

11. Bhattacharjee R, Sawatkar G, Vinay K.Platelet-rich fibrin dressings in treating nonhealing leg ulcers.J Am Acad Dermatol. 2019;80:e31–e32.
12. Ghatge A, Jawade S, Madke B, Singh A. Efficacy of platelet-rich fibrin in the treatment of trophic ulcer in leprosy. Skinmed. 2021;19:362–8.
13. Nagaraju U, Sundar PK, Agarwal P, et al. Autologous Platelet-rich fibrin matrix in nonhealing trophic ulcers in patients with Hansen's disease. J Cutan Aesthet Surg. 2017;10:3–7.
14. Sehgal VN, Prasad PV, Kaviarasan PK, Rajan D. Trophic skin ulceration in leprosy: evaluation of the efficacy of topical phenytoin sodium zinc oxide paste. Int J Dermatol. 2014;53:873–8.
15. Prakoeswa C, Oktaviyanti R, Indramaya D, et al. Efficacy of topical Epigallocatechin gallate (EGCG) 1% on the healing of chronic plantar ulcers in leprosy. J Dermatolog Treat. 2020;32:134–40.
16. Abdelmaksoud A, Bonamonte D, Giudice G, et al. Topical 1% propranolol in liposomal gel: A new adjuvant tool for chronic leprosy ulcers. Open Dermatol J. 2018;12:59–64.
17. Singh M, Pawar M. Efficacy of topical insulin therapy for chronic trophic ulcers in patients with leprosy: A randomized interventional pilot study. Adv Skin Wound Care. 2020;33:1–6.
18. Urso B, Ghias M, John A, Khachemoune A. Neuropathic ulcers: a focused review. Int J Dermatol. 2021;60:e383–e389.
19. Batista KT, Monteiro GB, Y-Schwartzman UP, et al. Treatment of leprosy-induced plantar ulcers. Rev Bras Cir Plást.2019;34:497–503.
20. Kadam D. Limb salvage surgery. Indian J Plast Surg. 2013;46:265–74.
21. Crowe CS, Cho DY, Kneib CJ, et al. Strategies for reconstruction of the plantar surface of the foot: A systematic review of the literature. Plast Reconstr Surg. 2019;143:1223–44.

Chapter 32

Rehabilitation of Leprosy Affected Persons with Disabilities and Management of Deformities

• Jerry Joshua • Sathish Paul • David Prakash

INTRODUCTION

Preceding chapters of this sections have dealt with the principle and role of physiotherapy for the management of deformities in leprosy. On part of the dermatologist, it is important to know about the potential risk factors for development of deformities and devise a pro-active plan. Identifying and designing such a customized rehabilitation plan for individual patient's needs would be vital in the reduction of deformities in leprosy.[1] The baseline assessment and planning for rehabilitation for the same is described in chapter (principles of physiotherapy) followed by self-care activities in a patient with nerve function impairment (Chapter 29, Section 5) and usage of various physical aids and splints for the same. This chapter shall deal with remaining aspects of prevention of worsening of deformities and disabilities.

GOOD PRACTICES FOR PREVENTION AND MANAGEMENT OF DEFORMITIES

Early Diagnosis of Leprosy

The earliest sign of leprosy is an insensitive patch of hypo-pigmented skin. If leprosy is diagnosed at this stage, it can be treated with multidrug therapy and further progress of the disease can be prevented without any risk of deformity or disability. At the time of diagnosis of leprosy, deformities and disabilities, if present, should be recorded and noted. Worsening of deformities and disabilities are prevented by regular monitoring, timely action and in some cases deformity correction procedures and physical therapy.

Counseling, Early Detection of Reactions and Neuritis and their Medical Management

Patients may not adhere strictly to treatment and discontinue treatment. They may also discontinue treatment if, in the course of taking MDT regularly, they develop symptoms of type 1 or type 2 reaction or if they develop symptoms of neuritis. They may attribute these symptoms and signs to improper treatment and not report the symptoms to the clinician. This can be avoided by counseling the patient at the time of diagnosis, explaining that such symptoms are likely to occur during the course of the disease or treatment and these symptoms are a result of the disease process itself. They need to know that they have to report the symptoms and take additional courses of treatment such as steroids (Box 32.1).

This information will help them repose faith in the clinician, if they should encounter such symptoms, and they will come back to receive steroids in time to prevent the chances of further nerve damage. This helps in early detection and treatment of reactions. If the patient is diagnosed with type 1 reaction, it is usually managed with a course of steroids. Neuritis,

Box 32.1: Patients need to report back, if they develop any of these symptoms

Report back, if there is

i. An increase in the number of patches
ii. Increase in size of patches
iii. increase in the thickness of patches (The patches become raised and reddish)
iv. There are new areas of loss of sensation
v. Radiating pain at the elbow, wrist, behind the knee or ankle
vi. If there is deformity of the fingers/thumb/toes; Or loss of control over action of the fingers, thumb, wrist, ankle or eyelids
vii. Redness of the eye or watering of the eyes
viii. Fever >3 days
ix. Multiple painful nodules of the skin

whether silent or painful, is managed with steroids as well.[2] Type 2 reactions, depending on the severity score are managed with NSAIDs, steroids and or thalidomide.

If there is continuing pain along the site of thickening of the nerve due to neuritis, or if there is worsening of nerve function despite adequate steroid management, or if there is formation of nerve abscess, surgical neurolysis is to be considered. If the neuritis is because of external nerve compression, freeing the nerve from its fibro-osseous tunnel will suffice. If the neuritis is because of internal compression of the nerve fibers (inflammation within the epineurium sheath) hemicircumferential epineurotomy[2] can be performed, in addition to then external decompression.

Health Education and Management of the Nerve Damaged Extremity or Eye to Prevent Secondary Deformity

Once nerve function impairment is established in form of loss of sensation (anesthesia) or loss of motor function and/or loss of autonomic function regulation (loss of sweating and sebaceous secretions) the patients need to be educated on how the above loss of function can affect them adversely.[3, 4]

i. Loss of sensation causes the patient to ignore open and concealed injuries to the affected limb. These injuries may be due to continuous trauma due to the body weight resting on the foot (increased pressure caused by standing for long duration),
ii. Continuous repetitive trauma due to the body weight landing repeatedly on the foot as in walking or running (the force the foot is subjected to while bearing the body weight multiplied by the acceleration).
iii. Direct sudden single injury, such as the forceful turning of a key in a lock or forcefully shutting a tight padlock. Ignoring tissue injury because of the loss of pain can cause dislocations or fractures or cut injuries to the fingers of the hand; burns can also occur to the sole while the patient walks barefoot on a hot road.
iv. Wounds caused by high shearing stresses (friction between ground and foot, friction between tissue planes and the movement of the tissues over the metatarsal heads, when the metatarsophalangeal joint is passively hyperextended during the push off phase of the gait cycle; or on the hand because of repetitive movement and friction as in using a crowbar, axe or spade between the hand and the tool being used).

When excessive tissue damage is caused by these mechanisms, it is reported to the brain as pain. When the sensory pathway is blocked by nerve damage, as in leprosy, the person is not aware of this tissue trauma and therefore continues to repeat this action leading to trauma again and again. This leads to irreversible damage in the form of tears to ligaments and tendons, fractures to the tarsal, metatarsal, metacarpal or phalangeal bones (Charcot's limbs) and trophic ulcers (patchy areas of necrosis of plantar or palmar skin and subcutaneous tissues).

A. Loss of motor function causes atypical distribution of forces in the limbs.[3,4]

In the foot an atypical distribution of weight over the foot occurs due to motor paralysis of the foot. In leprosy, it can be because of one of two reasons or both. The common peroneal nerve (lateral popliteal nerve) when affected just behind the neck of the fibula causes foot drop and the tibial nerve when affected just behind the medial malleolus causes "claw toes".

Foot drop alters the stress loading pattern on the foot during gait. The foot does not have a normal heel strike, but the forefoot hits the ground first, followed by the lateral border of the foot and then the heel followed by a reversal of the process in the same cycle. Thus we have a *forefoot–lateral border-heel–lateral border–forefoot* stress pattern rather than the normal *heel strike–lateral border-forefoot* pattern. This causes the forefoot to bear the weight twice during each gait cycle increasing the chances of damage. If there is associated plantar anesthesia the chances of damage is further increased. Further, if there is associated inversion of the foot, the lateral border of the forefoot strikes the ground first leading to damage over the lateral toes and lateral metatarsals and varus deformity of the toes.

Posterior tibial nerve paralysis causes wasting of the muscles of the foot and claw toes, causing increased prominence of the weight bearing metatarsal heads and tips of the toes. As this nerve damage in leprosy is always associated with plantar anesthesia, the chances of plantar ulcers over the metatarsal heads and toe tips is very high.

Muscle paralysis also leads to lax skeletal stability of the foot causing the ligaments and bones to take on more of the stresses of the body weight. This leads to damage to the ligaments, bones and joints. Strains, joint instability, subluxations and fractures occur with or without associated ulcers.

In the hand, the muscle imbalance can be because of any or a combination of these reasons mentioned below. The ulnar nerve when diseased above and below the elbow, as it passes through the fibro-osseous tunnel between the olecranon and the medial epicondyle, can be compressed and or demyelinated and this causes the characteristic hyperextension of the metacarpophalangeal joints and flexion of the interphalangeal joints; (a muscle imbalance resulting in the "claw hand". This results in in-coordinated grasp, and also abnormal distribution of pressures over the metacarpal heads and finger tips.

The median nerve when damaged, just proximal to the carpal tunnel, causes inability of opposition of the thumb, and loss of abduction of the thumb, resulting in the muscle imbalanced position of "ape thumb". This does not permit grasp and pinch, and results in abnormal pressures over the ulnar aspect of the thumb and ulnar aspect of the interphalangeal joint leading to ulceration in these areas and joint disruptions.

The radial nerve paralysis, causes "wrist-drop" and also loss of the ability to extend the fingers and thumb, resulting in a totally unstable hand.

When the triple nerve paralysis occurs in the same limb, it leaves the hand totally incapable of any function whatsoever, except with functioning long flexors and pronators and supinators of the forearm.

B. Loss of autonomic function regulation in these nerves causes vasodilatation with increased blood supply, loss of sweating and loss of sebaceous secretions. While the vasodilatation can be of benefit to the patient and the surgeon, (no interference with wound healing and the vessels do not go into spasm as a result of surgical trauma), the loss of sweating and loss of sebaceous secretions is a problem for the patient. Loss of sweating causes the skin to become dry and crack, leading to open fissures, which frequently get infected. Reduced sebaceous secretions leads to inability of the skin to trap the moisture and its loss by evaporation.

Once the patient understands these problems, it becomes easy for them to follow the instructions. Self-care for the anesthetic limbs has been mentioned in Chapter 29, Section 5.

The eye is usually damaged in one of three ways.[5]

i. Loss of sensation of the cornea leads to an absence of the stimulation to blink (All of us blink 15–20 times per minute). This is because the movement of the air in front of the cornea and conjunctiva stimulates the blink reflex. The blinking causes the lachrymal gland to be squeezed and the tears are expressed at the upper lateral corner of the palpebral fissure and wash down to the lower medial corner so that the cornea is washed clean. The tears then drain through the nasolachrymal duct). Due to loss of sensation of the moving air in front of the cornea, the stimulus to blink is removed. Hence the patient does not blink. This causes exposure keratitis of the cornea. Further, in case a foreign body settles on the palpebral conjunctiva, the sensation of the foreign body is not present. This leads to ulceration of the cornea as and when the person blinks. This could lead to infections or healing with scarring, which causes the cornea to lose its transparency and become opaque. The person thus loses some amount of visual acuity.
ii. Lagophthalmos or inability to close the eye because of paralysis of the facial nerve. Leprosy, usually during the type 1 reactions of the disease, involves and damage usually only the zygomatic branch of the facial nerve. Rarely, it can cause damage to all branches of the facial nerve. This can cause lagophthalmos alone or pan facial paralysis in leprosy. Lagophthalmos prevents the ability of the patient to close the eye completely. During waking hours, attempts to blink or close the eyes, by virtue of Bell's phenomenon (rolling of eyeball upwards), helps protect the cornea despite the inability to close the eye completely. However, during sleep, when the eye is not completely closed and Bell's phenomenon does not roll up the eyeball, the lower third of the cornea is exposed. This causes drying and exposure keratitis and consequent opacity of the lower third of the cornea, resulting in diminished vision. With the paralysis of the lower lid causing eversion of the lower eyelid, epiphora also results.
iii. Type 2 reaction can manifest as iridocyclitis with circum-corneal congestion. The iridocyclitis, causes closed angle glaucoma, synechiae (adhesions between the iris and the lens) and coloboma with irregularities of the iris. All these can lead to diminished vision and progressive damage to the eyes.

The usual health education to prevent further disability in vision are:[5]

a. Protect the eye with goggles
b. Think and blink (make blinking a habit)
c. Inspect the eyes daily with a mirror. Look for redness and watering of eyes. If there is redness, seek help of ophthalmologist, as it could be indicative of scleritis, corneal ulceration, exposure keratitis in lagophthalmos and also of iridocyclitis.
d. Use lubricating eyedrops.
e. Tape the eyes closed at night.

Management of the Ulcerated Feet or Hands

This has been described in detail in the preceding chapter of this section (Chapter 31).

Management of Disintegration of the Extremity

Nerve damage also causes insensitivity of the internal structures of the hands and feet. This can be with or without ulceration. Excessive use of the extremities subjects them to repeated forces. This causes damage to the ligaments, joint surfaces and bones. This can cause collapse of mid tarsal joints, ankle, sub-talar joint and even the wrist and metacarpophalangeal joints. In the foot, this can lead to reversal of the arch of the foot and cause rocker-bottom feet. These are progressive in nature and can lead to repeated acute episodes leading to chronic disintegration ("Charcot's limbs").

This is more common in the feet than in the hands. The patient presents with swelling of the foot. Pain is usually absent. On touching the foot, the clinician perceives warmth. An X ray may or may not reveal bone damage or disruption of the architecture of the joint. This is the first stage of the acute Charcot's foot. It is commonly referred to as the "hot foot". If ignored, this will lead to rapid disintegration of the foot. It is managed by immobilization.

Management of the 'Acute Disintegration of the Foot' (Hot Foot)[2,4]

The patient is provided bed rest and the foot is elevated. A total contact cast is applied and the patient is not permitted weight bearing for a month. After a month, the total contact cast is usually found to be loose because the swelling due to oedema has subsided. The cast is removed and reapplied. The patient is now fitted with a *Bohler* iron to permit weight bearing with an off-loading mechanism for the sole. The patient continues with the cast for 4 months. After that, the cast is removed and measurements are taken for a patella tendon bearing brace. The cast is reapplied for one more month while the brace is being prepared. At the end of the month, the cast is removed and the patient is fitted with the patella tendon bearing brace, which he or she has to wear for at least a year and a half, before other forms of less bulky customized protective footwear are permitted.

Repeated episodes of acute disintegration, without adequate attention and management in the acute stage, can lead to progressive disintegration and a chronically deformed foot. Such feet may be flail or stiff, depending on the type of damage. Both types need to be stabilized by surgery, so that the foot can continue to bear weight and provide adequate stability while walking. Such salvage procedures try to restore the architecture of the foot as much as possible. Often, this may not be possible and amputation may be the last resort.

CORRECTION OF DEFORMITIES IN LEPROSY BY SURGERY[2]

Deformities in leprosy that can be corrected by surgery are

i. Ulcers and tissue defects
ii. Disintegration of the feet and hands
iii. Muscle imbalance because of motor function loss in hands, feet and eyelids
iv. Face deformities

Ulcers lead to tissue defects, which need replacement. In some cases, the tissue defect can be restored by skin grafts. In areas where skin grafts are inadequate to replace lost tissue, soft tissue flaps are needed to replace the defects. This is done in the hands and feet, over specific weight bearing areas, such as the base of the big toe, the metatarsal heads, the lateral border of the foot, the heel, the lateral malleoli, the palmar aspect of fingers and palm and the first web space of the hand.

Disintegration of the hands and feet because of damage to ligaments, bones and joints, requires stabilization procedures such as repairs of ligaments, reconstruction of ligaments and arthrodesis, salvage of the mitten hand by pollicization of available stumps, etc.

Muscle imbalance causing deformities due to motor paralysis of nerves in leprosy results in "claw hand" deformity, inability to oppose the thumb, wrist drop, foot drop, "claw toes" and lagophthalmos. All these can be corrected by various static and dynamic procedures. Static procedures could be capsulodesis or capsulorrhaphy and pulley advancement for the hands, tarsorrhaphy for the eyelids. Dynamic procedures are usually tendon transfers for the various paralysis of the hands, feet and eyelids.

Facial deformities, such as collapsed nose, need staged reconstruction with tissue replacement. Madarosis or loss of eyebrows requires replacement of eyebrows by hair grafting. Loose and lax skin of the face, because of the loss of elasticity of the skin following treatment of lepromatous infiltration of the face skin, can be corrected by facelift surgery.

ROLE OF TECHNOLOGY IN MANAGEMENT OF DEFORMITIES

Advancements in technology have provided health workers an array of options in rehabilitating individuals challenged with impairments and disabilities and has brought a paradigm shift in making health care more appropriate and affordable. Technologically driven design and fabrication techniques of assistive devices have helped the physically challenged individuals lead independent lives overcoming the challenges that they had faced with impairments.

Though technology have facilitated in rehabilitating people with various impairments across the globe,[6] the leprosy affected patients have not benefited much through the technological advancements due to various reasons, although the customization and the fabrication time of the assistive devices have reduced considerably. Moreover, in some users, the aversion towards the use of technologically advanced devices is still present. Stigma of using assistive devices and the lacunae in considering user's opinion in the designing process were considered to be the key factors in abandoning the assistive devices by the users.[7,8] Nonetheless, it is important to counsel and offer these assistive devises to all leprosy affected with deformities.

CONCLUSION

In conclusion, it needs to be said that prevention of deformity and disability needs a lifelong motivation and effort by the patient and the healthcare providers. Measures such as early diagnosis and treatment of the disease and its complications, recognition of nerve function impairment and management are constantly required. Such measures help prevent primary deformities from progressing to secondary deformities. In case secondary deformities do occur, management with aids and appliances, footwear and surgery are necessary.

REFERENCES

1. Serranno-Coll H, Vélez JD, Trochez D, et al. Effectiveness of an individual physical rehabilitation programme in a group of patients with Hansen's disease. Lepr Rev. 2016; 87:355–67.
2. Fritschi EP. Ulcers of the foot and their sequelae. In: Surgical Reconstruction and Rehabilitation in Leprosy. 2nd ed. New Delhi: The Leprosy Mission; 1984. p.182–226.

3. Brand P. Insensitive Feet: A practical handbook on foot problems in leprosy. The Leprosy Mission; 1981.
4. Joshua J. Leg and foot ulcers in leprosy. In: Agrawal K.; Textbook of Plastic, Reconstructive and Aesthetic Surgery Vol IV; Thieme Medical and Scientific Publishers Pvt Ltd. 2020. p.551–66.
5. Brand M. Watch Those eyes: Eye Complications in Leprosy The Leprosy Mission; 1970.
6. Lancioni GE, Mantini M. A corrective-feedback system for helping a person with multiple disabilities during indoor travel. Percept Mot Skills. 1999;88:1291–5.
7. Kintsch, A. and DePaula, R. A Framework for the Adoption of Assistive Technology. SWAAAC 2002: Supporting Learning Through Assistive Technology. 2002. E3 1–10.
8. Parette P, Scherer M. Assistive Technology Use and Stigma. Education and Training in Developmental Disabilities. 2004;39:217–26.

Annexure 1

Model Leprosy Patient Card*

(Country) National Leprosy Programme

1. Registration data

Country	
State/Province	
Health facility (Name and address)	
Patient registration number	
Date of registration	

2. Personal data

Patient name	
Father's/husband's name	
Sex	☐ Male ☐ Female
Year of birth (or age)	
Place of birth	
Present address	
Number of years of residence at present address	
Nationality	
Telephone/mobile number	
Occupation	
Marital status	☐ Single ☐ Married ☐ Divorced ☐ Widow(er)
Contact person (Name, address, phone/mobile)	
Mode of detection	☐ Voluntary ☐ Referred ☐ Other ☐ Contact survey ☐ Other survey
Previous treatment details	(specify drug regimen, duration, year of treatment)
Type of patient	☐ New ☐ Transferred-in ☐ Replase after PB-MDT ☐ Relapse after MD-MDT ☐ Re-admission after dapsone monotherapy ☐ Treatment after default
Any known leprosy case in family?	☐ Yes ☐ No

*Pre-formatted leprosy patient record *Taken from* Leprosy/Hansen Disease: Management of reactions and prevention of disabilities. Technical guidance. New Delhi: World Health Organization, Regional Office for South-East Asia; 2017.

Details of household contacts

S.No.	Name	Sex	Year of birth (or age)	Relationship with patient
1.				
2.				
3.				
4.				
5.				
6.				

3. Disease status (Initial)

Presenting symptom(s)	☐ Patch(es) ☐ Visible impairment ☐ Reaction ☐ Other (specify):
Duration of presenting symptom(s)	________months/years

Number of skin patches	☐ 1	☐ 2–5	☐ >5
Reaction	☐ No		
	☐ Yes	☐ Type 1 reaction (reversal reaction)	
		☐ Type 2 reaction (ENL)	

Nerve status

Status	Ulnar		Median		Radial		Lateral popliteal		Posterior tibial	
	Right	Left	Right	Left	Right	Left	Right	Left	Right	Left
Thickening	☐	☐	☐	☐	☐	☐	☐	☐	☐	☐
Pain	☐	☐	☐	☐	☐	☐	☐	☐	☐	☐
Tendemess	☐	☐	☐	☐	☐	☐	☐	☐	☐	☐

WHO disability grading

	Eye	Hand	Foot
Right	☐	☐	☐
Left	☐	☐	☐

EHF score

Disease type

☐ PB
☐ MB

Body charting (Date:____/____/20____)

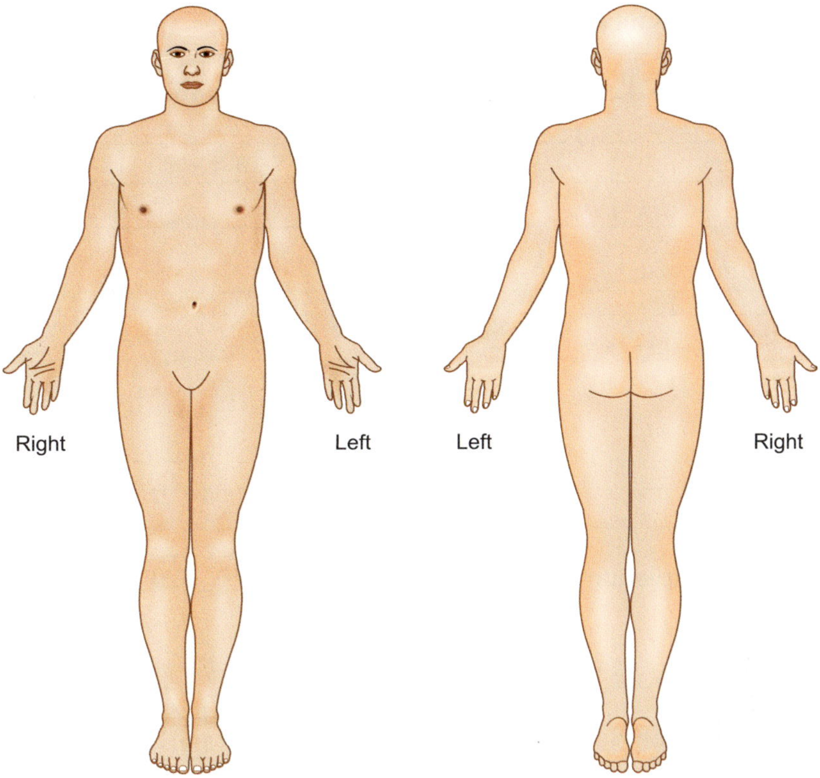

4. Details of other conditions

Medical history	☐ Diabetes ☐ Hepatitis ☐ Tuberculosis ☐ HIV/AIDS ☐ Any other disease (specify):
Duration of presenting symptom(s)	________months/years

Other conditions	☐ Pregnancy ☐ Drug allergy

☐ Pregnancy ☐ Drug allergy

Body weight	________kg

5. Treament details

Drug regimen prescribed	☐ PB-MDT ☐ 3-drug MDT ☐ 2-drug MDT
	☐ MB-MDT (3-drug MDT)
	☐ Any other regimen (specify):

Treatment monthly attendance

Dose (pulse)	1	2	3	4	5	6
Date						
Dose (pulse)	7	8	9	10	11	12
Date						

Treatment outcome

Type of outcome	☐ Treatment completed ☐ Defaulted ☐ Died ☐ Transfer out ☐ Change of classification
Date	____/____/20____

Body charting (at completion of treatment). Date: ____/____/20____

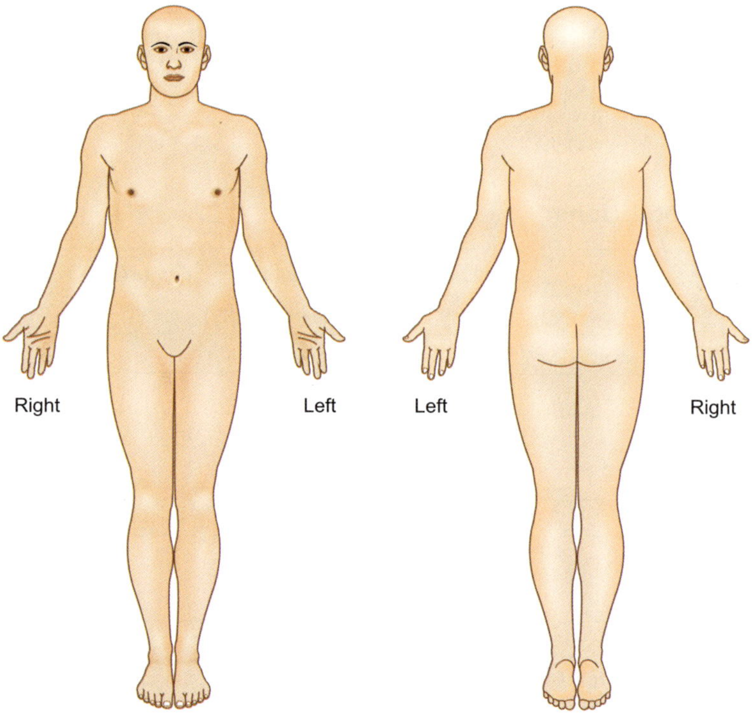

6. Bacteriological examination (slit-skin smear)

Date	1	2	3	4
Number of sites taken				
Slit-skin smear result	7	8	9	10
Date				

Sensory testing

Date/ Assessor	Palm		Sole		Comments
	Right	Left	Right	Left	
	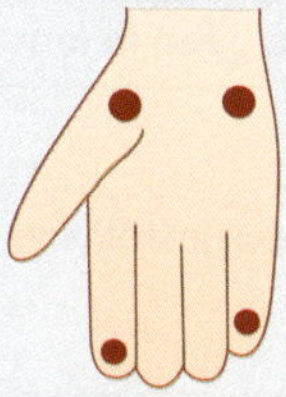	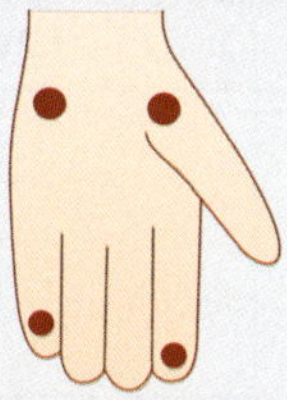	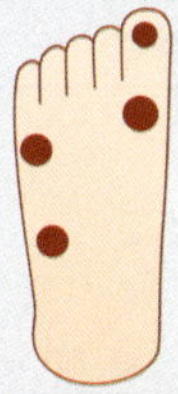	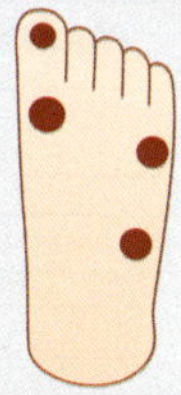	
	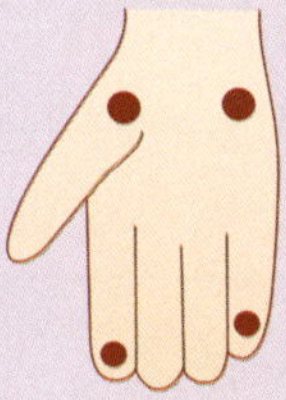	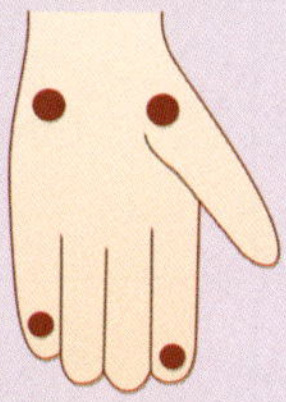	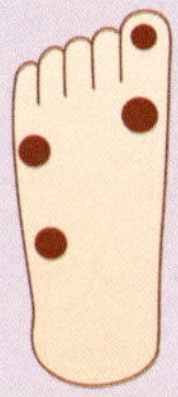	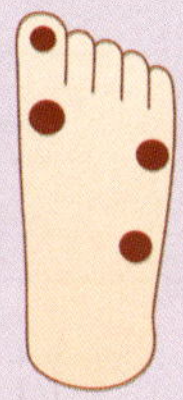	
	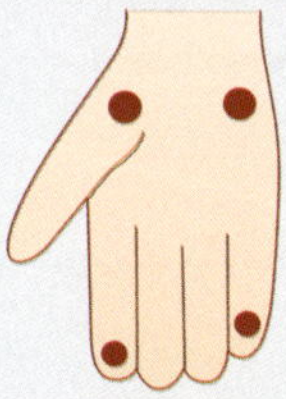	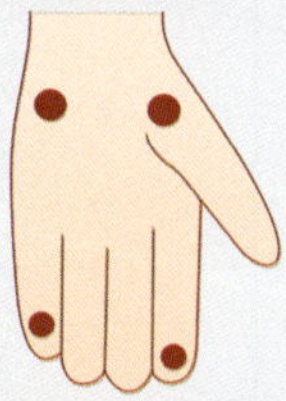	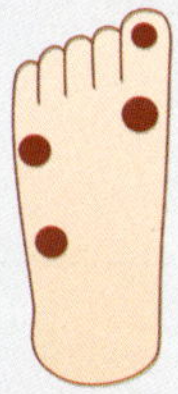	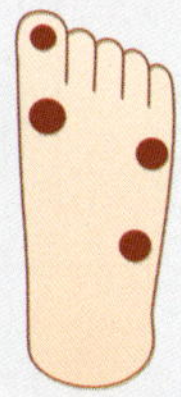	
	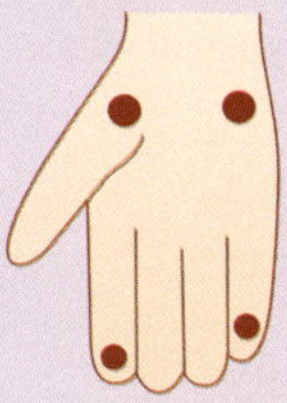	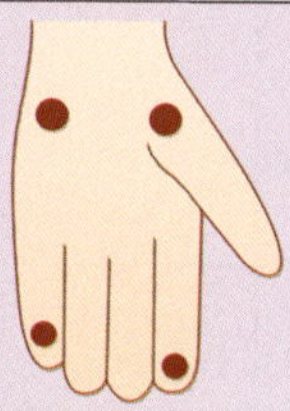	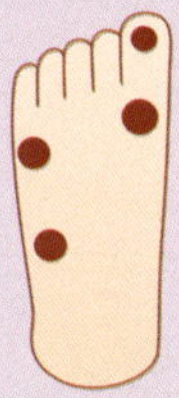	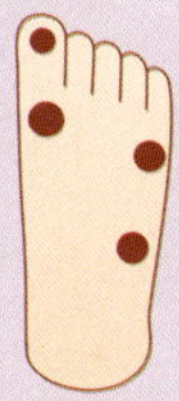	
	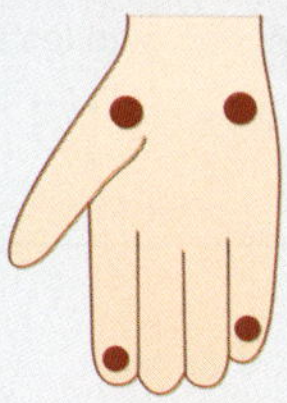	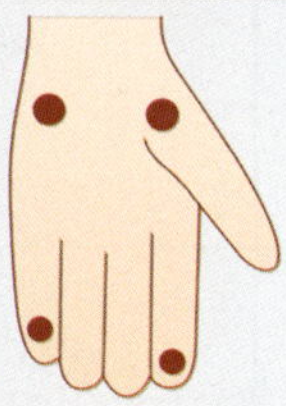	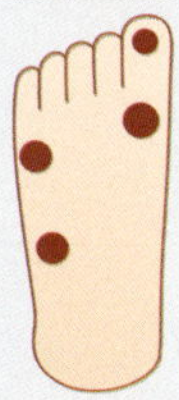	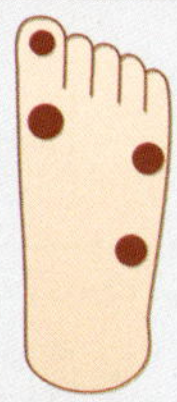	
	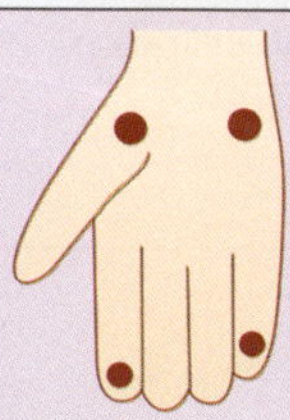	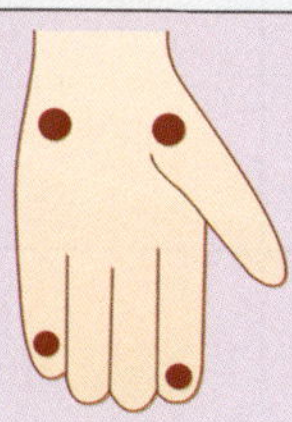	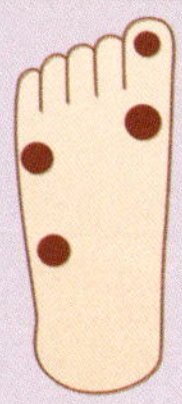	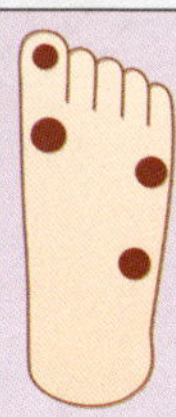	

Key: (Put these marks scors on the site where lession is seen)

Sensation Present within 3 cm ✓ contracture 5 Scar/Callus ⬭

Anaesthesia X Wound ⊗ Shortening level ✚ Crack ═

Annexure 2

Diagrammatic codes used in charting of lesions seen in leprosy*

	Diagramatic codes	Lesions seen in leprosy
1	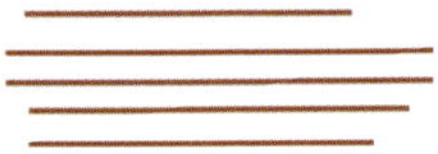	Hypopigmentation
2	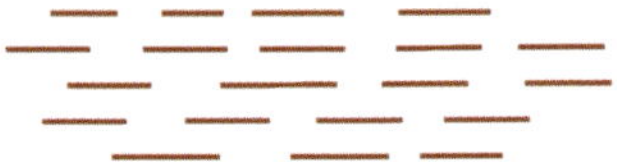	Residual hypopigmentation
3	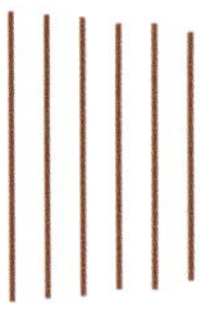	Anesthesia
4	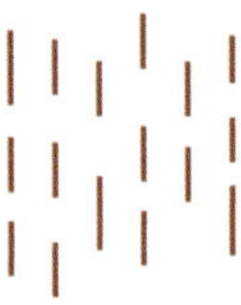	Hypoesthesia
5	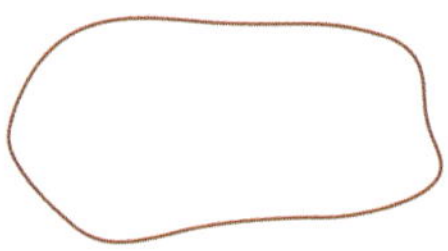	Well-defined skin lesion
6	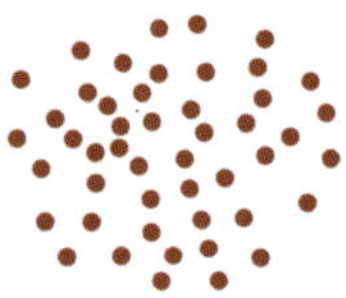	Fine infltration
7	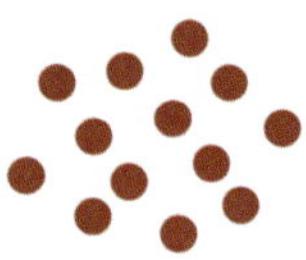	Marked infltration

(Contd.)

**Taken from* Model patient card/record, ILEP technical commission–advisory paper. Lepr Rev 2014;85:232–47.

(Contd.)

Diagramatic codes		Lesions seen in leprosy
8	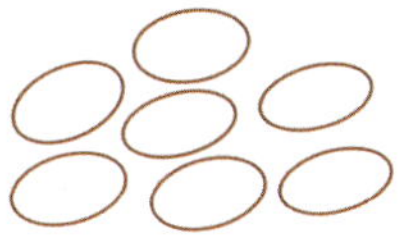	Nodules
9	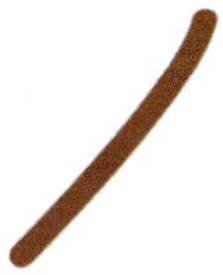	Nerve thickening
10		Nerve abscess
11	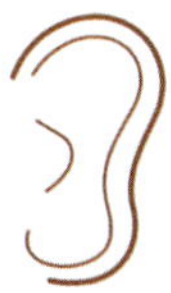	Thickening of ear margins
12	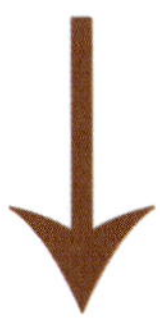	Foot drop/wrist drop
13	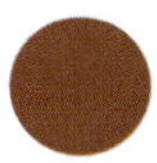	Gynecothelia
14	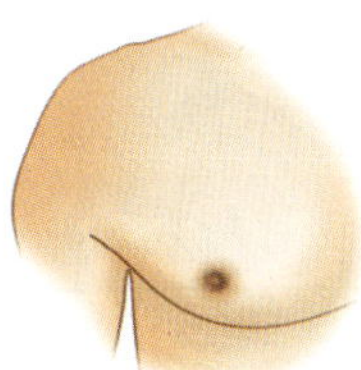	Gynaecomastia

(Contd.)

(Contd.)

Diagramatic codes		Lesions seen in leprosy
15	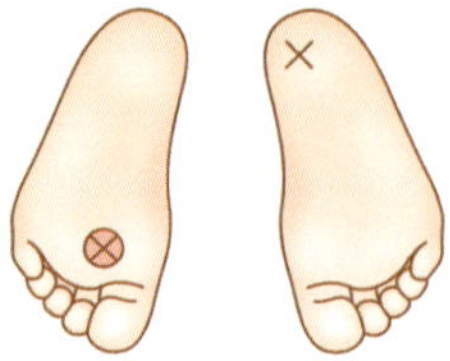	Plantar ulcer, scar
16	Sparse eyebrows	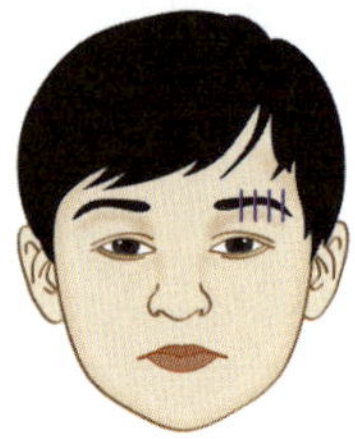
17	Loss of eyebrows	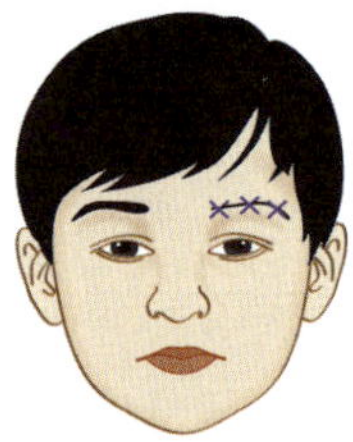
18	Collapse of nose	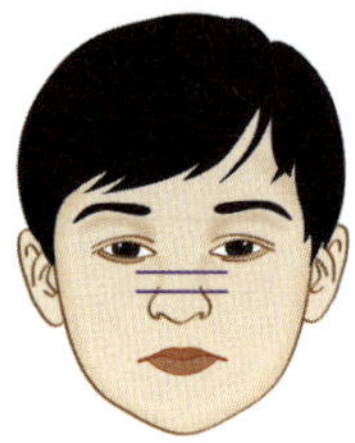
19	Loss/absorption of digits	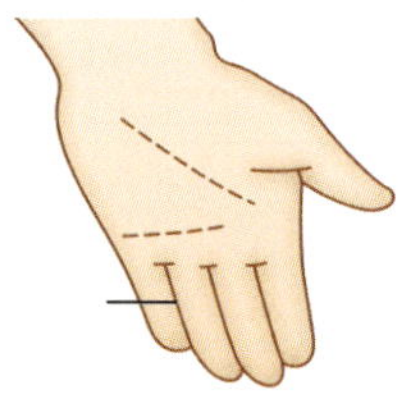
20	Flexion deformity of finger and toes	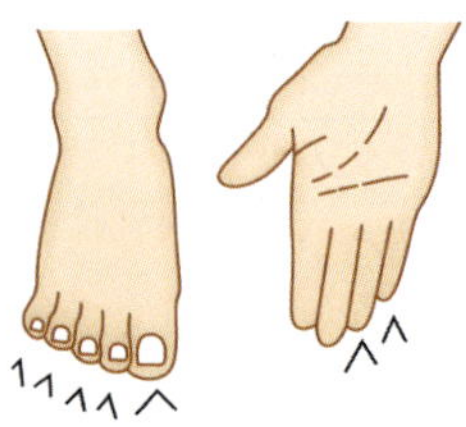

Index